Dietary
Fiber
In
Health
&
Disease

Edited by

David Kritchevsky and Charles Bonfield

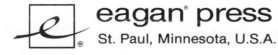

eagan® press

St. Paul, Minnesota, U.S.A.

Library of Congress Catalog Card Number: 94-62014
International Standard Book Number: 0-9624407-6-0

Printed in the United States of America on acid-free paper

Eagan Press
3340 Pilot Knob Road
St. Paul, MN 55121-2097, USA

Dedication
Denis Parsons Burkitt
1991–1993

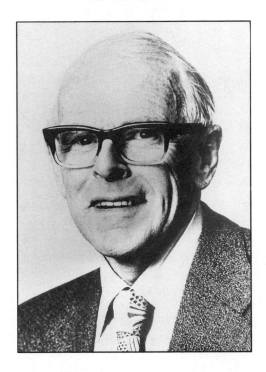

This book is dedicated to the memory of Dr. Denis Burkitt who championed the cause of dietary fiber and whose indefatigable program of writing and lecturing brought the value of fiber to the world.

Dr. Burkitt's opening chapter may be one of his last publications in the area of fiber research. His scientific insight and personal warmth touched everyone who knew him. Beyond any question he left this world a better place than he found it. His personal credo was:

Attitudes are more important than abilities
Motives are more important than methods
Character is more important than cleverness
The heart is more important than the head

Table of Contents

iii   **Dedication**

ix   **Preface**

I. Health Benefits

3   **Historical Aspects**
Denis Burkitt

11   **Dietary Fiber in Health and Disease: The South African Experience**
Alexander R. P. Walker

26   **The Structure of Dietary Fibre**
D. A. T. Southgate

37   **Fiber in Foods**
Edwin R. Morris

46   **Fiber as Energy in Man**
Geoffrey Livesey

58   **The Physiological Effects of Dietary Fiber**
Christine A. Edwards

72   **Modulation of Intestinal Development by Dietary Fiber Regimens**
Marie M. Cassidy and Leo R. Fitzpatrick

II. Lipids and Nutrient Metabolism

87   **Effect of Dietary Fiber on Alimentary Lipemia**
Barbara O. Schneeman

95 Dietary Fiber and Lipid Absorption: Interference of Chitosan and Its Hydrolysates with Cholesterol and Fatty Acid Absorption and Metabolic Consequences in Rats
Ikuo Ikeda, Michihiro Sugano, Katsuko Yoshida, Eiji Sasaki, Yasushi Iwamoto, and Kouta Hatano

106 The Role of Viscosity in the Cholesterol-Lowering Effect of Dietary Fiber
Daniel D. Gallaher and Craig A. Hassel

115 Fat/Fiber Interactions: Effect on Colon Physiology and Colonic Cytokinetics
Joanne R. Lupton

126 Cholesterol-Lowering Effects of Soluble Fiber in Humans
James W. Anderson

137 Dietary Fiber, Carbohydrate Metabolism and Diabetes
David J.A. Jenkins, Alexandra L. Jenkins, Thomas M.S. Wolever, Vladimir Vuksan, A. Venket Rao, Lilian U. Thompson, and Robert G. Josse

146 Dietary Fiber and Protein Digestion and Utilization
Bjørn O. Eggum

III. Fiber and Cancer

159 Fiber and Cancer: Prevention Research
Peter Greenwald and Carolyn Clifford

174 Fiber and Cancer: Historical Perspectives
John Higginson

183 Dietary Fiber and Colon Cancer Risk: The Epidemiologic Evidence
Tim Byers

191 Your Mother was Right—Eat Your Vegetables: The Role of Plant Foods in Cancer
John D. Potter and Kristi Steinmetz

219 The Polyp Prevention Trial: Rationale and Design
Arthur Schatzkin, Elaine Lanza, and Laura Kruse

226 ECP Trial of Fibre in Precancerous Lesion of the Large Bowel
Michael J. Hill

IV. Fiber's Nutritional Effects

237 **Dietary Fiber and Digestive Tract Disorders**
Albert I. Mendeloff

243 **Dietary Fiber and the Pattern of Energy Intake**
Victoria J. Burley and John E. Blundell

257 **Effect of Dietary Fiber on Intestinal Microflora and Health**
A. V. Rao

267 **Dietary Fiber and Mineral Nutrition**
Dennis T. Gordon, Dan Stoops, and Vicki Ratliff

294 **Effects of Lignans and Other Dietary Estrogens**
Kenneth D. R. Setchell

305 **Phytic Acid and Other Nutrients: Are They Partly Responsible for Health Benefits of High Fiber Foods?**
Lilian U. Thompson

V. Fiber Effects/In Vivo and In Vitro Laboratory Models

321 **Comparative Aspects of Animal Models**
P. J. Van Soest

340 **Propionate as a Mediator of the Effects of Dietary Fiber**
David L. Topping

346 **In Vitro Methods That Anticipate the Colonic Influence of Dietary Fibre**
W. Gordon Brydon

353 **Fiber and Aspects of Lipid and Cholesterol Metabolism**
David Kritchevsky

360 **In Vitro and In Vivo Models for Predicting the Effect of Dietary Fiber and Starchy Foods on Carbohydrate Metabolism**
Thomas M. S. Wolever

378 **Animal Models of Obesity: Diet, Inactivity, and Genetics**
Linda J. Magrum, Barbara A. Horwitz, and Judith S. Stern

406 **Animal Models of Colon Cancer**
David M. Klurfeld

Workshop Summaries

419 **Summary Report of Dietary Fiber Analysis Workshop**
Judith A. Marlett

423 **Fiber and the GI Microflora**
Abigail A. Salyers

433 **Dietary Fiber and Gastrointestinal Function**
Martin A. Eastwood

438 **Design of Human Studies to Determine the Effect of Fiber on
Serum Lipids in Relation to Blood Lipids, Fecal Bulking,
Glycemic Control or Bodyweight**
David J. A. Jenkins

441 **Short-Chain Fatty Acids—Research and Clinical Updates**
John L. Rombeau and Jonathan A. Roth

450 **Bile Acids**
Jon A. Story

453 **Resistant Starch**
Alison M. Stephen

459 **Dietary Fiber and Body Weight Management**
Charles T. Bonfield

Public Aspects

467 **Food Industry Perspective: Functional Properties and Food
Uses of Dietary Fiber**
Mark L. Dreher

475 **Future Research in Dietary Fibre?**
Martin Eastwood

481 **Index**

Preface

The Fourth Washington Symposium on Dietary Fiber was organized as a continuing memorial to our late friend and colleague George V. Vahouny who conceived and initiated this series of meetings in 1981. It was his belief that the conference provide an informal atmosphere for open discussion and deliberation on various aspects of new knowledge and research of the role of dietary fiber in human physiology. It is in this spirit that the conveners of the 1992 symposium attempted to set the stage for a free exchange of information and ideas.

The 1992 Vahouny Fiber symposium was organized with major contributions by many colleagues working in the field of dietary fiber. These suggestions and ideas were sincerely appreciated and contributed substantially to the overall success of the conference.

Among new areas explored in this conference was that of energy value of fiber, an aspect of fiber nutrition that is often overlooked. The interactions of fiber with other dietary components such as fat and protein were also explored. The roles of materials other than fiber which are present in a high fiber diet were discussed as were models for the study of effects.

To stimulate informal discussions and provide a forum whereby all attendees might share their own work and experiences in dietary fiber research, eight unstructured workshops were scheduled during the symposium. The enthusiastic participation and discussions which evolved during these workshops was lively and animated and made this particular format one of the highlights of the conference. Summaries of these discussions are reported in this volume.

The conference is deeply grateful to the following sponsors and contributors for their continuing interest in dietary fiber research and for their generous support of this symposium:

Sponsors

The Kellogg Company, The Proctor & Gamble Company, Ferrosan A/S and Madaus AG.

Contributors

American Cyanamid (Lederle), Campbell Soup Company, Carnation Nutritional Products, Delta Fibre Foods, General Mills, Inc., Kraft General Foods, Nabisco Brands, Inc., Protein Technologies International, Quaker Oats Company, Sandoz Pharmaceutical Corporation.

It is through these collaborative efforts between industry, academia, and government organizations and individuals that advances will be made in defining the role of dietary fiber in human health and disease.

David Kritchevsky
Charles T. Bonfield

I. Health Benefits

Historical Aspects

Denis Burkitt
Hartwell Cottage Bisley, Glos., GL6 7AG

Analogy of a River

The historical aspects of the fiber saga resemble the gradual and initially imperceptible growth of a river from its first trickle to the development of a stream and subsequent convergence with numerous other streams to eventually constitute a mighty river bearing no resemblance to its humble origins. From my experience and travels in Africa I cannot but compare it to the great River Nile, which commences as a small stream in the hills of Rwanda, and becomes the Kahera River flowing into the west side of Lake Victoria. From the north of this lake flows the Victoria Nile which connects with Lake Albert, supplying water to Lake Kioga on the way. After leaving Lake Albert it becomes the White Nile as far as Khartoum, where it is joined by the Blue Nile, which rises in the mountains of Ethiopia, to become just the Nile, which flows into the Mediterranean, watering The Sudan and Egypt on its way.

Just as the Nile changes its name en route, so what is now referred to as dietary fiber has had many previous names. It was first viewed as merely the less digestible constituent of food which exerted a laxative action by irritating the gut. It thus acquired the designation "roughage" which was later replaced by "crude fiber" and ultimately "dietary fiber." At times fiber has been considered almost synonymous with bran.

References from the Distant Past

What was to become fiber first appeared in the medical literature in the 6th century BC when Hippocrates made the observation that "to the human body it makes a great difference whether the bread be made of fine flour or coarse, whither of wheat; with the bran or without the bran."

Some twelve centuries later a Persian physician wrote: "wheat is a beneficial cereal. Chuppatis are made from wheat flour. The chuppatis containing more bran come out of the digestive tract quicker, but are less nutritious."

In the sixteenth century Shakespeare in his play Coriolanus (Act 1, scene 1) put the following words at the end of a speech made by the belly to all the other organs of the body to assert its unselfishness with the food put into it. "Yet I can make my audit up that all from me do back receive the flour of all and leave me but the bran."

The concept surfaces again, although not specifically named, in a book published in Dublin in 1733 under the title "Human Odure." This was a treatise on human excreta or stools written by no other than the author of "Gulliver's Travels," Dean Jonathan Swift, one of the most famous graduates of my old university, Trinity College, Dublin. Wishing to conceal his identity he was merely referred to on the title page as Dr. S...t. He graphically described the appearances of stools he observed as he traveled the Irish countryside, classifying them in botanical fashion as "species." These varied from the first, the soft relatively unformed stool resembling "boy's top reversed," and having a broad base below and an apex above, to the fifth and final form. This consisted of "small, round, distinct balls, buttons or bullets" observed to occur only "around institutes of higher education," and were presumably ascribed to more refined, roughage-depleted diets.

Nineteenth and Early Twentieth Centuries

In the second half of the 19th century, a British physician T. R. Allinson became convinced that many common ailments could be attributed to a deficiency of roughage in the diet, and that this could best be supplied in the form of whole-meal bread (1). He not only recommended this but went further and sold the flour. Allinson's whole-meal flour can still be purchased in Britain today. His marketing of bread was considered unethical and consequently his name was erased from the medical registry, and the brass plate outside his consulting room was henceforth inscribed Dr. T. R. Allinson, Ex. L.R.C.P.

At around the turn of the century the still-renowned Kellogg brothers John and William, started their healthy diet sanitorium and breakfast cereal company at Battle Creek, Michigan. This company has popularised breakfast cereals ever since.

Two decades later a British surgeon Sir Arbuthnot Lane, eponymously remembered by the surgical forceps he designed, became obsessed with the concept that a wide variety of common diseases varying from rheumatism to thyrotoxicosis could be attributed to a sluggish colon. Consequently he recommended the formidable operation of hemicolectomy for both the treatment and prevention of these and other disorders. Later he recognised that the prescription of bran could be equally effective, and certainly less traumatic, so he abandoned the surgical approach and routinely prescribed bran instead.

A British physician who was a contemporary of Lane served in the Indian Medical Service. Among the hill tribes in North India he observed and recorded an almost total absence of many of the diseases which today are numbered under the inclusive name "Western Diseases." He did not specifically refer to fiber, or even to diseases of western culture, although he attributed the rarity of these disorders to the diet consisting largely of local unrefined plant foods. Unconsciously he was laying the foundations for a later understanding not only of fiber but also of Western Diseases to be referred to below.

Other pioneers that must be mentioned in this period include the American gastroenterologists Cowgill and Anderson (2), and also Olmsted and his colleagues (3) who appreciated the deficiency of fiber in the diet as causative of several gastro-intestinal complaints.

In 1936 Ted Dimmock (4), a young English physician, published a paper providing evidence that the addition of miller's bran to the diet not only cured and prevented constipation, but was also beneficial in the treatment of haemorrhoids. I first met him and learned of his work at Mengo Mission Hospital in Kampala, Uganda in 1970. I had carried to this hospital samples of stools from a bush hospital serving a pastoral tribe over 300 miles away. These had to be x-rayed in connection with my intestinal transit-time studies referred to below.

The Post-War Period

Fiber only began to "take off" as of real value to nutrition after the 1939–45 war. Three names stand out from the two decades after the war, Alexander Walker, who was a contributor to the conference reported in this publication, began during the war to study the diets of prisoners in South Africa in relation to their health. He came to the conclusion that the high fiber diet of the black population was positively beneficial, and as long ago as 1955 (5) considered the low fat and high fiber content of their diets to be partly responsible for their almost complete immunity to coronary heart disease. In particular he demonstrated with very extensive studies that populations subsisting largely on fiber-rich plant foods passed much larger and softer stools, and had much shorter intestinal transit times.

Thomas (generally known at Peter) Cleave (6) very successfully treated constipated British sailors by administering bran when Senior Medical Officer on a battleship during the war. Subsequently he made much more important studies that will be referred to below under Western Diseases.

Hugh Trowell in 1960 (7) published a book which in retrospect was of seminal importance, but which was almost totally ignored at the time. In his "Non-infective disease in Africa" he listed over 30 diseases common in western countries, but rare or even non-existent in Africans. Evidence was provided from his own 30 years experience in Africa and a very extensive search of the African medical literature. He considered that the fiber-rich foods, resulting in the passage of bulky stools, was a protective factor against many of these disorders. It was my meetings with Cleave and Walker that prompted me, over 20 years ago, to make an almost worldwide study of stool weights and intestinal transit times (8). In the late 1960's and early 70's Martin Eastwood, Ken Heaton, Neil Painter, David Southgate, and John Cummings were making major contributions in Britain while the work of the fiber chemist Peter van Soest, and the contributions of Jim Anderson and David Jenkins and many others, was becoming widely recognised in North America.

It was not until 1974 (9) that Hugh Trowell recommended that the no-longer acceptable term "crude fiber" be replaced by the name "dietary fiber."

The dramatic explosion in interest in fiber that occurred during the 1970's is well demonstrated by the fact that published papers on the subject soared from around ten a year in the late 1960's to over 500 by 1980. The very word fiber other than "fiber optics" did not even appear in the Cumulative Index Medicus until the mid seventies and then it was followed by the words "see cellulose," assuming that fiber and cellulose were synonymous terms.

The low value ascribed to fiber two decades ago is illustrated by some controversy Trowell and I had with the British millers. In a major lecture delivered in London I had suggested that some of the common gastrointestinal problems in western countries might be attributed to the fact that we had removed much of the fiber from our diets not recognising its value. This was taken up by the press and so naturally worried the flour millers, who hurriedly issued a press release for use by any newspaper. This was forwarded to me by a friend when I was on holiday in Scotland. They wanted to refute what they considered totally untenable suggestions that were being made to the effect that a deficiency in fiber might play a role in the causation of any disease. Their scientists, reputed to be the best in the land, had assured them that such suggestions were ridiculous. A request for the names of these advisers was rejected but the milling authorities agreed to have a series of discussions on the matter with Trowell and myself. We failed to convince them but managed to keep the discussions amicable, with the result that I was invited to address the annual meeting of British Millers, the annual meeting of British Bakers, and one of the annual meetings of a large American group of millers on the subject. This demonstrated to us that one never persuades an opponent by attacking him.

Eventually we agreed that the matter be discussed by an important government nutrition committee who after long deliberation ruled that fiber in the diet could in fact have nutritional value. How dramatically things have changed within twenty years with the USA's Surgeon General's Report on "Nutrition and Health" (10), the WHO report on "Diet, Nutrition, and the Prevention of Chronic Diseases" (11), and the British Government NACNE Report—all recommending a large increase in the fiber content in foods in more industrialised countries. In fact similar recommendations have been made in over sixty reports on diet from eleven countries. It certainly could not have been foreseen in the early 1970's that less than two decades hence a series of international conferences would be dedicated to the implications of the dietary fiber content of foods.

The Concept of Western Diseases

Of infinitely greater importance than the emergence of fiber as an important component of nutrition has been the concept of Western Diseases (12), which was largely the outcome of investigating the epidemiology of fiber-related disorders. The recognition of the extremely important fact that many of the commonest diseases affecting more economically developed populations were rare; and, in some instances, unknown in communities whose life-styles differed little from that of their ancestors suggested the importance of environmental factors in their etiology. This conclusion was strengthened by the observation that these diseases were apparently rare even in North America and Western Europe before the first quarter of the present century, and yet had comparable prevalence in both black and white Americans. The inescapable conclusion that life-style was to blame rather than genetic inheritance was further underlined by the speed at which the descendants of Japanese immigrants to the USA exhibited diseases patterns similar to other ethnic populations in North America. Similar changes have been taking place in Japan since 1950, as the introduction of western-type diets has been followed by increased prevalence of many western diseases (13).

It was Cleave who first fired my enthusiasm for what appeared to me of outstanding importance. The evidence that he had accumulated, mainly by extensive long-hand correspondence throughout the world, that many of our commonest diseases were man-made, and consequently potentially preventable, was obviously of enormous importance. This was, I believe, his greatest contribution, far exceeding his incrimination of refined carbohydrate foods as a causation of disease.

At that time, the late 1960's, I was receiving information regularly on certain selected types of cancer from over 150 mainly rural mission hospitals throughout much of Africa (14), but also from Asia. I was able to collect, with the assistance of various agencies from over 600 Third World hospitals, information regarding the rarity of such common diseases in the west as gall-stones, colon cancer, diabetes, coronary-heart-disease and varicose veins; and to obtain from more major medical institutions evidence on the virtual absence of diverticular disease of the colon and hiatus hernia.

Although my name has been linked with the Western Diseases concept I disclaim any credit for originality. I just happened to be in a particularly favourable situation to collect data to substantiate the brilliant observations of men like Cleave and Trowell whose work had not been taken seriously.

The Concept of Maladaptation

Another revolutionary concept now widely accepted was the conclusion that the diseases which only occur commonly in populations whose life-styles have altered dramatically from that in which their ancestors evolved, must be viewed as manifestations of maladaptation to a new environment to which western man is not genetically adapted. We have made more changes in our life-style, and in our diet in particular, during the past 200 years than our ancestors made over the previous 2000 years. There are enormous contrasts between the life-styles of so-called Third World populations and that of the west, but much smaller contrasts between that of the Third World and the life-style of our Paleolithic ancestors. Although the contrasts are many, nutrition and activity appear to be the ones most likely to be linked with the extreme contrasts in the prevalence of Western Diseases. The major nutritional changes that have accompanied economical development have been a great reduction in consumption of fiber-rich starch foods and a compensatory increased intake of fat, animal protein, salt and sugar (15). Some of the early fiber pioneers—Walker, Trowell, and Cleave—helped formulate the concept of Western Diseases. The concept of maladaptation, hinted at by Cleave and Trowell, was later enormously strengthened by Thomas McKeown (16) and by Boyd Eaton and his colleagues (17). An appropriate analogy for the concept of Western Diseases being manifestations of maladaptation and one which illustrated the only sound approach to prevention, is the manner in which two wheels with equally spaced cogs engage smoothly with one another. If the size or number of cogs in either wheel is altered, there is no longer smooth engagement. Our life-style is represented by the arrangement of cogs on one wheel, and our genetically determined constitution by the cogs on the other. In the past our genes were adapted to their environment and the cogs on each wheel were the same. We have so changed our environmental cogs that they no longer engage harmoniously with our genetic constitution which cannot be changed. Consequently the only solution is to alter the pattern of our life-style towards that to which we are genetically adapted, using all the tricks of modern food technology to make our more Paleolithic diets as attractive and tasteful as possible.

If McKeown's judgment is right, which I believe it is, then some of those who contributed to this observation like Peter Cleave, Alexander Walker, and Hugh Trowell must be included among our major medical pioneers.

References

1. T. R. Allinson. The Advantages of Whole-meal Bread. Reprints from "Food." Published by F. N. Fowler, London (1889).
2. G. R. Cowgill and W. E. Anderson. Laxative effects of wheat bran and washed bran in healthy men. J. Amer. Med. Assoc. 98:1866-1875 (1932).
3. W. H. Olmsted and O. K. Timm. Cause of laxative effects of feeding bran, pentosan and cellulose to man. Proc. Soc. Exper. Biol. and Med. 32:141-142 (1937).
4. T. M. Dimmock. The prevention of constipation. Brit. Med. J. 1:906-909 (1937).
5. A. R. P. Walker. Diet and atherosclerosis. Lancet, 565-566 (1955).
6. T. L. Cleave and D. G. Campbell. Diabetes, Coronary Thrombosis and the Saccharine Disease. Wright, Bristol (1966).
7. H. C. Trowell. Non-infective Disease in Africa. Edward Arnold, London (1960).
8. D. P. Burkitt, A. R. P. Walker and N. S. Painter. Dietary fiber and disease. J.A.M.A. 229, 1078-1074 (1974).
9. H. C. Trowell. Definition of fiber. Lancet, 503 (1974).
10. Surgeon General's Report on Nutrition and health. U.S. Department of Health (1988).
11. Nutrition and the Prevention of Chronic Diseases. WHO, Technical Report Series 797, Geneva (1990).
12. H. C. Trowell and D. P. Burkitt. Western Diseases, Their Emergence and Prevention. Edward Arnold, London (1981).
13. Tsuneyuki Oku. The Epidemiological Significance of Dietary Changes in Japan. Proceedings of Kellogg International Symposium on Dietary Fiber. Center for Academic Publications, Tokyo, Japan (1990).
14. D. P. Burkitt. Some diseases characteristic of modern western civilization. Brit.

Med. J. 1:174-178 (1973).
15. D. P. Burkitt. Putting the wrong fuel in the tank. Nutrition 5:189-191 (1989).
16. T. McKeown. The Origins of Human Disease. Basil Blackwell, Oxford, pp. 140-141 (1988).
17. S. B. Eaton, M. Shostack and M. Konner. The Paleolithic Prescription. Harper and Row, New York (1988).

Dietary Fiber in Health and Disease: The South African Experience

Alexander R. P. Walker

Human Biochemistry Research Unit, Department of Tropical Diseases, School of Pathology of the University of the Witwatersrand, and the South African Institute for Medical Research, Johannesburg, South Africa

Introduction

This contribution provides past and present information on fiber and health/disease in the South African black population. South Africa, about four times the size of the UK, has roughly 25 million blacks, 5½ million whites, 3 million coloureds (Eur-African-Malay), and 2 million Indians. Approaching half of blacks, and most of the other populations live in urban areas.

Populations range from traditionally living rural blacks, through urban blacks in transition, to the Western-like white population. In diet and life-style, rural blacks resemble Western ancestors; black urban dwellers resemble whites of yesteryear; present whites resemble those in prosperous Western populations.

2. Historical Epidemiology of Diets, Disorders, and Diseases, with Special Reference to South Africa

From early historical times, there was a fair appreciation of what to eat and to avoid. The first ever list of essential nutrients was that put forward by Ben Sirach, in *Ecclesiasticu*—water, flour, milk, oil, salt, wine, honey. Presumably, the availability of vegetables and fruit was

11

taken for granted. In Biblical times, Josephus marvelled at the good health of the Essenes; he noted their "unfailing sobriety and the restriction of their food and drink to a simple sufficiency ... They are long lived, most of them passing the century, owing to the simplicity of their daily life ... and the regular routine' (Williamson, 1969). Hippocrates, about 450 BC, maintained 'And this I know, moreover, that to the human body it makes a great difference whether the bread be fine or coarse; of wheat with or without the hull ...' (Adams, 1939). The great Moses Maimonides in the 12th century wrote, 'Bread ... should not be sifted thoroughly'...'One should take before the meal whatever fruit softens the stools ...' (Leibowitz and Marcus, 1974).

In brief, from 6000 BC, when crop cultivation and animal husbandry started, until the 19th century, Western populations' diets consisted mainly of plant foods; intakes of dairy produce and meat tended to be low (Den Hartog, 1980).

In past times, chief causes of sickness and death were diseases of poverty—malnutrition, nutritional deficiency diseases (especially rickets), and infectious diseases (early childhood infections, smallpox, and tuberculosis in later years). Many infants and very young children died. In the few well circumstanced, common disorders and diseases were obesity, diabetes, gout, and apoplexy. As to fiber-related diseases, constipation, appendicitis, gallstones, colon cancer, and coronary heart disease, either were very uncommon or were far less common than at present.

Nowadays, diets are higher in energy, fat and protein, mineral salts, and to a variable extent, vitamins. Deaths in infancy and childhood are near negligible. But diseases of prosperity, principally coronary heart disease, cancer, and stroke, are 'killers,' accounting for over half of total deaths (Mortality Statistics, 1989). All chronic bowel disorders and diseases are common. As to non-dietary factors, physical activity is low, and smoking practice, although decreasing, remains high, as does alcohol consumption. Nothwithstanding, vital statistics have improved tremendously; whereas life expectancy was 50 years in 1900, now it is 70–75 years.

2.2. Traditionally living Third World populations

Dietarily, there is preponderant dependence on plant foods. Malnutrition and infections are major causes of sickness and death (Trowell, 1960). People are very physically active; and, in the masses, there is relatively low smoking practice and alcohol consumption. Westernization of diet, with higher intakes of energy, fat and protein, but less fiber, is associated with variable rises in the diseases of prosperity. There are only small rises in chronic bowel diseases, but marked rises in dental caries, obesity, hypertension and stroke. However, there is greatly reduced mortality in the young and increased expectation of life (Trowell and Burkitt, 1981).

3. War-time Experimental Studies: Brown Bread and Mineral Metabolism

3.1. Studies on standard war bread in the UK.

In 1942, war conditions caused white bread to be replaced by a National Wheatmeal Loaf, of 85% extraction rate. McCance and Widdowson (1942), in Cambridge, carried out balance studies in which subjects first ate 450 g (1 lb) of white bread daily for 3–4 consecutive weeks, and then likewise the same amount of the national loaf, with observation periods of everyday diet before and after. Brown bread reduced retentions of calcium, magnesium and iron, attributed largely to the precipitating effect of the higher intake of phytic acid contained in the branny portion of the wheat meal.

3.2. Studies on standard war bread in South Africa.

In 1941, a national war loaf made from 95–100% extraction wheat meal was introduced. The National Nutrition Council decided that the studies made by McCance and Widdowson should be repeated locally, in part because the large black population had, and still has, a low calcium intake.

Studies were carried out by the author and helpers on white volunteers, not for 4, but for 6- to 10-week periods. Consumption of 450 g of white bread daily was followed by a period of 450 g daily of national war bread. On the latter regimen there were initial negative balances of calcium, magnesium, and iron. These became less with time, equilibrium was reached, followed by positive balances. The implication is that the body, given time, adapts to an increased phytic acid intake, so that, in the long-term, mineral absorptions and retentions are not meaningfully reduced (Walker et al., 1948).

Next, in a study conducted in a prison, five black subjects were studied, first on their everyday high-fiber diet, high in maize meal (of 80% extraction rate) and beans (jugo beans, cowpeas), then on white bread, followed by a period on the national brown bread diet. Periods of observation were 4, 4, and 10 weeks. Subjects, in equilibrium on their everyday diet, went into negative balance on the brown bread regimen, but in time they reached equilibrium again. Hence, in this context, apparently the body satisfactorily adapts to an increased intake of phytic acid, despite blacks' calcium intake being habitually low, about 350–400 mg daily. In harmony, the black subjects had excellent teeth, and the X-ray appearance of hands and wrists were similar to those of white counterparts accustomed to a much higher calcium intake. Furthermore, in subsequent studies it was found that the average compositions of ribs and vertebral bodies of blacks and whites were closely similar. Thus, among the black population, a high-fiber, high phytic acid, low-calcium diet does not appear to meaningfully prejudice their calcification and general well being (Walker, 1951; Walker 1987).

4. War-time Black Prisoners' Diet, Disorders, and Diseases

4.1. Fiber intake.

Their diet included maize meal porridge, brown bread, beans, vegetables, and meat four times per week. From weighed portions of foodstuffs over a week period, mean daily crude fiber intake was 9.5 g daily, i.e., about 33 g of dietary fiber daily.

4.2. Stool size.

Feces voided over one-week collections averaged 285 g wet feces, and 70.2 g dry feces *per diem* for black prisoners. That of white prisoners on their everyday diet, averaged 28.8g.

4.3. Transit time.

Using carmine, transit time averaged 16.5 hours for blacks. That of young white prisoners averaged 28.7 hours, and of young white men in this Institute, 32.6 hours.

4.4. Defecation frequency.

Over a 7-day period for blacks, average daily frequency was 2.1; for white prisoners 1.2, and for the young men on their everyday diet, 0.9. The latter value is similar to those of like populations (Connell *et al.*, 1965). Hippocrates said that defecation should be 'twice or thrice daily' (Adams, 1939).

4.5. Passage of stool on request.

Four of the five black subjects produced a stool on request, within half an hour, collections ranging from 15 to 241 g. The passage of stools on request has been noted for black schoolchildren (Walker, 1961a).

4.6. Bowel behavior and constipation.

In a month period, 3% of black prisoners, but 18% of white prisoners asked for a laxative. However, 45% of the young white men on their everyday diet took a laxative once or more per month.

4.7. Appendicitis.

Over a ten-year period, out of a thousand or so of black prisoners only one developed appendicitis. The disease was then rare in blacks admitted to hospital (Erasmus, 1939).

4.8. Colon cancer.

No case had occurred over a ten-year period; however, only 13% of black prisoners were aged 50 years or over. This cancer was rare amongst urban patients admitted to hospital (Isaacson *et al.*,1978).

4.9. Coronary heart disease.

No case had occurred in older prisoners. The disease was very rarely seen in hospital.

5. The Beginnings of the Fiber Hypothesis in South Africa

In the early 1950's, the question obtruded—what is it in the diet of blacks which keeps them relatively free from degenerative diseases? Walker and Arvidsson (1954) suggested, 'Of the dietary factors, our impression is that, apart from low fat intake, there is a factor or factors in the pattern of diet of the Bantu possibly related to its high fibre content, which bears some responsibility for the low serum cholesterol values observed.' Subsequently, in a letter to *Lancet* (Walker, 1955), it was advanced that a low fat intake is only one feature of their pattern of diet; furthermore, a low incidence of atherosclerosis is but one feature of their disease pattern. Their diet, while probably adequate in calories and gross protein, is low in animal protein, fat, cholesterol, sugar, certain mineral salts and vitamins, yet high in carbohydrate and crude fibre. Among these people there is a high incidence of liver disease, though a low incidence not only of atherosclerosis, but of appendicitis, eclampsia, peptic ulcer, diabetes, gallstones, urinary stones, and certain forms of cancer.

Accordingly, clearly, a traditional diet low in fat but high in fiber inhibits development of western diseases; there are no exceptions. In the 1960's and later, Burkitt (Burkitt, 1969; Burkitt *et al.*, 1972; Burkitt, 1988), Trowell (1960, 1976), Cleave (1974), and others, advanced further evidence that definite patterns of diet evoke particular patterns of disorders and diseases.

6. Experimental Studies: Recent Observations and Research on Blacks' Diet, Disorders, and Diseases

6.1. Fiber intake, with change in diet, has fallen.

As to general dietary changes from the 1940s to the 1980's and later, in black populations there have been increased intakes of energy, fat, and protein, especially of animal origin, mineral salts, especially of calcium, and certain vitamins (Manning *et al.*, 1974; Richter *et al.,* 1984). Consumption of maize products has fallen, and there is a much greater reliance on bread, a ready-to-eat foodstuff. Increase in meat consumption is slight; it is so expensive. Sugar intake has risen, as it has with all developing populations. Vegetables and fruit consumptions have increased, although these foodstuffs are also expensive. Less wild 'spinaches' are now eaten. The mean daily total vegetable and fruit consumption noted in a series of elderly women, 133 g, is low (Walker *et al.,* 1992a), less than half of that eaten by elderly whites (Elwood *et al.* 1990). An intake of 400 g has been is urged (Report of a Study Group of World Health Organization, 1991). The low intake of calcium in children and adults is consistent with satisfactory bone dimension indices (Walker *et al.* 1971). In urban areas, frequency of hip fracture in black women is a *tenth* of that in elderly white women (Solomon, 1979).

6.2. Feces voided daily has decreased.

Among 15 young adult males, feces voided daily averaged 120 ± 45 g wet feces, and 32 ± 11 g dry feces.

6.3. Transit time longer.

Using carmine, time of first appearance averaged 22 ± 8 hours, longer than that reported for black prisoners.

6.4. Defecation less frequent.

Frequency over a 7-day period was 1.5 ± 0.9 times daily.

6.5. Stool consistency, now mainly formed stools.

Of subjects, 40% voided unformed stools; it was 80% in the case of the prisoners.

6.6. Passage of stools on request: the capacity remains.

On 100 each of rural and urban black school pupils, 94% and 86%, respectively, could comply within an hour.

6.7. Constipation.

Laxative use by blacks has increased, from enquiries made at chemists, clinics, and hospitals. Interestingly, in the UK, Goodhart, in 1910, who wrote of the diet's falling bulk-forming and laxation capacity, 'regretted the change of the occasional pill of our forefathers to the excess of the present day.'

6.8. Appendicectomy incidence in children.

Annual incidences of appendicectomy in urban black and white children of 0–14 years for 1985–1987 were estimated from questionnaires filled in by pupils and parents. Rates per 10,000 children were low for blacks, varying from 0.5 to 1.9; but high for whites, 21.5 to 39.5 (Walker *et al.*, 1989a). The latter rates are similar to those published for western child populations (Addiss *et al.*, 1990).

6.9. Diverticular disease.

The number of patients with the disease, as seen at Baragwanath Hospital (3,000 beds), Soweto, was 18 in 1970, but 43 in 1982.

6.10. Colon cancer.

The rate in 1986 (Cancer Registry of South Africa, 1988), adjusted for world population, was 1.8 per 100,000; i.e., 5–10% of that reported for white populations (Whelan *et al.*, 1990).

6.11. Gall stones in elderly urban black women.

In developed populations, a third of elderly women have gall stones, as assessed from ultrasonography. In South Africa, cholelithiasis is rare in those blacks consuming their low-fat high-fiber diet. Recently, ultrasonography studies were carried out in association with workers at Baragwanath Hospital, on 100 urban black women aged 55–85 years. Ten (10%) were positive (Walker *et al.*, 1989b). There was no association with parity. Mean Body Mass Index of those positive was significantly higher than that of those negative. No significant differences were noted between the dietary intakes of those positive and negative, respecting energy, protein, fat, carbohydrate, dietary fiber nor sugar.

6.12. Coronary heart disease.

The disease is absent in rural blacks. Even in urban blacks it is still relatively rare (Walker and Walker, 1985; Walker *et al.* 1992c). Intriguingly, rates of all local populations save blacks are now falling despite near negligible avoiding action.

7. Reasons for Slowness of Rises in Blacks' Fiber-Related Disorders and Diseases

7.1. Fecal pH remains low.

Early studies made on rural black schoolchildren aged 10–12 years, of homogeneous socio-economic level and village environment, revealed wide ranges in bowel behavior, including transit time and fecal pH values. It was considered that a constitutional determinant of fecal pH could be in operation (Walker *et al.* 1986, 1987, 1988). A constitutionally set low or set high pH value, evident in early life, could be a major determinant of whether the subject in later life will or will not develop certain chronic bowel diseases including colon cancer (Walker *et al.*, 1992d). Thornton (1981) postulated that 'it may be possible to eat a high fat (and low fiber) diet with impunity provided one's colon is sufficiently acidified.'

7.2. Transit time still shorter.

In crude studies using first appearance of a meal of sweet corn as marker (studies using carmine or pellets are no longer favoured), transit time averaged 21 ± 12 hours for rural black pupils, 25 ± 14 hours for urban black pupils, and 31.5 ± 14 hours for white pupils.

7.3. High breath methane excretion.

At Baragwanath Hospital, breath methane was measured in 1,016 people from four populations at widely different risks of bowel cancer and other colonic diseases. Percentages of producers were—rural black 84%, urban black 72%, white 52%, Indian 41% (Segal *et al.*, 1988). Bowel cancer risk was least in the population with the highest proportion of methane producers, so that methanogenesis is not a risk factor as previously suggested, but could reflect healthy colonic function.

7.4. Polyps remain rare.

According to Segal and co-workers (1981), intestinal polyps are virtually absent. Current colonoscopy observations indicate the colon even of elderly blacks to have the same appearance and elasticity as that of white adolescents.

7.5. Fecal mutagens.

Over a decade ago, mutagens in the feces of three populations at different risk levels for colon cancer were determined, using the *Salmonella mammalian* microsome mutagenicity test (Ehrich *et al.*, 1979). Nineteen percent of the samples from urban white adults were mutagenic using *Salmonella typhimurium* strain TA 100. This frequency was far greater than that in the low-risk populations of urban blacks 2%, and rural blacks 0%.

7.6. Comment.

The foregoing observations may help to explain why urban blacks still have relatively low frequencies of chronic bowel diseases (Segal and Walker, 1986). However, contrastingly, there is the experience of Japanese immigrants to Hawaii and California (Shimizu *et al.*, 1987).

With changes including a rise in fat intake and a fall in fiber intake, these people soon experience tremendous increases in polyps and colon cancer. The first-generation of immigrants attain almost *double* the frequency of sigmoid colon cancer, also of rectal cancer, compared with the rates in their white host neighbors. The investigators concluded 'the patterns of risk in relation to migration are complex and defy simple dietary or other interpretations.'

8. Other African Black Populations' Experience

8.1. Comment.

Evidence indicates that in African countries to the north, the changes in diet, behavior and diseases described are analogous to those noted in urban populations in South Africa.

9. Future Outlook of Blacks Regarding Diet, Disorders, Diseases

9.1. South African Blacks wish for total adoption of the life-style of whites.

Urban blacks in transition, and to a lesser extent rural blacks, are eager to attain the economic advantages and lifestyle characteristics of whites. The impact of a 'prudent' life-style message will be near nil. Even in US blacks, response to dietary and non-dietary guidelines has been disappointingly small.

9.2. Urban blacks are racing ahead with rising frequencies of some disorders and diseases.

Currently, 12-year-old urban black children have higher decayed-missing-filled-teeth scores than contemporary white children (Steyn and Albertse, 1987). Obesity frequency, also that of hypertension in urban blacks (more especially among women) exceed proportions prevailing in white populations (Walker *et al.*, 1990; Seedat and Seedat, 1982; Walker and Walker, 1991).

9.3. Experience of immigrant blacks in the UK.

Hospital admission studies made in Birmingham, UK, indicate that Caribbean and West African immigrants have lower occurrences of diet-related cancers and coronary heart disease, than the local white population (Potter *et al.*, 1984).

9.4. Experience of blacks in the US.

Currently, blacks' and whites' intakes of dietary fiber are very low, and averaging 9 and 11 g daily, respectively (Block and Lanza, 1987).

Nowadays, appendicitis, formerly rare, is common (Addiss *et al.*, 1990). Diverticular disease, once infrequent, has now increased (Heaton, 1990). Intestinal polyps are common (Williams *et al.*, 1975); moreover, colon cancer is now somewhat more common in the black than in the white population (Whelan *et al.*, 1990). Diabetes is now more common in blacks than in whites (Roseman, 1985). Coronary heart disease prevalence, previously low in blacks, is now much the same as that in whites (Watkins, 1984).

9.5. Outlook for Africans in the far future.

Although world production of food is approximately sufficient, this is not the case in Africa. The food situation will become even more acute in the future (Calvani, 1992). The annual increase in population in Africa is now 3.1%, in western populations it is 0.2% (Sadik, 1991). Hence, the relatively low intake of animal products could tend to even decrease, with increasing reliance on plant foods.

10. Limitations of the Dietary Fiber Hypothesis.

From the African viewpoint, the fiber hypothesis maintains that among habitual consumers of a diet *very* high in fiber and low in fat, non-infective bowel diseases (and other degenerative diseases) are rare or uncommon. In the African context there are *no* exceptions. With prosperity, when fiber intake (especially cereal fiber intake) falls and fat intake rises, the diseases mentioned emerge or become more common. However, incidence rise then becomes governed by many factors (dietary and non-dietary), some understandable, others not so. In the changed context, because fiber intake and, say, appendicitis rate, are not associated, many regard the fiber hypothesis as having been put out of court. This is unfortunate and incorrect. By analogy, in coronary heart disease there are many puzzling facets. These include not only the epidemiology, but the weight of dietary and non-dietary risk factors, their disappointingly low predictive capacity, and, moreover, the recent falls in mortality rate. Yet the uncertainties are still compatible with certain nutrient intakes having important causal roles (Walker and Segal, 1985b). The same applies regarding the limited role of sugar in caries development.

11. Current Research

11.1. Fecal pH value in blacks with Western diseases.

Values are being determined in patients with appendicitis, diabetes, and other western diseases.

11.2. Short-chain fatty acids and contrasting diseases in blacks and whites.

Concentrations are being measured, in association with Professor I Segal (Baragwanath Hospital, Soweto, Johannesburg), in the feces of outwardly healthy blacks and whites, young and old, and in patients with various bowel diseases.

11.3. Fecal mutagen changes.

Questions being tackled are—in persons positive, how much and for how long must supplementary fiber foods be given to render feces negative for mutagens? What proportion of affected persons respond? Are there interethnic differences? Once fiber supplementation stops in responders, for how long do the feces remain negative? Again, in the studies described, what are the acccompanying changes in bowel behavior and in short chain fatty acid concentrations?

11.4. Coagulation and fibrinolysis.

Major advances have been made by Vorster and co-workers, at University of Potchefstroom, who have examined effects of different dietary fiber components on coagulation and fibrinolytic systems (Vorster *et al.*, 1988). This group has demonstrated that soluble dietary fiber lowers plasma fibrinogen levels in the hyperfibrinogenemic Zucker fatty rat (Vorster *et al.*, 1985; Venter *et al.*, 1991), the android obese baboon model (Venter *et al.*, 1990b), and in diabetic patients (Vorster *et al.*, 1988). Also being investigated are the effects of high fiber diets on coagulation profiles and fibrinolytic activity of hypercholesterolemic patients, and also in subjects in different ethnic groups.

11.5. Fiber, phytic acid and hip fractures.

Studies are being made on the antecedents, dietary and non-dietary, of elderly black women with hip fractures.

11.6. Colonic microbiology of rural and urban blacks.

Collaborative studies on this important, but little researched subject, have been commenced.

12. Summary

In African urban dwellers, there have been decreases in intakes of cereals (mainly refined) and other plant products, but increases in animal products. In such populations the diseases under discussion have increased, although only slightly so, and that variably. The possible mechanisms of protective factors are discussed.

While blacks are avid to adopt more Western-like lifestyles, in general, only slight, not major, changes in diet are likely to eventuate, largely because of Africa's ubiquitous impoverishment.

Accordingly, increases in chronic bowel diseases and diet-related cancers will tend to be limited. Advice to those moving to a Western-like lifestyle regarding a 'prudent' diet, is unlikely to be heeded.

Certainly, there are limitations in explanations from the fiber hypothesis, especially concerning relationships with disease occurrence when fiber intakes are low. The not uncommon overclaiming of fiber's implication is unproductive. Yet the hypothesis's origin and development have been highly stimulatory in the quest for diet-disease relationships. Emphasis on eating more fiber-containing foods is as relevant now as it was when the hypothesis was propounded. Doubters should appreciate the universal commonness of perplexing epidemiological situations which caution against over-expectancy from *any* hypothesis on disease causation, prevention or control.

References

Adams, F., 1939, *The Genuine Works of Hippocrates,* Baltimore: Williams and Wilkins.

Addiss, D. G., Shaffer, N., Fowler, B. S., and Tauxe, R. V., 1990, The epidemiology of appendicitis and appendectomy in the United States, *Am. J. Epidemiol.* 132:910-925.

Block, G., and Lanza, E., 1987, Dietary fiber sources in the United States by demographic group. *J. Natl. Cancer Inst.* 79:83-91.

Burkitt, D. P., 1969, Related disease—related cause? *Lancet* ii:1229-1231.

Burkitt, D. P., Walker, A. R. P., and Painter, N. S., 1972, Effect of dietary fiber on stools and transit times, and its role in the causation of disease, *Lancet* ii:1408-1412.

Burkitt, D. P., 1988, Dietary fiber and cancer, *J. Nutr.*118:531-533.

Calvani, S., 1992, Health crisis in African countries, *Lancet* 339:126.

Cancer Registry of South Africa, 1986, Johannesburg: South African Institute for Medical Research, 1988.

Cleave, T. L., 1974, *The Saccharine Disease,* Bristol: John Wright.

Connell, A. M., Hilton, C., Irvine, G., Lennard-Jones, J. E., and Misiewicz, J. J., 1965, Variation of bowel habit in two population samples, *Brit. Med. J.* 2:1095-1099.

Den Hartog, A. P., 1980, The beginning of the modern dietary pattern in the Netherlands. Food and nutrition in the years 1850-1914. A survey, *Voeding* 41:334-342.

Ehrich, M., Aswell, H. E., van Tassell, R. L., Wilkins, T. D., Walker, A. R. P., and Richardson, N. V., 1979, Mutagens in the feces of 3 South African populations at different levels of risk for colon cancer, *Mutation Res.* 64:231-240.&2.

Elwood, P. C., Bird, G., Hughes, S. J., and Fehily, A. M., 1990, The nutrient intakes of women: dietary surveys in 1966 and 1983 compared, *J. Hum. Nutr. Dietet.* 3:33-37.

Erasmus, J. F. P., 1939, The incidence of appendicitis in the Bantu, *S. Afr. Med. J.* 13:601-606.

Goodhart, J. F., 1910, The treatment of chronic constipation, *Lancet*, 2:468-472.

Heaton, K. W., 1990, Other colonic diseases. *Med. Internat.* 4:3305-3307.

Household Food Consumption and Expenditure. 1983. Annual report of the national food survey committee. London: Her Majesty's Stationery Office, 1983.

Isaacson, C., Selzer, G., Kaye, V., Breenberg, M., Woodruff, J. D., Davies, J., Ninin, D., Vetten, D., Andrew, M., 1978, Cancer in urban blacks of South Africa, *S. Afr. Cancer Bull.* 22:49-84.

Leibowitz, J. O., and Marcus, S., 1974, *Moses Maimonides on the Causes of Symptoms*, London: University of California Press.

Manning, E. B., Mann, J. I., Sophangisa, E., and Truswell, A. S., 1974, Dietary patterns in urbanized blacks, *S. Afr. Med. J.* 48:485-497.

McCance, R. A., and Widdowson, E. M., 1940, The Chemical Composition of Foods, Med. Res. Coun. Spec. Rep. Ser. No. 235, London: Her Majesty's Stationery Office.

McCance, R. A., and Widdowson, E. M., 1942, Mineral metabolism of healthy adults on white and brown bread dietaries, *J. Physiol.* 101 44-85.

Mortality Statistics, 1989, General. Review of the Register General on deaths in England and Wales, 1989. Series D H I No. 23. Her Majesty's Stationery Office, 1991.

Potter, J. F., Dawkins, D. M., Pandha, H. S., and Beevers, D. G., 1984, Cancer in Blacks, Whites and Asians in a British hospital, *J. R. Coll. Physicians Lond.* 18:231-235.

Quin, P. J., 1959, *Foods and Feeding Habits of the Pedi,* Johannesburg: Witwatersrand University Press.

Richter, M. J. C., Langenhoven, M. L., du Plessis, J. P., Ferreira, J. J., Swanepoel, A.S.P., and Jordaan, P.C.J., 1984, Nutritional value of diets of Blacks in Ciskei. *S. Afr.* Med. J. 65:338-345.

Roseman, J. M., 1985, Diabetes in black Americans. In: *Diabetes in America.* Washington: U.S. Department of Health and Human Services, Public Health Service. National Institutes of Health, Chapter VIII 1-24.

Sadik, N., 1991, Healthy people—in numbers the world can support, *World Health Forum* 12: 347-355.

Seedat, Y. K., and Seedat, M. A., 1982, An inter-racial study of the prevalence of hypertension in an urban South African population, *Trans. Roy. Soc. Trop. Med. Hyg.* 76:62-71.

Shimizu, H., Mack, T. M., Ross, R. K., and Henderson, B. E., 1987, Cancer of the gastrointestinal tract among the Japanese and white immigrants in Los Angeles County, *J. Natl. Cancer Inst.* 78: 223-228.

Segal, I., Cooke, S. A., Hamilton, D. G., and Ou Tim, L., 1981, Polyps and colorectal cancer in South African blacks, *Gut* 22: 653-657.

Segal, I., and Walker, A. R. P., 1986, Low-fat intake with falling fiber intake commensurate with rarity of non-infective bowel diseases in blacks in Soweto, Johannesburg, South Africa, *Nutr. Cancer* 8:185-191.

Segal, I., Walker, A. R. P., Lord, S., and Cummings, J. H., 1988, Breath methane and large bowel cancer risk in contrasting African populations, *Gut* 29:608-613.

Solomon, L., 1979, Bone density in ageing Caucasian and African populations. *Lancet* ii:1326-1330.

Steyn, N. P., and Albertse, E. C., 1987, Sucrose consumption and dental caries in twelve-year-old children residing in Cape Town, *J. Dent. Ass. S. Afr.* 42:43-49.

Thornton, J. R., 1981, High colonic pH promotes colorectal cancer, *Lancet* i:1083-1087.

Trowell, H. C., 1960, *Non-Infective Diseases in Africa*, London: Edward Arnold.

Trowell, H. C., 1976, Definition of dietary fiber and hypothesis that it is a protective factor in certain diseases, *Am. J. Clin. Nutr.* 29:417-427.

Trowell, H. C., and Burkitt, D. P., 1981, *Western Diseases: their emergence and prevention*, London: Edward Arnold.

Venter, C. S., Vorster, H. H., Smuts, M., *et al.*, 1990b, Effect of weight changes on plasma fibrinogen and serum insulin levels in the baboon (Papio Ursinus). (Abstr.). *S. Afr. J. Food Sci. Nutr.* 2(1) Suppl: 15A.

Vorster, H. H., Kruger, H. S., Frylinck, S., Botha, B. J., Lombard, W. A., De Jager, J., 1985, Physiological effects of the dietary fibre component konjac-glucomannan in rats and baboons. *J. Plant Foods* 6(4):263-274.

Vorster, H. H., Venter, C. S., Silvis, N., Van Eeden, T. S., Huisman, H. W., and Walker, A. R. P., 1988, Dietary influences on haemostasis may affect risk for coronary heart disease. *S. Afr. J. Sci.* 84:289-293.

Walker, A. R. P., 1947, The effect of recent changes of food habits on bowel motility, *S. Afr. Med. J.* 21:590-596.

Walker, A. R. P., Fox, F. W., and Irving, J. T., 1948, Studies in human mineral metabolism. The effect of bread rich in phytic acid phosphorus on the metabolism of certain mineral salts with special reference to calcium, *Biochem. J.* 42:452-462.

Walker, A. R. P., 1950, *Calcification in the Bantu: calcium balance experiments*, Annual Report of the South African Institute for Medical Research, Johannesburg, p.15.

Walker, A. R. P., and Arvidsson, U. B., 1954, Fat intake, serum cholesterol concentration, and atherosclerosis in the South African Bantu. Part I. Low fat intake and the age trend of serum cholesterol concentration in the South African Bantu, *J. Clin. Invest.* 33:1358-1365.

Walker, A. R. P., 1955, Diet and atherosclerosis. *Lancet* i:565-566.

Walker, A. R. P., 1959, Some aspects of the endocrinological picture of the South African Bantu. A population relatively free from mortality from coronary heart disease, In: Pincus G, ed. *Hormones and Atherosclerosis,* Chapter 28. New York: Academic Press, p. 385.

Walker, A. R. P., 1961a, Crude fiber, bowel motility, and pattern of diet, *S. Afr. Med. J.* 35:114-115.

Walker, A. R. P., 1961b, Fibrinolytic activity of whole blood from South African Bantu and White subjects, *Am. J. Clin. Nutr.* 9:461-472.

Walker, A. R. P., Walker, B. F., and Richardson, B. D., 1971, Metacarpal bone dimensions in young and aged South African Bantu consuming a diet low in calcium, *Postgrad. Med. J.* 47:320-325.

Walker, A. R. P., and Walker, B. F., 1985, Coronary heart disease in blacks in underdeveloped populations, *Am. Heart J.* 109:1410.

Walker, A. R. P., Walker, B. F., and Walker, A. J., 1986, Faecal pH, dietary fibre intake, and proneness to colon cancer in four South African populations, *Br. J. Cancer* 53:489-495.

Walker, A. R. P., 1987, Dietary fiber and mineral metabolism, *Molec. Aspect Med.* 9:69-87.

Walker, A. R. P., Walker, B. F., and Walker, A. J., 1987, Reply to selected summary. Fecal pH, dietary fiber, and colon cancer risk, *Gastroenterology* 92:1277.

Walker, A. R. P., Walker, B. F., Segal, I., 1988, Faecal pH: a constitutional characteristic? *S. Afr. Med. J.* 73:672.

Walker, A. R. P., Shipton, E., Walker, B. F., Manetsi, B., Van Rensburg, P. J. S., and Vorster, H. H., 1989a, Appendicectomy incidence in black and white children aged 0-14 years, with a discussion on the disease's causation, *Trop. Gastroenterol.* 24:42-46.

Walker, A. R. P., Segal, I., Posner, R., Shein, H., Tsotsetsi, N.G., and Walker, A. J., 1989b, Prevalence of gall stones in elderly black women in Soweto, Johannesburg, as assessed by ultrasonography, *Am. J. Gastroenterol.* 84:1383-1385.

Walker, A. R. P., Walker, B. F., Manetsi, B., Tsotetsi, N. G., and Walker, A. J., 1990, Obesity in black women in Soweto, South Africa: minimal effects on hypertension, hyperlipidaemia, hyperglycaemia. *J. Roy. Soc. Health* 110:101-103.

Walker, A. R. P., and Walker, B. F., 1991, Diabetes prevalence in elderly rural blacks in South Africa, *S. Afr. J. Food Sci. Nutr.* 3:68-71.

Walker, A. R. P., Adam, A., and Küstner, H. G. V., 1992c, Changes in total death rate and in ischaemic heart disease death rate from 1978 to 1989 in South African interethnic populations. *S. Afr. Med. J.* In press.

Walker, A. R. P., Walker, B. F., and Segal, I., 1992d, Faecal pH and colon cancer, *Gut.* In press.

Watkins, L. O., 1984, Coronary heart disease and coronary disease risk factors in black populations in underdeveloped countries: The case for primordial prevention, *Am. Heart J.* 108:850-862.

Whelan, S. L., Parkin, D. M., and Masuyer, E., 1990, *Patterns of Cancer in Five Continents*. Lyon: International Agency for Research on Cancer.

Williams, A. O., Chung, E. B., Agbata, A., and Jackson, M. A., 1975, Intestinal polyps in American Negroes and Nigerian Africans, *Br. J. Cancer* 31: 485-491.

Williamson, G. A., 1969, *Josephus: The Jewish War*. London: Penguin Classics.

The Structure of Dietary Fibre

D. A. T. Southgate

AFRC Institute of Food Research, Norwich Laboratory, Norwich Research Park, Norwich, UK

Introduction

The plant foods in the diet provide, in dietary fibre, a range of different types of polysaccharides exhibiting a variety of primary, secondary, and tertiary structures (Morris, 1980). In addition to these structural features characteristic of most biopolymers these polysaccharides are combined in the supramolecular structures of the plant cell wall (Albersheim, 1965), plant tissues (Cutter, 1971), and plant foods (Masefield *et al.*, 1969). These confer additional levels of structure which, together with the physico-chemical structural features, characterise dietary fibre. All of these levels of structure act as determinants of the physiological properties of dietary fibre and contribute to the interactions with the aetiology of various disease processes and therefore to the postulated protective role of dietary fibre (British Nutrition Foundation, 1990).

The evaluation of the "Dietary Fibre Hypothesis" and the development of understanding of the functions of dietary fibre from different sources is thus dependent on the study of the various levels of structure/function relationships.

Primary Structure

The polysaccharides of the plant cell walls in foods and the range of analogous extrinsic polysaccharides, derived for the most part from plant cell wall polysaccharides, together make up dietary fibre, include a range of different monosaccharide components and many contain uronic acids. The monosaccharides of the pentose series, arabinose and xylose, are present together with the hexoses glucose, galactose, and mannose. Two uronic acids, galacturonic and glucuronic, are found in the poly-saccharides in most cell walls, and mannuronic and guluronic are found in the alginates used as polysaccharide food additives. Desoxy sugars are present in some polysaccharides with rhamnose being the most common in cell wall materials. The hexoses are characteristically present in the pyranosyl ring form and the pentoses in the furanosyl form. These ring structures result in the hydroxyls on carbon-1 having either an axial or equatorial orientation so hemi-acetal bonds at this carbon are of two types beta and alpha corresponding to the steric orientations.

The carboxylic groups of the uronic acids are capable of forming salts with cations and esters with alcohols and are the major functional groups on most polysaccharides. Sulphated ester groups are found in some algal polysaccharides with strong cation-binding properties. The hydroxyl groups on the pyranosyl and furanosyl rings take part in the formation of hemi-acetal bonds with other monosaccharide units of the polymers and also in hydrogen bonding between polysaccharides.

Secondary Structures

These monosaccharide components are combined in a number of different types of polymer. The basic structural feature is a backbone chain usually involving links between carbon-1 and carbon-4 with branches or side chains from the hydroxyls on the other carbons. The polysaccharides may be homo-polysaccharides containing only one monosaccharides species or hetero-polysaccharides with two or more monosaccharide units in linear or branched structures. The branches may be many monosaccharide units long or be limited to few residues in a side chain.

The configuration of the hemi-acetal bonds is a major determinant of the form of the polysaccharide chain so that in the alpha configuration the chain adopts a helical form, whereas in the beta configuration the chain is a flat ribbon-like structure. These are important determinants of polysaccharide structure in two respects; firstly, the configuration is a major determinant of binding to proteins especially the hydrolytic enzymes (British Nutrition Foundation, 1990). Second the configuration of the molecule determines the extent of intermolecular associations with other polysaccharides with the same or different structures, which are important in determining solubility and colloidal behaviour in solution (Morris, 1980, 1992).

Intermolecular associations are also determined by the extent of branching and the distribution of side chains. In polymers with regions of the backbone free from side chains intermolecular associations can occur, whereas so-called "hairy" regions where side chains are frequent may not associate (Rees, 1972). Branching has the effect of limiting hydrogen bonding between polysaccharides so that highly branched polymers tend to be more soluble than less branched and linear polymers.

Tertiary Structures

One of the more important tertiary structures seen in the polysaccharides of the plant cell wall is the formation of fibrous structure by the association and hydrogen bonding of parallel cellulose molecules. Many chains may be involved leading to the development of microscopic fibrils and macroscopic cellulose fibres such as found in cotton. These have a high degree of ordering and many preparations of cellulose have pronounced crystallinity (Meyer and Misch, 1927). In this state the polysaccharide is virtually insoluble in aqueous solutions and resistant to all but the most vigorous chemical treatments. Cellulose is a 1-4 beta glucan and is unusual in being a natural linear homopolymer; mannose and xylose chains share a similar configuration and potential to associate in insoluble fibrils, but most of the naturally occurring mannans have galacto- or gluco-side chains which prevent the necessary hydrogen-bonding as do the branching and side chains of the naturally occurring xylans.

The numerous types of non-cellulosic polysaccharide found in the matrix of the plant cell wall have other properties due to their tertiary structures in the capacity to form hydrated colloidal sols and gels, usually by association between several different molecules. The effects of the tertiary structure in the wall itself are probably secondary to higher levels of structural organisation discussed below and most of our current experimentally based understanding relates to the behaviour of isolated polysaccharides (Rees 1969; Morris, 1992).

Polymers of Uronic Acid

Polymers of galacturonic acid are widely distributed in plant cell walls, especially the undifferentiated walls of fruits and vegetables where they form part of the water-soluble pectic fraction. Pectin itself is a polymer of galacturonic acid extracted from fruits under conditions which may lead to some depolymerisation and loss of labile side chains. The galacturonyl residues are linked 1-4 alpha and the chain is characteristically interrupted with rhamnose residues which produce a kink in the molecule. When the uronic acid carboxyl groups are free, the chains of the polymer can chelate divalent ions such as calcium and form gels at acid pHs; in most natural pectic materials the uronic groups are methoxylated and these polmers form gels in acid solutions when the concentration of solutes is increased. The concentrations of solute required are high, for example, sucrose concentrations of the order of 65% are required for the setting of jams. Acetyl groups sterically hinder the formation of gels in pectins derived from sugar beet.

Alginates which are co-polymers of mannuronic and guluronic acids widely used as polysaccharide additives also form gels with divalent ions which appear to form intermolecular bridges. The physical characteristics of the gels formed are dependent on the cation used (Glicksman, 1969).

Neutral Polysaccharides

Many polysaccharides without significant levels of uronic acid also form gels or viscous solutions under appropriate conditions and are widely used in foods as additives to control the physical properties of processed foods. One group of polymers that have been widely studied, and also used in studies of the physiological effects of polysaccharides are the galacto-mannans, locust bean and guar gums. These are linear 1-4 beta mannans with single unit galacto-side chains usually on C 6. The distribution of side chains differs in the two gums with guar having about half the mannose residues bearing galactosyl residues and locust bean gum about one in three.

The galactomannans produce viscous solutions in water and are used as thickening agents in foods where they are commonly used in combination with other polysaccharides to utilise synergistic effects, often with carrageenans which are suphated galactose and anhdro-galactose polymers. In these viscous solutions intermolecular association limits the mobility of the chains and "traps" water molecules within the interstices of the sol or gel.

A second group of polymers that have recently attracted attention are the beta-glucans which, unlike cellulose, are branched structures with 1-2 and 1-3 linkages, these polysaccharides form viscous solutions in water.

Critical Influence of Molecular Size

In these and many other polysaccharides, the side chains (and branches) are critical for solubility and colloidal properties. Partial hydrolysis to remove the side chains of guar gum, for example, reduces the viscosity of the solution very significantly. The degree of polymerisation is also critical, presumably because more potential associating sites are available to form an interlocking network. These tertiary properties therefore require a critical number of residues for their expression, for example association between uronic acid chains require at least seven residues but the strength of gel increases with molecular size (Rees and Wright, 1971).

Organisation in the Plant Cell Wall

The major proportion of the polysaccharide components of dietary fibre are not consumed in the form of isolated substances but are consumed in the structures of the plant cell wall; this imposes a higher level of structural organisation on the components of dietary fibre (Southgate, 1976). In this paper I do not propose to discuss how the plant food sources determine the composition of the dietary fibre in foods (Selvendran, 1984) but to focus on the structural feature that needs to be considered if we are to understand the relation between the effects of consuming dietary fibre and the dietary sources. The objective is to reach the point where we can predict with confidence the effects of particular diets and to explain how dietary fibre influences the aetiology of disease.

Basic Features of Cell Wall Organisation

The organisation of the plant cell wall changes as the wall develops and matures; these processes are essential to accommodate the needs of growth in the plant and the development of specialised functions of tissues in the plant (Muhlethaler, 1961). When a new cell wall forms after division the first visible structure is a cell-plate which is rich in uronans and becomes the middle lamella of the cell wall. Cellulose fibrils are deposited on this plate initially in a random network to form the primary wall. The fibrils are embedded in a matrix of non-cellulosic polysaccharides; initially these are soluble pectic substances in which arabino-galactans are major components. As the wall thickens the cellulose fibrils are laid down in a more orientated arrangement, possibly in response to physical stresses on the plant. The matrix non-cellulosic polysaccharides become richer in the hemicelluosic type of polysaccharides such as the various xylans often with highly branched and substituted molecules. This undifferentiated type of wall is found in parenchymatous tissues which make up the major part of the flesh of fruits and vegetables (Selvendran, 1984). Such walls are rich in soluble pectic substances (rhamno-galacturonans and arabino-galactans). The walls contain significant levels of protein (about 10%) and are relatively thin and elastic. The tissue maintains its form by the turgour of the cells.

Further growth of the wall occurs as the tissue matures; the wall becomes thicker by the deposition of more layers of matrix polysaccharide and cellulose fibrils. These walls are stiffer and the collenchyma tissue which contains cells with these walls contributes structural strength to stems and leaf structures.

Vascular conducting tissue develops within the plant; in the xylem regions the walls thicken and become lignified; the lignin polmer infiltrates the wall matrix which expands. Initially the lignin forms in discrete regions of the wall producing spiral or annular lignified bands but in the mature plant the walls of the xylem conducting vessels are completely lignified (Cutter, 1971). In woody tissues the cell contents disappear in the xylem vessels. The walls of other cells also become lignified in mature plants as sclerenchyma where they contribute to the rigidity of the plant body.

On the epidermal surfaces of the plant other substances are formed and these are virtually integral parts of the wall structure. Leaves and stems become cuticularised with the deposition of the substance cutin, a complex internal ester of long chain hydroxy aliphatic acids. In the subepidermal layers of roots and tubers an analogous material, suberin, is often deposited. Suberin is also deposited in the epidermal tissues of some fruits and in the outer layers of mature plants. These two types of waxy materials act as barriers to prevent water loss.

In the outer layers of many seeds the walls are lignified and in the case of nuts very thick lignified layers are present. The lignification serves to protect the seeds from desiccation and more importantly from being eaten by animals.

The Structure of Plant Foods

Our diet contains a wide range of different parts of the plant (Masefield *et al.*, 1969), and each of these parts contains a range of different types of tissue and cell wall types. The plant foods that we choose to cat and the products derived from plant foods therefore act as the determinants of the structure of the dietary fibre in the diet. Although every plant food has some special characteristics it is posssible to make some generalisations.

Cereal foods: Most of these are consumed in the form of flours or products derived from flours. In these the process of grinding the cereal has disrupted much of the cell wall architecture and the types of cell walls present are further modified by the screening and sieving processes (Kent, 1983). In low extraction, highly refined flours the walls are thin-walled structures from the endosperm and extensively broken. The thicker more lignified tissues are sieved out as bran. In whole grain flours these seed coat structures are present as discrete pieces of cellular mattter usually with small amounts of endospermal walls attached. Some grains are consumed virtually intact, for example, immature maize seeds, whereas other grains such as rice, where the seed coat is fused to the grain the outer layers are removed by abrasion or by parboiling; in these cereals cellular structures are retained into the foods consumed.

Fruits: The wide range of types of fruit consumed consist for the most part of undifferentiated parenchymatous tissues with very small amounts of lignified vascular tissues. The outer skins are usually cutinised and sometimes suberinised. Many fruits are eaten with the lignified seeds that they contain.

Leafy vegetables: These consist of leaves, petioles, and stems and associated structures such as buds and flowers. These contain parenchymal tissues with variable amounts of vascular and supporting tissues. The major parts of the cell wall materials are therefore thin-walled structures. The outer tissues are often cutinised and may be suberinised. The lignified tissues are small in proportion to the whole. Heat treatment of these tissues results in some loss of cellular structure due to softening of the walls as soluble polysaccharides are dissolved out.

Seed legumes: These seeds have thick seed coats which are cutinised but not lignified but may have polyphenolic materials deposited in them. The cotyledons or endospermal tissues which form the major part of these foods have thicker walls than the corresponding tissues in cereals. Vascular lignified tissues represent a very small part of these foods.

Tubers: These often have suberinised skins; the major proportion of the tuber consists of thin-walled undifferentiated cells usually filled with storage polysaccharides. The amounts of vascular tissue are very small.

Roots: As with most vegetables the bulk of the tissues are undifferentiated although in mature roots the vascular tissues may be significantly developed, producing a cylinder of densely lignified cells. The outer tissues are often suberinised.

The Implications of Structure
for the Physiological Effects of Dietary Fibre

In the final part of this paper I would like to discuss the implications of these structural features for the physiological effects of consuming dietary fibre. In this I will confine myself to considering the effects of the cell wall material as the source of dietary fibre, this is the dietary fibre that is intrinsic or endogenous to foods and the diet. In preparing this review I am conscious that there are many aspects of structure where the experimental evidence is lacking and I have had therefore to speculate somewhat, it may be that some of these speculations may be worthy of experimental examination.

The first structural feature of importance in the polysaccharides in the plant cell wall is the linking of the monosaccharide residues itself since by being non-alpha-glucosidic bonds (Non-Starch Polysaccharides) renders the polysaccharides resistant to the hydrolytic enzymes secreted into the mammalian digestive tract (Trowell *et al.*, 1976). Thus structure at this level is the primary defining characteristic of dietary fibre.

The second factor that is of importance relates to the secondary and tertiary levels of structure which determine solubility (Table 1). The preparation of many plant foods involves the application of moist heat, and this results in the loss of turgour in the tissues. Other techniques and practices used in preparation such as mechanical mixing further disrupt the tissue structures and, where thin cell walls are present, leads to cellular breakage. The ingestion of foods and chewing continues this disruption of the cellular organisation of the tissues. In many vegetables and the more firmly textured fruits, such as, apples and pears, discrete pieces of cellular tissue are passed into the oesophagus and into the stomach, further disintegration of tissue organisation occurs as a result of gastric activity. These processes combine to reduce the particle size of the plant tissues and expose the surfaces of the cellular structures to digestive enzymes and the other constituents of the small intestine, leaching of the more soluble components will occur progressively as the contents move down the tract. The action of the proteolytic and amylolytic enzmes on the cellular contents further expose the cell wall surfaces. Many of the matrix non-cellulosic polysaccharides are relatively insoluble because of the supramolecular structures present and the pH of

Table 1. Physico-chemical structure attributes of dietary fiber and its components

Structure level	Variable attributes	Effects on properties	Physiological implications
Primary	Monosaccharides and Uronic acid species	Hydroxyl functional groups Carboxyl	Hydration Hydrogen-bonding cation binding
	Hemiacetal bonds	Anomeric steric configuration of polymeric chains	Specificity of enzymic susceptibility
	Pyranosyl and Furanosyl conformation		
Secondary	Linear Molecules Branched Molecules Side chains	Configuration imposed by anomeric bonds Solubility	Specificity of hydrolysis by enzymes Ease of degradation by bacteria
Tertiary	Intermolecular hydrogen bonding Intermolecular helical coiling	Solubility Colloidal properties in solutions or gels	Ease of degradation by bacteria Increased viscosity of intestinal contents Reduced bulk mixing and rates of diffusion Increase unstirred layers at mucosal surface

the intestinal contents is not sufficiently high to solubilise the "hemi-cellulose" fraction (Timell, 1965; Selvendran and O'Neill, 1987). Gums and mucilages and some of the pectic components would, however, be expected to dissolve and increase the viscosity of the intestinal contents. It is probable that effects analogous to those observed when isolated soluble polysaccharides are consumed are also exhibited—but to a lesser extent—by the soluble intrinsic components (Judd and Truswell, 1981).

The functional groups of the intrinsic pectic substances are probably not sufficiently exposed in the small intestine, but the large surface areas provided by the disrupted plant tissues may be significant in binding by adsorption, or more specifically, and the matrix with its complex cellular structure may be expected to be a potent potential binder of any substances with surface activity and/or ionic properties.

In the large bowel this spongy character may serve to bind water and solutes (Eastwood, Brydon, and Anderson, 1986) and the surface properties of the cellular residues will determine the adhesion of bacteria which is the essential requirement for bacterial degradation of insoluble material. The hydrophobic character of cutinised and suberinised surfaces serves to inhibit degradation of the external walls and the hydrophobic regions of the lignified walls prevent or slow bacterial degradation. The lower polyphenolic material present in many walls also serve to inhibit the rate of degradation. Surface active degradation will degrade thinner walls more rapidly than thicker walls of the same com-

Table 2. Structural attributes of plant cell wall material and plant foods

Structure level	Variable attributes	Effects on properties	Physiological implications
Plant Cell Wall Molecular Architecture	Cellulose fibrils in Non-Cellulosic Matrix Differentiation Lignification	Elastic thin walled structures with large surface area Composition of matrix; thicker walls More rigid walls with hydrophobic regions	Soluble components contained in matrix structure Particle size increases Cell walls become stronger Resistant to bacterial degradation
Plant Tissue Structures	Parenchymatous (undifferentiated) Vascular tissues Lignified support tissues	Thin-walled; pectic substance-rich Lignified discrete particles Resistance to disruption by processing and mastication	Highly degradable by bacteria Resistant to degradation Larger particles in intestinal contents
Plant Food Structure	Range of tissues Surfaces cutinised or suberinised	Range of composition Physical properties Hydrophobic surfaces	Patterns of SCFA produced Particle size distribution Resistance to bacterial degradation

position and since the thicker walls are usually those that are more lignified it is clear that the structural organisation of plant tissues is a major determinant of the rate and extent of degradation (Van Soest 1973) (Table 2).

The composition of the polysaccharides being degraded does appear to influence the patterns of fermentation products (Mortensen, Holtug and Rasmussen, 1988), although as yet differences found in different fermentation systems make the formulation of the effects of polysaccharide composition difficult.

Conclusions

The structure of dietary fibre at several levels of organisation determines the pattern of physiogical effects and the effects of consuming polysaccharides within cell wall structures are different from those of isolated polysaccharides. While studies of isolated polysaccharides provide valuable information on the behaviour of the components of dietary fibre in the intestine; a proper understanding of the role of high fibre diets depends on the study of defined cellular materials and the properties of the cell wall surfaces, both internal and external may, I suspect, be very important for binding of constituents in the intestine and in controlling bacterial degradation in the large.

References

Albersheim, P., 1965, Biogenesis of the plant cell wall, *in*: Plant Biochemistry, J. Bonner and J. E. Varner, eds., Academic Press, New York, 298-321.

British Nutrition Foundation, 1990, Complex Carbohydrates in Foods, Chapman and Hall, London.

Cutter, E. G., 1971, Plant Anatomy-Experiment and Interpretation, Part 2 Organs, Arnold, London.

Eastwood, M. A., Brydon, W. G., and Anderson, D. M. W., 1986, The effect of the polysaccharide composition and structure of dietary fibers on caecal fermentation and faecal excretion, *Amer. J. Clin. Nutr.*, 44:51-55.

Glicksman, M., 1969, Gum Technology in the Food Industry, Academic Press, New York.

Kent, N. L., 1983, Technology of Cereals, 3rd edition, Pergamon, Oxford.

Judd, P. A., and Truswell, A. S., 1981, The effect of rolled oats on blood lipids and fecal steroid excretion in man, *Amer. J. Clin. Nutr.*, 34:2061-2067.

Masefield, G. B., Willis, M., Harrison, S. G., and Nicholson, B. E., 1969, The Oxford Book of Food Plants, Oxford University Press, Oxford.

Meyer, K. H. and Misch, L., 1927, Positions des atoms dans le nouveau modele spatial de la cellulose, *Helv. Chim. Acta*, 20:232-244.

Morris, E. R., 1980, Polysaccharide structure and conformation in solutions and gels, *in*: Polysaccharides in Foods, J.M.V. Blanshard and J.R. Mitchell, eds., Butterworths, London, 15-31.

Morris, E.R., 1992, in press.

Mortenson, P. B., Holtug, K., and Rasmussen, H. S., 1988, Short chain fatty acid production from monosaccharides and disaccharides in a faecal manbation system, Implications for the colonic fermentation of dietary fiber in humans, *J. Nutr.* 118:321-325.

Muhlethaler, K., 1961, Plant cell walls, *in*: The Cell, Vol 2, J. Brachet and A. E. Minsky, eds., Academic Press, New York, 85-134.

Rees, D. A., 1969, Structure, conformation and mechanism in the formation of polysaccharide gels and networks, *in*: Advances in Carbohydrate Chemistry, M.L. Wolfrom and R.S. Tipson, eds., Vol.24, Academic Press, New York, 267-332.

Rees, D. A., 1972, Shapely polysaccharides, *Bichem. J.*, 16:257-273.

Rees, D. A., and Wright, A. W., 1971, Polysaccharides conformation, Part VII, Model building computations for alpha 1-4 galacturonans and the kinking function of L-rhamnose residues in pectic substances, *J. Chem. Soc.*, Ser.B, 1366-1372.

Selvendran, R. R., 1984, The plant cell wall as a source of dietary fiber: chemistry and structure, *Amer. J. Clin. Nutr.*, 39:320-327.

Selvendran, R. S., and O'Neill, M. A., 1987, Isolation and analysis of cell walls from plant material, *in*: Methods of Biochemical Analysis, Vol. 32, D.Glick, ed., John Wiley, New York, 25-153.

Southgate, D. A. T., 1976, The chemistry of dietary fiber, *in*: Fiber in Human Nutrition, G. A. Spiller and R. J. Amen, eds., Plenum Press, New York, 31-72.

Timell, T. E., 1965, Wood hemicelluloses, *in*: Advances in Carbohydrate Chemistry, M. L. Wolfrom and R. S.Tipson. (eds) Vol 19. Academic Press, New York. 247-307.

Trowell, H. C., Southgate, D. A. T., Wolever, T. M. S., Leeds, A. R., Gassul, M. A. and Jenkins, D. J. A., 1976, Dietary fibre redefined, *Lancet*, 1:967.

Van Soest, P. J., 1973, The uniformity and nutritive availability of cellulose, *Fed. Proc*, 32:1804-1808.

Fiber in Foods

Edwin R. Morris

Department of Food Research and Technology,
Cranfield Institute of Technology, Silsoe College,
Silsoe,
Bedford MK45 4DT, UK.

Introduction

About the Author

I am a physical chemist who has spent over twenty years working in and around the food industry on the structure-function relationships of polysaccharides. For the last five or six years I have had a peripheral involvement with the dietary fiber area, as an unofficial 'consultant' to a couple of research groups working on different aspects of physiological action, and as a participant in several meetings like the present Symposium. One thing I have learned is that a lot of otherwise meticulous clinical research neglects basic principles of polysaccharide behaviour that are well known in the food industry, and have been reviewed comprehensively.

About this Paper

The intention of the present paper is not to duplicate the content of such previous reviews[1-5], but to highlight a few 'take-home messages' for the dietary fiber audience. Readers who require more detailed information are encouraged to refer to the publications cited in the reference list, or indeed to contact me directly.

The style of this article is deliberately informal and provocative, to focus attention on the importance of taking into account the physical properties of polysaccharides when planning clinical studies of their physiological action. The same considerations are at least as important when dealing with 'natural' fiber. I of course realise that the structures may be more complex, but the basic principles remain the same. Complex systems demand greater rigour in experimental design, not less.

General Principle

Order and Disorder

The starting point is to realise that polysaccharides, which are the basic building blocks of dietary fiber, can exist in either ordered or disordered forms[1]. The ordered structures can have quite different geometries. Common motifs include assemblies of flat ribbons (cellulose fibrils), double helices (starch) and buckled chains with cavities occupied by bound ions (pectin).

Hydrated Networks Need Both

Swollen networks (which can include anything from a simple jelly to plant tissue or complex food products) are held together by ordered junctions. Too much order, however, will give a packed solid. A three-dimensional network that can hold water also requires some disordered sequences to interrupt the packing and stretch between the junctions. Co-existence of ordered and disordered regions in the same polysaccharide chain usually involves a change in primary sequence. Some polysaccharides (such as alginate) have a block structure, with only one type of block forming ordered junctions. In others the association is broken by 'rogue' residues in the polymer backbone, or by sidechains that cannot pack within the ordered structure.

Solubility and Melting

It is the relative stabilities of the ordered and disordered forms that determine whether or not a polysaccharide will dissolve. Packed order maximises enthalpically-favourable interactions (non-covalent bonding) between the chains. Conversion to disordered, fluctuating coils in solution takes out the bonding but maximises the entropy (freedom of movement). The balance between the enthalpic disadvantage of dissolving (ΔH) and the entropic advantage (ΔS) is given by the difference in 'free energy' (ΔG), and can be tipped by temperature (T):

$$\Delta G = \Delta H - T\Delta S = 0 \text{ at } T_m$$

Entropy becomes more important at higher temperatures. That is why some materials that are insoluble in cold water will dissolve on heating.

It is also the reason why some gel networks melt (quite sharply) on heating. The 'transition-midpoint temperature', T_m, is the point at which the enthalpy and entropy effects just balance:

$$T_m = \Delta H / \Delta S$$

Higher temperatures promote conversion to a soluble, disordered coil; lower temperatures favour the ordered structure (either as 'insoluble fiber' or as part of a hydrated network, depending on the structure of the rest of the chain).

In 'natural' fibres (i.e., intact plant tissue), these non-covalent associations may be augmented by covalent attachment of polysaccharides to proteins or, more rarely, to other polysaccharides. Covalent linkages will normally survive high temperatures (e.g., during cooking), but may be broken down during digestion and colonic fermentation.

Structure–Function Relationships

Carbohydrate Analysis Doesn't Tell Us Much

The type of ordered structure (if any) that a polysaccharide chain will adopt does not depend on which sugars are present, but on how they are linked together. The same sugar linked in different ways can give entirely different structures with entirely different properties (e.g., starch, cellulose, and dextran). Conversely, different sugars linked in the same way often give similar structures with similar properties (e.g., cellulose, chitin, and mannan).

Small Differences Can Have Big Effects

Knowing the linkages between the sugars is an enormous improvement, but it is still not enough to predict physical properties. Because the non-covalent bonds between sugar residues are weak, ordered junctions are stable only when they exceed a critical length. This can vary enormously from one polysaccharide to another, and for the same polysaccharide under different conditions (e.g., of ionic environment), but typical values are in the range 6–20 residues. Structural irregularities spaced more closely than this may totally abolish ordered packing. For example, methyl ester substituents on pectin have little effect on its ability to form gels with calcium if they are grouped together in blocks, leaving long runs of unesterified residues. The same proportion of ester distributed randomly along the chain can have a profound effect, by splitting the unesterified regions into runs that are too short to form ordered junctions. Determination of the 'fine structure' of polysaccharides (i.e., the distribution of irregularities) is often impossible, and is certainly never easy enough to be carried out routinely.

Charge Blows Chains Apart

About the only useful general relationship that can be drawn between polysaccharide composition and physical properties is that charged groups, by repelling one another, inhibit ordered packing and promote solubility. In the disordered coil form in solution, electrostatic repulsions between different segments of the same chain expand the coil and therefore, as described later, increase the solution viscosity.

Counterions Let Them Come Together

Ions of opposite charge can reduce or eliminate the electrostatic repulsions within and between charged polysaccharide chains. They can do this in two ways. The first is by clustering round the polymer chain as an 'ion atmosphere'. The second is by direct binding to specific sites along the chain.

Atmospheric binding depends almost entirely on charge. Specific site-binding also requires the ions to be the right size to fit in the binding site. Since the charged groups on natural polysaccharides are invariably negatively charged (carboxyl or sulphate) the relevant counterions are metal cations (e.g., Na^+, K^+, Ca^{2+}).

The effect of atmospheric binding in solution is to allow the coil dimensions to collapse towards those of the equivalent uncharged polysaccharide. The effect on conformational ordering is to increase T_m, making ordered structures stable to higher temperature. Site-binding, allowing counterions to become part of the ordered structure, can have even more dramatic effects, often converting disordered coils to structures that are stable to above 100 C.

Ordered Packing Inhibits Enzymic Digestion

Although the presence of appropriate enzymes is, of course, essential for digestion of polysaccharides, the physical form of the polymer can also be of major importance. Enzymes that readily cleave disordered coils may act much more slowly, or not at all, if the same polysaccharide is present in a packed, ordered structure. In particular, retrograded amylose and the amylopectin molecules in native starch both exist as packed assemblies of double helices, and are resistant to human digestive enzymes, in contrast to freshly gelatinised starch where the same molecules are present in the disordered form. The same principle will, of course, apply to the susceptibility or resistance of dietary-fiber poly-saccharides to bacterial fermentation in the colon.

Solution Properties

Viscosity Is Not One Number

For simple fluids such as oils or syrups, pushing twice as hard will make them move twice as fast. More formally, the shear-rate (γ) generated increases in direct proportion to the applied shear-stress (τ), so that the viscosity ($\eta = \tau/\gamma$) remains constant. This is known as Newtonian behaviour. Most polysaccharide solutions are not Newtonian. Pushing twice as hard will normally make them move more than twice as fast (often a lot more). In other words, the higher the shear-rate the lower the viscosity. For moderately concentrated solutions this 'shear-thinning' behaviour can often change the viscosity by two or three orders of magnitude over the range of rates encountered on standard viscometers. *It is meaningless to quote viscosity at one shear rate,* particularly if that rate is not defined. Solutions of disordered polysaccharide coils do, however, have a constant, maximum viscosity (η_o) at low shear rates, before the onset of thinning, providing a valid basis for comparing different solutions.

Molecular Size is as Important as Concentration

The viscosity generated by a disordered polysaccharide in solution [1,2] depends on two things: how much is there (i.e., concentration, c) and how much space each coil occupies. Coil volume can best be characterised by intrinsic viscosity, [η]. This is not a difficult number to obtain. It involves measuring the viscosity of a few very dilute solutions, and carrying out a simple extrapolation to zero concentration. The product of concentration and intrinsic viscosity then gives a measure of the total amount of space occupied by the polymer. The maximum viscosity, η_o, depends on this 'degree of space occupancy', c[η], not on concentration alone.

Double-logarithmic plots of η_o *vs.* c[η] for different disordered poly-saccharides, or different molecular weights of the same polysaccharide, are virtually identical[1]. Up to a viscosity about ten times that of water, doubling c[η] increases η_o by about a factor of 2.5. Beyond that point the increase is much steeper, so that doubling c[η] gives about a ten-fold increase in η_o. The sharp change in behaviour occurs when the coils just occupy the whole of the available space. At higher degrees of space-occupancy they are forced to interpenetrate one another, to form an entangled network with much greater resistance to flow than isolated coils moving through the water. The onset of entanglement occurs when c[η] ≈ 4, and the concentration at this point is known as c* (i.e., c* ≈ 4/[η]).

The main point to note is that increasing the size of the coils (i.e., in-

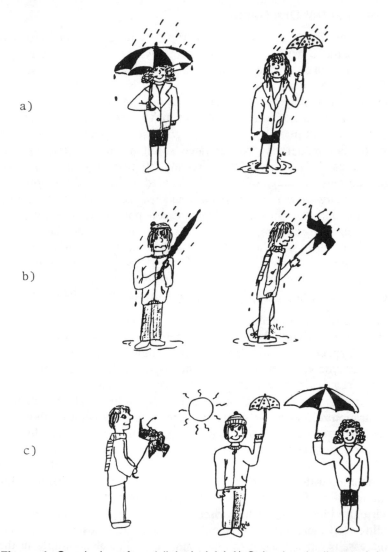

Figure 1. Conclusions from 'clinical trials' A) Striped umbrellas work better than spotted ones. B) Black umbrellas don't work at all. C) None of them has much effect! The illustrations are by courtesy of Miss Michelle Gothard, a graduate student in my research group.

creasing [η]) has exactly the same effect as increasing the concentration. In any clinical trial where viscosity is likely to be an important factor it is just as important to make sure that different 'soluble fibres' are matched for molecular size as it is to administer them at the same dosage. Differences in performance *may* mean that one material is more effective than another; it may equally well mean that the molecular weights of the two particular samples used were different (Fig. 1A).

Characterising Shear Thinning

At concentrations below c* polysaccharide solutions are virtually Newtonian. The further we go above c* the greater the extent of shear thinning. At low shear rates the viscosity remains constant (at η_o) because entanglements pulled apart to allow the solution to flow are replaced by new entanglements between different chains.

At higher rates there is less time for re-entanglement; that is why the viscosity drops. The form of shear-thinning for disordered polysaccharides is entirely general[6], and follows the empirical relationship:

$$\eta = \eta_o /[1 + (\gamma/\gamma_{c_{1/2}})^{0.76}].$$

where $\gamma_{1/2}$ is the shear-rate required to decrease the viscosity to $\eta_o/2$. Thus the two parameters η_o and $\gamma_{1/2}$ are sufficient to characterise the viscosity of a particular solution at any shear rate. Both can be derived by measuring viscosity at a few accessible shear rates and plotting η against $\eta\gamma^{0.76}$. The intercept on the vertical axis is η_o and $\gamma_{1/2}$ can be calculated from the value of $\eta\gamma^{0.76}$ half way up.

Some 'Solutions' Are Gels

Some polysaccharide preparations that look like solutions are actually very weak gels[2,7]. The distinction is that the chains are linked together through ordered junctions rather than simply entangling, but the junctions are weak enough to break down very easily and allow the 'solution' to flow. One way of detecting this is by severe curvature in the plots of η *vs.* $\eta\gamma^{0.76}$ described above. In these 'weak gel' systems, log η normally decreases linearly with log γ, and the slope and intercept can again be used to characterise viscosity at any shear rate.

In the food area, the best characterised example of 'weak gel' behaviour is the bacterial polysaccharide xanthan. A notable example in the dietary fiber area is ispaghula husk. In both cases the network is formed by tenuous association of ordered structures: between rigid molecules in xanthan, and between micron-sized fibrils in ispaghula.

Some 'Gels' Are Solutions

Some workers unfortunately use the word 'gel' to refer to very viscous concentrated solutions of disordered coils. This is totally misleading. A high degree of entanglement (i.e., high $c[\eta]$) is quite different from association of ordered structures, and gives entirely different properties[2]. 'Weak gels' may look more fluid than concentrated solutions, but it requires a finite stress to break them down, unlike entanglements where all that is needed is enough time to allow them to come apart.

'Soluble' Is Not the Same as 'Dissolved'

Because a polysaccharide is soluble does not imply that it will dissolve as soon as it is exposed to water. Dissociation of the ordered assemblies of polysaccharide chains in solid powders to allow them to go into solution takes time. The larger the particles, and therefore the smaller their total surface area, the longer it takes.

The disappointing performance of some commercial guar granulates in lowering post-prandial levels of blood glucose and insulin simply reflects their inability to dissolve within their transit time through the foregut[8]. Soluble fibers cannot confer their full viscosity until they are properly dissolved (Fig. 1B).

Overview

The main point of this paper has been to stress that polysaccharides are structural materials. How they behave depends on how they are handled. I was horrified at a previous dietary fiber meeting to hear a fellow participant arguing that pectin would not be of much clinical use because he had tasted a spoonful and found it revoltingly gummy. That makes about as much sense as opening a bag of cement and concluding that it would not be much use in building because it is too soft and powdery. Network structures may obviously have profound effects on the physical properties of digesta, but they need to be assembled first.

I was equally dismayed, at the same meeting, to hear another participant arguing that fiber was unlikely to be useful in long-term control of diabetes because of the ineffectiveness of wheat bran and other similar insoluble materials. The issue here, of course, is that 'dietary fiber' embraces a wide spectrum of different materials with, as discussed above, correspondingly wide differences in molecular organisation and physical properties. There is not much point in studying specific fibers in situations where there is no realistic expectation of them having any effect (Fig. 1C).

References

1. D. A. Rees, E. R. Morris, D. Thom, and J. K. Madden, Shapes and interactions of polysaccharide chains, in "The Polysaccharides", G. O. Aspinall, ed., Academic Press, New York, Vol. 1, pp. 195-290 (1982).
2. A. H. Clark and S. B. Ross-Murphy, Structural and mechanical properties of biopolymer gels, *Advan. Polym. Sci.*, 83:57 (1987).
3. I. C. M. Dea, Industrial polysaccharides, *Pure Appl. Chem.*, 61:1315 (1989).
4. E. R. Morris, Physical properties of dietary fibre in relation to biological function, in "Dietary Fibre: Chemical and Biological Aspects", D. A. T. Southgate, K. Waldron, I. T. Johnson and G. Fenwick, eds., Special Publication No. 83, Royal Society of Chemistry, Cambridge, pp. 91-102 (1990).
5. E. R. Morris, Physico-chemical properties of food polysaccharides, *in* "Dietary Fibre—A Component of Food—Nutritional Function in Health and Disease", T. Schweizer, ed., Springer-Verlag, London, pp. 41-56 (1992).
6. E. R. Morris, Shear-thinning of "random coil" polysaccharides: characterisation by two parameters from a simple linear plot, *Carbohydr. Polym.*, 13:85 (1990).
7. E. R. Morris, Pourable gels: polysaccharides that stabilise emulsions and dispersions by physical trapping, *Int. Food Ingredients*, 1:32 (1991).
8. P. R. Ellis and E. R. Morris, Importance of the rate of hydration of pharmaceutical preparations of guar gum; a new *in vitro* monitoring method, *Diabetic Medicine*, 8:378 (1991).

Fiber as Energy in Man

Geoffrey Livesey

AFRC Institute of Food Research Norwich Research Park Colney Norwich NR4 7UA United Kingdom

Introduction

Dietary fiber is poorly defined, but is complex and mostly plant cell wall carbohydrate or non-starch polysaccharide (NSP). No longer is NSP thought of as non-nutritive in humans. At the very least, some is fermented in the large intestine: mainly to small organic acids (mixtures of acetic, propionic, butyric, and lesser amounts of lactic and succinic acids). Absorption of these acids followed by their oxidative metabolism yields energy, a contribution to fuel the metabolic processes of the human tissues. Carbohydrates which escape digestion and absorption in the small intestine, which yield short-chain fatty acids in the large intestine, and which are found in human foodstuffs are mainly the non-starch polysaccharides (NSP) and the 'resistant starches' (RS). The latter refers to the sum of starch and maltodextrins escaping small intestinal digestion. It is the energy density value (kJ/g) of these two classes of carbohydrates that concerns this paper. Other carbohydrates which may be metabolised in a similar manner are certain oligosaccharides and sugar alcohols, considered elsewhere (1,2).

Maximum Energy

The maximum amount of energy to be obtained from the metabolism of any carbohydrate is the chemical energy released as heat during complete combustion to CO_2 and H_2O and is usually measured by bomb calorimetry (3). The isolation of NSP and RS from foodstuffs to purity is not usually practical. However, the composition of NSP in terms of

46

neutral sugars and uronic acids, and RS in terms of glucose can be determined. The heats of combustion of the polymers, NSP and RS, may then be calculated using knowledge of the energy content of the monomers. Heats of combustion (or gross energy, GE) of NSP from three groups of foods are shown in Fig. 1. GE tends to decline with increasing uronic acid content, so decline in the order cereal, vegetables, and fruit. In all cases, however, a value of about 17 kJGE/g applies. Isolated NSP preparations may be contaminated with cutins, lignins, and protein, all

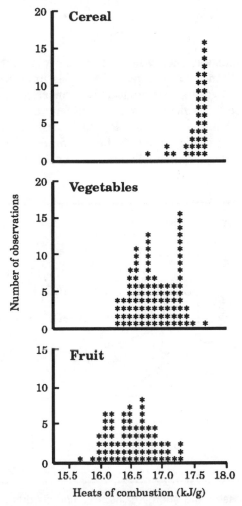

Figure 1. Heats of combustion of non-starch polysaccharides, based on NSP compositions in references 31 and 32. Each point represents an individual food item.

of which have higher heats of combustion (>23 kJ/g). The heat of combustion of RS is identical to that of all starches, about 17.5 kJGE/g.

Intakes of RS and NSP vary with both the amount and composition of food eaten. The highest sum intake of such materials in experimental energy balance studies with humans is approximately 0.14 kJGE per kJGE from the total diet, i.e., about 14% of the diet (4,5,6). More usually amongst Western subjects it is about 3%. Precise values are unknown, largely because methods to assay RS are only just reaching development and are unapplied in epidemiological work.

Energy Losses

Not all the combustible energy in RS and NSP is absorbed as short-chain fatty acids. Some may escape to faeces as unfermented carbohydrate. Other losses are the end products of fermentation, as shown in Fig. 2. End products other than the short-chain fatty acids represent energy losses and are: micro-organisms lost to faeces, molecular hydrogen, and methane lost to the air and the heat of fermentation lost to the environment via the body (potentially useful in a cold environment). An

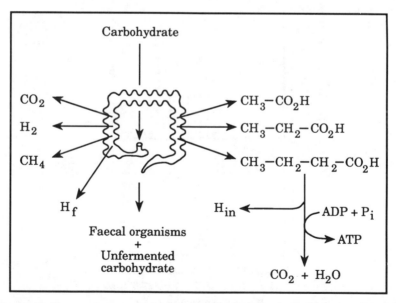

Figure 2. Energy losses and energy gains from carbohydrates undergoing fermentation. Hf and Hin are the heat of fermentation and heat of inefficiency of short-chain or volatile fatty acid (VFA) metabolism compared with an equicaloric amount of glucose.

additional loss of energy arises when shortchain fatty acids are oxidised in the mammalian tissues; their oxidation is inefficient by comparison with an equicaloric (absorbed energy) amount of available carbohydrate, eg., glucose. This additional energy loss is as heat to the environment (again energy potentially useful in a cold environment).

The faecal losses of microbial matter (protein and fat) explain, at least in part, the elevated losses of protein and fat in faeces on increased ingestion of NSP and RS.

Energy Gains

It is difficult to directly determine the quantities of short-chain fatty acids that arise during fermentation in man. The energy losses are, however, related to the extent of fermentation of NSP (4) and very probably RS. Consequently, energy gains may be calculated by difference between maximum energy (GE) and the energy losses arising from the fermentation process (Fig. 2). This energy gain has been termed the net energy value (7,8).

Net Energy Value

The energy gained from NSP and RS (unavailable carbohydrates) may be calculated by formula as show in Fig. 3 (7,9). A similar approach is used for estimating the net energy values of sugar alcohols, taking cognisance also of differences in small intestinal absorption amongst the sugar alcohols and the partition between oxidation and loss to urine (10). With RS and NSP, small intestinal absorption does not occur, nor are losses of energy to urine associated with NSP (and RS?) intake. Net energy values may be calculated (Fig. 3) from determinations of the proportion of the NSP or RS which is fermented. In conventional nutritional nomenclature this proportion for NSP and RS in vivo is the apparent digestibility. The calculation assumes factors that are difficult to determine on a routine basis. As shown in Fig. 3 these factors are expressed as fractions of NSP and RS fermented: 0.05 as combustible gasses (in practice it is slightly less), 0.05 as heat of fermentation (may actually be slightly higher), 0.30 as faecal microorganisms (may be slightly less, but made up to 0.3 when including some induced losses of non-microbial protein and fat). The gain of ATP from each kJ or kcal of short-chain fatty acid is only 0.85 times that from an equal kJ or kcal of glucose (may be 0.87, and slightly higher when the fermentation produces large amounts of butyric acid). All factors in the formula are rounded to the nearest 0.05 and have been considered in detail previously (1).

Mixed Diets

The average apparent digestibility of unavailable carbohydrates (NSP and RS together) in humans eating mixed diets is about 0.7, as reviewed previously (4), so the calculated net energy value is about 6 kJ/g (Fig. 3). This value remains apparently unchanged with diets of increasing unavailable carbohydrate intake from about 7 to 70 g daily. Analyses of NSP and RS which are more specific than the unavailable carbohydrate analyses used in the studies reviewed previously (4,11), will allow more appropriate energy values to be assigned to each class of carbohydrate in the mixed diet. In a reported study (12) with humans where NSP intake was increased from 19 to 52 g daily the calculated net energy value of the NSP may also be calculated to be about 6 kJ/g, similar at both intakes (Fig. 3).

Specific NSPs and RSs

The findings that the energy values of unavailable carbohydrates may be related to their apparent digestibilities (4,9) opened the way to the calculations of net energy values for specific NSPs and RSs. With NSPs selected for study in humans and rats, and reaching publication, there is a broad range of apparent digestibilities, and so too of the calculated net

---

Hybrid Factorial Calculation of the 'Energy Value' of Unavailable Carbohydrates

$$E = (1 - A - B - C) * D * G * H$$

E =	energy value (kJ/g)	~ 6.1 kJ/g (1.5 kcal/g)
A =	additional fecal energy that is non-UC	~ 0.30
B =	additional gaseous energy	~ 0.05
C =	additional heat of fermentation	~ 0.05
D =	apparent digestibility of UC	~ 0.70
G =	$\dfrac{\text{ATP per kJ VFA}}{\text{ATP per kJ Glucose}}$	~ 0.85
H =	heat of combustion of UC	~ 17.2 kJ/g (~ 4.1 kcal/g)

Figure 3. Calculation of net energy values from determinations of apparent digestibility. The factors given to the right are described more fully in the text.

energy values (Fig. 3). The values shown in Fig. 3 are approximately similar in rat and man and are based on information on apparent digestibilities already available in the literature (12,17). But note, there are few data comparing humans and rats fed whole food diets and starches unprotected by cell walls.

Validation

While the net energy values of NSP and RS may be calculated using factors which are reasoned (1), the approach is presently not validated. perhaps the largest uncertainty has been attached to the influence of NSP and RS on the losses of faecal protein and fat; however, such losses

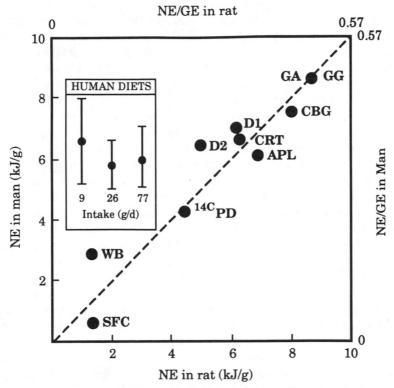

Figure 4. Net energy values (NE) of unavailable carbohydrates in mixed diets (Box) and of non-starch polysaccharides in humans and rats. NE/GE is the proportion of gross energy (GE) in the carbohydrates which is calculated to be available according to Fig. 3. Abbreviations used for NSPs are: GG for guar gum, GA for gum arabic, CBG for cabbage, CRT for carrot, A pL for apple, 14C pD for radiolabelled polydextrose, WB for wheat bran, SFC for Solka-floc cellulose, D1 and D2 for NSPs in two diets. References to original observations are given in the text. (Adapted from reference 1.)

are largely predictable: Using Solka-floc cellulose, seven fractions of sugar-beet NSP with widely varying apparent digestibility, guar gum and gum arabic in juvenile rats, we have found (14,15 and author, unpublished) that these energy losses are within a few percentage points of the indicated (Fig. 4) 0.3 kJ faecal fat plus protein per kJ carbohydrate fermented. Moreover, for one of the beet-fiber preparations, called Beta-fiber, the factor is appropriate at three intakes from approx. 0.05 to 0.15 g Beta-fibre per g diet. Further, the 0.7 apparent digestibility of unavailable carbohydrate for mixed diets fed to humans (4), and the energy losses to faeces on such diets (11) are observations consistent with the 0.3 kJ faecal fat plus protein energy per kJ carbohydrate fermented. Additional evidence is being obtained for five sources of NSP isolates fed to rats in a paneuropean interlaboratory study involving five independent laboratories sponsored by industry through the International Life Science's Institute (ILSI, Europe). The study is also examining the intake dependency (0.05 and 0.10 g NSP isolate/g diet intake). These ILSI studies are to assess the possibility of using the rat to assay fermentability and energy value of NSP isolates. A parallel study involving another 5 European laboratories is examining a batch in vitro fermentation system which is intended to be calibrated against the observations on fermentability and energy value in the rat studies. The latter would thus avoid use of animals and speed up the assessment.

The changes in body composition of rats when exchanging dietary sucrose for palatinit, a disaccharides sugar alcohol some of which undergoes fermentation, are agreeable with its net energy value (18). Similar rat studies with L-sugars give changes in body composition agreeable with their metabolisable energy values (author, unpublished). With several NSPs our current studies with the rat provide preliminary observations validating the net energy values obtained by calculation. All these materials (palatinit, L-sugars, and NSPs) have no unexpected substantial effects on the energy economy of the rat. A small effect which may be significant is the influences of certain carbohydrates on protein and fat losses from the small to the large intestine (19,20—see below). Another disaccharide sugar alcohol called lactitol, which is virtually completely fermented, influences body energy balance in man approximately in accord with its calculated net energy value (21). There are, however, no comparable studies with NSPs in man.

Discordant Observations

Interactions with Fat

In the human small intestine an interaction occurs between guar gum and fat to increase stomal fat losses in ileostomists (20). In the rat an interaction between dietary fat and guar gum occurs to increase faecal energy losses to an extent that such losses may be greater than the 0.3 kJ faecal fat plus protein per kJ guar gum fermented (author, unpublished). Some NSPs when ingested at high dose may therefore have effects on energy availability which differ from expectations based on the net energy calculation. It is interesting to note that interactions between guar gum and dietary fat elevate the rate of ileal mucosal cell proliferation (J. Pell and I. T. Johnson, unpublished).

By contrast with the mentioned interaction between fat and guar gum, there appears to be no marked interactions between NSP within flaked cereal grains (wheat, barley, oats) and dietary fat in the rat (author, unpublished). The observation with guar gum may be an extreme case, however, rolled barley grits elevate stomal fat losses in ileostomists (22). As fatty acids are generally unfermentable, any NSP induced small intestinal fat losses must contribute to the 0.3 kJ faecal protein plus fat per g NSP fermented, in man and in rat.

Body Composition

Additional to the effect of guar gum on faecal fat, the gum influences body composition of the rat. Thus, we find this influence to be consistent with a net energy value down to about −5 kJ/g gum (15). This is in discord with its calculated net energy value (8.4 kJ/g). As yet we have not established whether this is a metabolic effect of the gum or whether it is due to a marked effect of the gum on the time taken to eat a given amount of food. The effect is, however, very reproducible, and appears independent of intake of dietary fat (17 vs 35% energy) and of the ambient temperature (21 vs 28 C) (author, unpublished).

Cereal Diets

While the net energy values of mixed diets may be predicted, four diets high in whole grain cereals appear to elicit energy losses to faeces that are higher than expected on the basis of the reported intakes of gross energy and of unavailable carbohydrate (11). It may be noted that losses of energy to faeces for a high-cereal diet containing no whole grains (23) appear much as expected from the factors in Fig. 3. Similarly, a diet very high in polished rice results (24) in faecal energy losses no greater than expected. However, observations available in the literature (11,24–26) with brown rice, wheat, rye plus wheat together and barley suggest an intact endosperm, perhaps associated with a protective bran layer, is associated with elevated faecal energy losses. This has been postulated (4,11,26) as possibly due to some starch reaching the large intestine in addition to the NSPs of the cereal cell walls. In the case of oats cooked in the presence of much water, when cells are expected to separate during the cooking process, the physical protection of starch from digestion by cell walls is negligible (27). In the case of barley minimally cooked under low moisture conditions, the endospermal cells do not separate and the cell walls protect some starch from digestion in the small intestine. As much starch as NSP may then escape from the small to the large bowel (22). Starch may be released from such barley endospermal cells with a mixture of pancreatic enzymes in vitro (author, unpublished), a process which presumably happens in the small intestine in vivo. The physical protection of starch by such barley cell walls occurs much less in rat than man (22), either because of a higher degree of mastication to produce a digesta with smaller particles of endosperm or because pancreatic enzyme activity in the rat is more effective than in human ileostomists (or both). The losses of starch observed in our human ileostomy studies (22), nevertheless, is not sufficient to explain the large faecal energy losses as seen in the majority of studies feeding whole grain cereal diets. Moreover, in our own work (unpublished) the faecal energy losses from rolled barley grits fed to human volunteers is not much different from expectations based on the NSP and RS content. The factors causing high faecal energy losses in the majority of studies in humans receiving whole grain diets are presently elusive, high losses do not always seem to occur.

Three relevant observations in the rat are: Faecal energy losses on feeding rolled grits of wheat, barley, and oats are greater than expected based on their NSP content and the fermentability of that NSP. Cereal particle size influences faecal energy losses to a small extent and is apparently not related to cell-wall protection of starch. There are sometimes, but not always, differences in faecal energy losses between botanical sources of cereals when fed to rats (28). From the cereal studies with humans and rats one can only surmise that whole grain cereals sometimes increase faecal energy losses above our expectations; cooking, particle size, and botanical source each appear to be important.

Missing Data

The calculations of net energy values of NSP and RS (Fig. 3) are based on studies with adult subjects. It remains unclear whether the calculations are appropriate for young children, for the aged, and for people who eat predominantly from rice, as in Asia, or from boiled mixtures of cereals and beans, as in certain African and Central or South American countries. There remains also missing data from individuals eating low-energy high-complex carbohydrate diets while attempting to lose weight.

Assay Methods for Fermentable NSP and RS

In order to ascribe energy values to carbohydrates, it obviously helps to be able to assay them with some degree of accuracy. AOAC fiber is poorly defined. This paper refers to NSP and RS. The methods of Englyst for assaying NSP (29) and RS (30) currently find use in the author's energy evaluation studies. Subclasses of NSP and RS may be defined by physical or other means, a topic beyond the scope of this review. However, for precise energy evaluation there will be a need eventually for assays of fermentable NSP and RS. Presently no such methods have reached an advanced state of development. Potentially useful methods are being elaborated within the AFRC Institute of Food Research, UK, also by the International Life Science's Institute (Europe), Brussels and through a European Council research activity, EURESTA, and elsewhere.

Current Recommendations

Presently, in the USA, UK, Europe, and elsewhere no energy value has been assigned to NSP and RS. It is now clear that both provide energy. For mixed diets a net energy value of about 6 kJ/g NSP appears appropriate. Generally RS in mixed diets is completely fermented so a net energy value of 8.4 kJ/g RS might be used. Specific NSPs and RSs may be attributed a net energy value dependent on the extent to which they become fermented, with values ranging from 0 to 8.4 kJ/g. There would seem little reason to adopt these values until some of the missing data is made available and some discordant data are understood, in particular to establish the validity of these energy values with low-energy, high-complex carbohydrate diets as may be consumed during attempts to slim, and to more fully solve the mechanism by which some cereal diets apparently show unexpectedly low energy values.

Acknowledgments

The author is grateful to several researches working in his laboratory: R. M. Faulks, J. C. Brown, T, Smith, and J. A. Wilkingson for experimental work leading to many of the comments made presently, some of which have been referred to as "author, unpublished."

References

1. G. Livesey. The energy value of dietary fibre and sugar alcohols. Nutrition Research Reviews 5: submitted (1992).
2. N. Hosoya (editor). "Caloric Evaluation of Carbohydrates," Research Founda-

tion for Sugar Metabolism, Tokyo (1990).

3. C. Brown. Bomb calorimetry, in: Encyclopedia of Food Science, Food Technology and Nutrition, R. Mcreae, R. Robinson and M. Sadler eds., (in press for 1993).

4. G. Livesey. Energy values of unavailable carbohydrates and diets, Am. J. Clin. Nutr. 51:617 (1990).

5. H. Goranzon, E. Forsum and M. Thil_n, Calculation and determination of metabolisable energy in mixed diets to humans, Am. J. Clin. Nutr. 38:954 (1983).

6. D. H. Calloway and M. J. Kretsch, Protein and energy utilisation in men given a rural Guatemalan diet and egg formulas with and without added oat bran, Am. J. Clin. Nutr. 31:1118 (1983).

7. G. Livesey, Determinants of energy density with conventional foods and artificial feeds, Proc. Nutr. Soc. 50:371 (1991).

8. A. J. H. van Es, Dietary energy density on using sugar alcohols in place of sugars, Proc. Nutr. Soc. 50:383 (1991).

9. British Nutrition Foundation's Task Force on Complex Carbohydrates. "Complex carbohydrates in Foods," Chapman Hall, London (1990).

10. Dutch Nutrition Council, "The Energy Value of Sugar Alcohols. Recommendations of the Committee on Polyols," Vaedingsraad, The Hague (1987).

11. G. Livesey, Calculating the energy values of foods: Towards new empirical formulae based on diets with varied intakes of unavailable complex carbohydrates, Eu. J. Clin. Nutr. 45:1 (1991).

12. J. C. Mathers, Digestion of non-starch polysaccharide by non-ruminant omnivores, Proc. Nutr. Soc. 50:161 (1991).

13. M. Nyman, N.-G. Asp, J. H. Cummings, and H. Wiggins, Fermentation of dietary fibre in the intestinal tract: Comparison between man and rat. Br. J. Nutr. 55, 487 (1986).

14. C. J. Harley, I. R. Davies, and G. Livesey, Caloric value of gums in the rat— Data on gum arabic. Food Additives and Contaminants 6, 13 (1988).

15. I. R. Davies, J. C. Brown, and G. Livesey, Energy value and energy balance in rats fed guar gum or cellulose. Br. J. Nutr. 65, 415 (1991).

16. S. K. Figdor and J. R. Bianchine, Caloric utilisation of polydexrose in man. J. Agric. Food Chem. 31:389 (1983).

17. S. K. Figdor and H. H. Rennhard, Caloric utilisation of polydextrose in the rat. J. Agric. Food. Chem. 29:1181 (1981).

18. G. Livesey, On the energy value of sugar alcohols with reference to Isomalt, in: Caloric Evaluation of Carbohydrates. N. Hosoya, ed., Research Foundation for Sugar Metabolism, Tokyo (1990).

19. G. Livesey, The impact of the concentration and dose of palatinit in foods and diets on energy value, Food Science and Nutrition 42F:223 (1990).

20. S. E. Hingham, and N. J. Read, The effect of the ingestion of guar gum on ileostomy effluent. Br. J. Nutr. 67:115 (1992).

21. A. J. H. van Es, L. de Groot, and J. E. Vogt, Energy balance in eight volunteers fed on diets with either lactitol or saccharose. Br. J. Nutr. 56:545 (1986).

22. G. Livesey, The energy value of carbohydrate and fibre for man, Proc. Nutr. Soc. Aust. 16:79 (1991).

23. H. G_ranzon and E. Forsum, Metabolisable energy in humans in two diets.

Calculation and analysis, J. Nutr. 117:267 (1987).

24. H. Miyoshi, T. Okuda, Y. Oi, and H. Koishi, Effect of rice fibre on faecal weight, apparent digestibilities of energy, nitrogen and fat, and degradation of neutral detergent fibre in young men. J. Nutr. Sci. Vitaminol. 32:581 (1986).

25. P. A. Judd, The effects of high intakes of barley on gastrointestinal function and apparent digestibilities of dry matter, nitrogen and fat in human volunteers. J. Plant Foods, 4:79 (1982).

26. E. Wisker, A. Maltz, and W. Feldheim, Metabolisable energy of diets low and high in cereal when eaten by humans, J. Nutr, 118: 945 (1988).

27. H. N. Englyst and J. H. Cummings, Digestion of the polysaccharides of some cereal foods in the human small intestine, Am. J. Clin. Nutr, 42:778 (1985).

28. D. J. Naismith, G. S. Mahdi, and N. N. Shakier, Therapeutic value of barley in the management of diabetes, Ann. Nutr. Metab. 35:61 (1991).

29. H. N. Englyst and J. H. Cummings, Improved method for the measurement of dietary fibre as non-starch polysaccharides in plant foods, Assoc. Off. Anal. Chem. 74:808 (1988).

30. H. N. Englyst and S. M. Kingman, Dietary fibre and resistant starch. A nutritional classification of plant polysaccharides, in: "Dietary Fibre," D. Kritchevsky, C. Bonefield, and J. W. Anderson eds., Plenum Publishing Corp. New York (1990).

31. N. Englyst, S. A. Bingham, S. A. Runswick, E. Collins, and J. H. Cummings, Dietary fibre (non-starch polysaccharides) in fruits, vegetables and nuts. J. Hum. Nutr. Diet. 1:247 (1988).

32. H. N. Englyst, S. A. Bingham, S. A. Runswick, E. Collins, and J. H. Cummings, Dietary fibre (non-starch polysaccharides) in cereal products. J. Hum. Nutr. Diet. 2:253 (1988).

The Physiological Effects of Dietary Fiber

Christine A. Edwards

Department of Human Nutrition
Glasgow University
Yorkhill Hospitals
Glasgow, G3 8SJ
U.K.

Introduction

The physiological effects of dietary fiber depend not only on the type of fiber ingested or on the dose of fiber but also on the composition of the rest of the meal or diet and the idiosyncratic physiology of the subject.

Before considering the effects of dietary fiber on any physiological process it is important to clarify what is meant by the term dietary fiber. The characterisation of dietary fiber has been dealt with in a preceding chapter. However, it may be useful to re-emphasise the fact that no two polysaccharides which fall under the definition of dietary fiber are the same in the way they act in the gastrointestinal tract, and that physiological effects are difficult to predict from chemical structure. When considering the action of dietary fibers on the upper intestine it is useful to classify plant polysaccharides into those which when mixed with water form viscous solutions, those which do not, and those which are still contained within the plant cell wall matrix when ingested. Isolated polysaccharides are often classified as soluble or insoluble. This division is useful but may have limitations as solubility depends on the conditions used. Most but not all soluble fibers form viscous solutions in the gut. Gum arabic is an exception. Viscous polysaccharides have the greatest effect on gastric and small intestinal function. The viscosity of these fibers may explain their effect on upper gastrointestinal function as described below, but it is important to note that it is the viscosity in the gut that relates to action and not preingestion viscosity. The two may be very different for some polysaccharides (Edwards et al 1987). It is difficult to measure the viscosity in the gut and it may vary in different regions of the gut.

For the most part, isolated soluble fibers are ingested in significant quantities only as therapeutic agents and most dietary fiber is ingested as plant cell wall material. In this latter case it is important to determine whether the soluble dietary fiber components are released into the bulk phase and hence are able to increase luminal viscosity or whether they remain an integral part of the cell wall. The physical intactness of the cell wall in plant foods may in fact be the most important determinant of dietary fiber action in people ingesting a normal diet.

Another important factor in determining the effects of fiber is the adaptability of the gut. The gut is a finely tuned organ and responds quickly to any change in input to compensate and return to normal function and capacity. It is therefore very important to consider the long-term effects of dietary fiber and not to extrapolate too far from acute experiments.

In this chapter I will concentrate on the effects of dietary fiber on events occurring in the gut. The extent and rate of absorption of nutrients, which may be affected by dietary fiber, and the fermentation products from the colon may of course influence many other physiological processes in the body but these are dealt with in other chapters.

Slowing of Nutrient Absorption

It is now well established that soluble viscous polysaccharides can impede the absorption of nutrients such as carbohydrates (Jenkins et al 1978, Blackburn et al 1984) and lipids (Sandberg et al 1983, Higham and Read 1992) from the gut in acute studies. In most cases this is a slowing of absorption rather than an inhibition or reduction in total amount absorbed (Jenkins et al 1978). This will result in lower postprandial plasma levels as the nutrient load is absorbed across a larger area of the gut and sometimes an increase in delivery of material to the colon where it may be fermented to products which are then absorbed by the body.

This slowing of absorption is related to viscosity and may be due to a variety of mechanisms; slowing of gastric emptying (Holt et al 1979), physical entrapment of nutrients, resistance to the mixing movements of intestinal contractions (Edwards et al 1988), inhibition of enzyme activity and increase in mucin production (Satchithanandam et al 1990). The major mechanism is likely to be the resistance to the mixing action of intestinal contractions which is related to an increase in the theoretical unstirred water layer (Johnson and Gee 1981, Flourie et al 1984).

Studies looking at the role of a slowing of gastric emptying in determining the action of fiber on postprandial glucose have shown there to be no direct relation between delayed gastric emptying times and the decrease in postprandial glucose (Blackburn et al 1984) and some fibers which have no effect or even accelerate gastric emptying still reduce postprandial glycaemia (Edwards et al 1987). A recent study (Meyer et al 1988) in fistulated dogs attempted to separate the roles of the slowed gastric emptying and impaired small intestinal absorption in determining plasma glucose. In this model they were able to confine viscous contents to the stomach and prevent interaction of nutrients with the duodenal receptors, or to the small intestine with no action on gastric emptying. They concluded that both delayed gastric emptying and slowed small bowel absorption were important parts of the overall mechanism. The effect of viscous fibers on the emptying of solids is less clear, however. The emptying rate of poorly digestible solids was increased by guar gum (Meyer et al 1986) and larger pieces of digesta were found in the mid-gut of the dog (Meyer and Doty 1988), but fat absorption was still inhibited. Within the small intestine the interaction of enzymes and nutrients, the movement of small molecules to the mucosa and therefore absorption are all dependent on good mixing within the gut. Any agent which reduces the effectiveness of this mixing should therefore slow down digestion and absorption. In vitro studies suggest that enzyme activity is reduced by viscous fibers (Isaksson et al 1982) although in vivo more enzymes may be secreted by the pancreas to compensate (Ikegami et al 1990). We have shown in vitro that 1% guar gum will abolish the increase in movement of glucose caused by an increase in the contraction rate of paddles compressing and releasing a dialysis tube mimicking a small intestinal segment (Edwards et al 1988).

Although it is believed that these effects are due to increased luminal viscosity, attempts to measure the viscosity increase in the gut have not always met with success. A recent study by Higham and Read (1992) has shown that although guar gum reduced the absorption of lipids in ileostomy subjects, the viscosity of the ileal effluent was actually reduced. This may be due to a difference between ileostomy subjects and normal subjects. Increased viscosities have been reported in the rat gut after ingestion of guar and oatbran (Blackburn and Johnson 1981, Lund et al 1989). There may be some loss of viscosity due to fermentation in the terminal ileum in ileostomists, but these results may also indicate that the immobilisation of water in the gut is more important in determining the action of viscous polysaccharides than the viscosity itself.

Differences in the viscosity of luminal contents in different regions of the small intestinal have also been indicated in studies of transit in the small intestine. On the whole viscous polysaccharides tend to delay mouth to cecum transit (Jenkins et al 1978, Blackburn et al 1984, Brown et al 1988). Experiments in rats showed the biggest effects in the stomach and ileum (Leeds 1982, Brown et al 1988) and in cecal filling (ileal emptying) (Spiller et al 1987) with little effect in the jejunum. This is probably due to reduction in the viscosity of luminal contents by secretions in the upper small intestine.

Insoluble Fibers

Isolated insoluble fibers such as wheat bran or cellulose have very little effect on the absorption of nutrients in the small intestine.

Intact Plant Cells

When food is ingested as intact plant cells the release of nutrients can be related to the resistance of the cells to disruption. The nutrients are physically entrapped within the cellular structure and cannot be digested until the cell wall has been breeched. In the case of starch, the starch granule must also be disrupted. Raw starches, as found in raw potato and bananas, are resistant to amylase in the small intestine and enter the colon where they are fermented (Englyst and Cummings 1986). The factors that influence the disruptibility of the cell wall are cell wall structure, lignification, particle size (O'Dea et al 1981), cooking, processing (Traianedes and O'Dea 1986) and chewing (Read et al 1986). The glycaemic index (a measure of the increase in plasma glucose caused by a carbohydrate load see chapter) varies considerably between carbohydrate foods and part of this variation is due to differences in disruptibility of the cell wall although other factors such as lipid content may also play a role. The intactness of the cell wall may represent the major effect of a high fiber diet on absorption of nutrients and needs to be studied in more detail. The effects of phytate and other plants components which may also contribute in part to the action of high fiber diets on the small intestine are discussed elsewhere in this book.

Colonic Fermentation and Its Consequences

Material which enters the colon is subject to the metabolism of the colonic microflora. Dietary fiber by definition reaches the colon intact and is a major source of energy for the colonic bacteria. A whole range of other molecules also enter the colon; unabsorbed nutrients including resistant starch, unabsorbed lipids, biliary excretions, and mucus. The range of metabolism activities of the colonic bacteria is vast as are the many potentially bioactive products. I will concentrate on a few which relate directly to the action of dietary fiber.

The consequences of fermentation on dietary fiber are shown in Figure 1. Fibers which are extensively fermented lose their structure and water-holding capacity (McBurney et al 1985). The loss of water-holding capacity may prevent or reduce any action on stool output especially if the fermentation is rapid and occurs in the cecum and proximal colon. The fermentation may, however, be followed by an increase in bacterial cell mass with its own inherent water-holding capacity and this may play some role in increasing stool output (Stephen and Cummings 1980). Some dietary fibers with cation exchange properties may have bound mineral ions or bile acids in the small intestine. After fermentation these will be released and may be absorbed. Bile acids will be metabolised by the bacteria to secondary bileacids and may have a stimulating effect on secretion (Mekhjian et al 1971) and motility (Kirwan et al 1975). Hydroxy fatty acids produced from unabsorbed fats may have a similar effect (Ammon and Phillips 1973, Spiller et al 1986). The increased production of bacterial enzymes may have important implications in the toxicology of molecules in the colon (Rowland and Mallett 1990). The products of fermentation, short chain fatty acids (scfa), gases and acidity, may have effects on motility (Squires et al 1992), distension which may give rise to propulsive activity (Narducci et al 1985) and the stability and proliferation of the colonic mucosa (Lupton et al 1988, Sakata 1987).

Insoluble fibers such as wheatbran without a large water-holding capacity which escape fermentation may promote propulsion and reduce water absorption by stimulation of multimodal mechano receptors in the

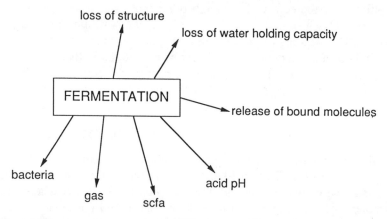

Figure 1. The consequences of bacterial fermentation of fiber.

colonic wall. Plastic particles have been shown to have a similar effect (Tomlin and Read 1988a).

The fermentation of carbohydrate including dietary fibers, is dependent on the solubility, particle size, lignification, the induction of enzymes, and on time. The fermentation of a dietary fiber may be characterised by rate of fermentation, extent of fermentation, sites of fermentation, and products (pattern) of fermentation. Each of these parameters may determine the action of a dietary fiber on stool output, colonic motility and cellular proliferation of the colonic mucosa.

Rate, Site, and Pattern, of Fermentation

Dietary fiber and other polysaccharides are fermented by the colonic bacteria to form short chain fatty acids (scfa) predominant acetic, propionic and n-butyric acid and gases such as methane, CO_2, H_2, and H_2S. Amino acid degradation gives rise to the branched scfa such as isovaleric and isobutyric acids (MacFarlane et al 1986).

It is difficult to study the fermentation of polysaccharides in vivo in man since most of the fermentation takes place in the proximal colon. Measurements of fecal material can give estimates of fermentability by measurement of undigested dietary fiber but fecal short chain fatty acids may not reveal any information about rapidly fermented polysaccharides. Much of our present knowledge is based on animal studies and in vitro fermentations. The rate of fermentation of a polysaccharides may be critical to its action in the colon. In studies where a variety of dietary fibers were fed to rats (Edwards et al 1990) for 4 weeks and stool output related to cecal and fecal short chain fatty acids, the fibers divided into one of three groups. Those which were rapidly fermented such as guar gum which increased cecal scfa but had no effect on fecal scfa or stool output. Fibers in group 2, such as Tragacanth, were more slowly fermented, had some effects on cecal scfa, increased fecal scfa concentration and increased fecal. Fibers in group 3, such as gellan, were very slowly fermented, had no effect on cecal scfa or fecal scfa concentration but increased total fecal scfa output and increased stool wet and dry weight. Slower fermentation with production of scfa in the distal colon and an increase in fecal scfa concentrations appeared to be associated with increased fecal water, whereas fibers which were rapidly fermented had no effect on fecal output at all.

If some fibers are fermented throughout the colon, they may have important influences on distal colonic scfa and hence distal colonic function. In another rat study (Edwards and Eastwood 1992) where we compared the in vivo effects of wheat bran and ispaghula, wheat bran appeared to have a rapidly fermentable portion which changed scfa in the cecum only and an unfermentable residue which had no effect on

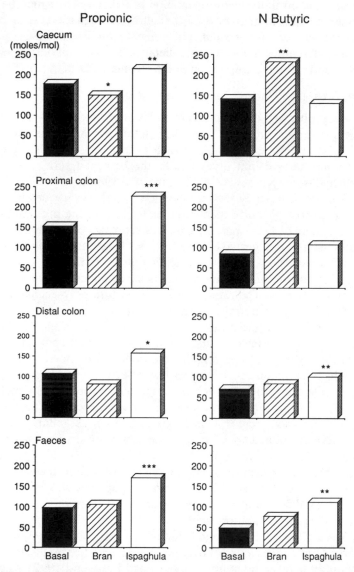

Figure 2. The proportions of propionic and butyric acids in the cecum, colon and feces of rats fed a basal low fiber diet or one supplemented with 5% ispaghula or 10% wheat bran. * $p < 0.05$, ** $p < 0.01$, *** $p < 0.001$. (Edwards and Eastwood 1992)

colonic contents but increased stool output, presumably by stimulating propulsion. Ispaghula, however, appeared to be fermented throughout the colon increasing colonic contents, retaining fluid in the colon and increasing scfa content in all parts of the colon. Wheat bran fermentation was associated with high butyrate in the cecum (Fig 2) and ispaghula with high propionate. However, in the distal colon ispaghula produced the highest proportion of butyrate. This may be of importance in light of the interest in the action of butyrate on cell proliferation (Sakata 1987) and differentiation (Augeron and Laboisse 1984) and the more common occurrence of distal colonic cancer.

Products of Fermentation

As stated above, polysaccharides in the colon are fermented to short chain fatty acids and gases. The microbial ecology fermenting these polysaccharides is very complex and different groups of bacteria are responsible for producing different short chain fatty acids (Macy and Probst 1979, Mandelstam et al 1982). This along with the diverse range of substrates fermented in the colon produces the variability of scfa found in human feces. In vitro studies have shown that although there is some variation in the proportions of scfa produced from an individual polysaccharide between laboratories due to different methodologies, an overall pattern is seen. (Table 1) Acetic acid is the major scfa produced from all substrates. Starch, wheat bran, and oat fiber are associated with large proportions of butyric acid while arabinogalactan, ispaghula (an arabinoxylan), guar gum, and starch are associated with large proportions of propionic acid. These patterns are also demonstrated in vivo in rats (Topping et al 1988, Mallett et al 1988, Goodlad and Mathers 1990, Edwards and Eastwood 1992). Since butyrate and propionate may have different roles in influencing the physiology of the colonic mucosa and liver, the pattern of scfa produced and the site at which they are produced may be very important factors in the physiological effects of a dietary fiber.

Physiological Actions of Short Chain Fatty Acids

There has been considerable interest in the effects of the scfa on the colonic mucosa and colonic function as well as postabsorptive actions on the liver and other tissues. In the gut, scfa are rapidly absorbed (McNeil et al 1987) and promote the absorption of water (Argenzio et al 1977). However, as discussed above in some cases where fermentation may continue in the distal colon they may be associated with an increase in fecal water (Edwards et al 1990). Scfa may have an effect of colonic motility. They have been shown to both stimulate (Yajima 1985) and inhibit (Squires et al 1992) motility in the colon in different in vitro preparations. The physiological consequence of these effects in vivo are difficult to assess as unless propagation or flow is measured an increase in colonic motor activity may in fact reflect in increase in non-propagating contractions which impede flow and slow transit (Bueno and Fioramonti 1981). Indirect evidence for the action of scfa, or at least fermentation, on motility and transit was shown by Tomlin and Read (1988b) who carried out fecal incubations of fibers using feces from human volunteers who had been fed the fibers and had their gut transit times and stool output measured. They found that some fibers which were fer-

Table 1. The patterns of SCFA production from the fermentation of various complex carbohydrates by human fecal bacteria *in vitro*

Carbohydrate	% Acetate	% Propionate	% Butyrate	Reference
Starch	50	22	29	1
Potato Starch	67	6	25	8
Corn starch	69.7	13.7	16.3	8
Resistant starch	41	21	38	7
Wheat bran	52	11.4	19.2	2
	61.4	19.1	19.5	3
	64	16.1	18.4	8
Pectin	84	14	2	1
	71	14.8	8.5	2
	69	13	17	6
	82	7	11	8
Cellulose	61	20	19	6
Gum arabic	68.2	19.6	8.2	2
Guar gum	57.7	27.2	8.0	2
	61.4	24.7	13.7	3
Tragacanth	67	18.5	8.2	2
Xanthan	71	18.6	3.2	2
Gellan	62.2	19.6	7.0	2
Karaya	63	9.9	9.5	2
Xylan	82	15	3	1
Arabinogalactan	50	42	8	1
	60	22.4	17.3	6
	55.1	32.1	11.4	8
	56.3	26.3	9.5	4
Ispaghula	56.3	26.3	9.5	4
Oat bran	57	20.8	22.5	3
	64.3	12.3	38.8	8
Lactulose	67	13	20	6

Reference: 1 - Englyst *et al.*, 1987; 2 - Adiotomre *et al.*, 3 - McBurney and Thompson, 1987; 4 - Edwards *et al.*, 1992; 5 - McBurney *et al.*, 1988; 6 - Vince *et al.*, 1990; 7 - Englyst and MacFarlane, 1987; 8 - Weaver *et al.*, 1992.

mented, speeded up transit and increased stool frequency without increasing stool output.

Short chain fatty acids have been shown to stimulate motility in the ileum (Kamath et al 1988) but not in the jejunum (Masliah et al 1992) and scfa infused into the ileum of rats accelerated stomach to cecum transit time (Richardson et al 1991).

There has been much recent interest in the effects of scfa on colonic cellular proliferation (Sakata 1987) and indeed ingestion of fermentable dietary fibers increases cellular proliferation in rats and when given in conjunction with carcinogens, increases colonic tumor yield (Jacobs 1990). In our studies, however, when rats were fed either elemental diet supplemented with fermentable fiber (Edwards et al 1992a), or low and high fiber diets (Edwards et al 1992b), although cellular proliferation was stimulated in the proximal colon, very little effect was seen in the distal colon despite large changes in luminal scfa. This emphasises the difference in the physiology of the proximal and distal colon and the importance of studying events at the site of interest and not extrapolating too much from in vitro fermentations or fecal contents.

Conclusion

Dietary fibers have a variety of actions on the gastrointestinal tract depending on their physical properties and fermentation characteristics. Studies of the physiological and fermentation actions of dietary fiber must take into account the differences in both the chemical and physical properties of the luminal contents and the reactivity of the gut at each relevant site.

References

Adiotomre, J., Eastwood, M. A., Edwards, C. A., and Brydon, W. G., 1990. Dietary fiber: in vitro methods that anticipate nutrition and metabolic activity in humans. Am. J. Clin. Nutr. 52:128-34.

Ammon, H. V., and Phillips, S. F., 1973. Inhibition of colonic water and electrolyte absorption by fatty acids in man. Gastroenterology 65:744-9.

Argenzio, R. A., Southworth, M., Lowe, J. E., and Stevens, C. G., 1977. Interrelationship of Na, HCO_3 and vfa transport by equine large intestine. Am. J. Physiol. 233:E469-78.

Augeron, C., and Laboisse, C. L., 1984. Emergence of permanently differentiated cell clones in a human colonic cancer cell line in culture after treatment with sodium butyrate. Cancer Res. 1984. 44:3961-9.

Blackburn, N. A., and Johnson, I. T., 1981. The effect of guar gum on the viscosity of the gastrointestinal contents and on glucose uptake from the perfused jejunum of the rat. Br. J. Nutr. 46:239-46.

Blackburn, N. A., Redfern, J. S., Jarjis, M., Holgate, A. M., Hanning, I., Scarpello, J. H. B., Johnson, I. T., and Read, N. W., 1984a. The mechanisms of action of guar gum in improving glucose tolerance in man. *Clin. Sci.* 66:329-336.

Brown, N. J., Worlding, J., Rumsey, R. D. E., and Read, N. W., 1988. The effect of guar gum on the distribution of a radiolabelled meal in the gastrointestinal tract of the rat. *Br. J. Nutr.* 59:223-31.

Bueno, L., and Fioramont, J., 1981. Patterns of colonic motility. Clinical Research Reviews 1 (Suppl 1)91-100.

Edwards, C. A., Blackburn, N. A., Craigen, L., Davison, P., Tomlin, J., Sugden, K., Johnson, I. T., and Read, N. W., 1987. Viscosity of food gums determined in vitro related to their hypoglycaemic actions. *Am. J. Clin. Nutr.* 46:72-77.

Edwards, C. A., Bowen, J., and Eastwood, M. A., 1990. The effect of isolated complex carbohydrates on cecal and fecal short chain fatty acids and stool output in the rat. *In*: Dietary Fiber: Chemical and Biological Aspects. eds., D. A. T. Southgate, K. Waldron, I. T. Johnson and G. R. Fenwick. Royal Society of Chemistry, Cambridge, pp. 273-6.

Edwards, C. A., Bruce, M., and Ferguson, A., 1992a. The effect of supplementing elemental diet with dextran on colonic short chain fatty acids and cellular proliferation in the rat. *Pro. Nutr. Soc.* In press.

Edwards, C. A., and Eastwood, M. A., 1992. Comparison of the effects of ispaghula and wheat bran on rat cecal and colonic fermentation. Gut. In press.

Edwards, C. A., Johnson, I. T., and Read, N. W., 1988. Do viscous polysaccharides reduce absorption by inhibiting diffusion on convection. *Eu. J. Clin. Nutr.* 42:307-12.

Edwards, C. A., Wilson, R. G., Hanlon, L., and Eastwood, M. A., 1992b. The effect of lifelong high fiber diet on colonic cellular proliferation in the rat. Gut. In press.

Englyst, H. N., and Cummings, J. H., 1986. Digestion of the carbohydrates of banana (Musa paradisa sapientum) in the human small intestine. *Am. J. Clin. Nutr.* 44:42-50.

Englyst, H. N., Ay, S., and MacFarlane, G. T., 1987. Polysaccharide breakdown by mixed populations of human fecal bacteria. Microbiology Ecology 95: 163-171.

Flourie, B., Vidon, N., Florent, C. H., and Bernier, S. J., 1984. Effect of pectin on jejunal glucose absorption and unstirred layer thickness in normal man. Gut 25:936-41.

Goodlad, J. S., and Matthers, J. C., 1990. Large bowel fermentation in rats given diets containing raw peas (Pisum Sativum). *Br. J. Nut.* 64: 569-87.

Higham, S. E., and Read, N. W., 1992. The effect of ingestion of guar gum on ileostomy effluent. *Br. J. Nutr.* 67:115-22.

Holt, S., Heading, R. C., Carter, D. C., Prescott, L. F., and Tothill, P., 1979. Effect of gel forming fiber on gastric emptying and absorption of glucose and paracetemol. Lancet 1:636-9.

Ikegami, S., Tsuchihashi, F., Harada, H., Tsuchihashi, N., Nishide, E., and Innami, S., 1990. Effect of viscous indigestible polysacchardies on pancreatic biliary secretion and digestive organs in rats. *J. Nutr.* 120:353-360.

Isaksson, G., Lundquist, I., and Ihse, I., 1982. Effect of dietary fiber on pancreatic enzyme activity in vitro. *Gastroenterology* 82:918-924.

Jacobs, L. R., 1990. Influence of soluble fibers on experimental colon carcinogenesis. *In:* Dietary Fiber Chemistry Physiology and Health Effects. eds., D. Kritchevsky, C. Bonfield, J.W. Anderson. Plenum Press: NY pp. 399-402.

Jenkins, D. J. A., Wolever, T. M. S., Leeds, A. R., Gassull, M. A., Haisman, P., Dilawari, J., Goff, D. V., Metz, G. L., and Albert, K. G. M. M., 1978. Dietary fibers, fiber analogues and glucose tolerance importance of viscosity. *Br. Med. J.* 1:1392-94.

Johnson, I. T., and Gee, J. M., 1981. Effect of gel-forming food gums on the intestinal unstirred layer and sugar transport in vitro. Gut 22:398-403.

Kamath, P. S., Phillips, S. F., and Zinsmeister, A. R., 1988. Short chain fatty acids stimulate ileal motility in humans. Gastroenterology 95:1496-1502.

Kirwan, W. O., Smith, A. N., Mitchell, W. D., Falconer, J. D., Eastwood, M. A., 1975. Bile acids and colonic motility in the rabbit and human. *Gut* 16:894-902.

Leeds, A. R., 1982. Modification of intestinal absorption by dietary fiber and fiber components. *In:* Dietary Fiber in Health and Disease. ed., G. V. Vahouny, D. Kritchevsky, pp. 57-71, NY Plenum Press.

Lund, E. K., Gee, J. M., Brown, J. C., Wood, P. J., and Johnson, I. T., 1989. Effect of oat gum on the physical properties of the gastrointestinal contents and on the uptake of D-galactose and cholesterol by rat small intestine in vitro. *Br. J. Nutr.* 62:91-101.

Lupton, J. R., Coder, D. M., and Jacobs, L. R., 1988. Longterm effects of fermentable fibers on rat colonic pH and epithelial cell cycle. *J. Nutr.* 118:840-5.

Macy, J. M., and Probst, I., 1979. The biology of gastrointestinal bacteroides. *Annu. Rev. Microbiol.* 33: 561-94.

Mallett, A. K., Bearne, C. A., Young, P. J., and Rowland, I. R., 1988. Influence of starches of low digestibility on the rat cecal microflora. *Br. J. Nutr.* 60:597-604.

Mandelstam McQuillen, K., and Davies, I., 1982. Eds., Biochemistry of Bacterial Growth 3rd ed. Blackwell Scientific, Oxford.

Masliah, C., Cherbut, C., Bruley des Varannes, S., Barry, J. L., Dubois, A., and Galmiche, J. P., 1992. Short chain fatty acids do not alter jejunal motility in man. *Dig. Dis. Sci.* 37:193-7.

Melkhjian, K. S., Phillips, S. F., and Hofmann, A.F., 1971. Colonic secretion of water and electrolytes induced by bile acids: Perfusion studies in man. *J. Clin. Invest.* 50:1569-77.

Meyer, J. H., and Doty, J. E., 1988. GI transit and absorption of solid food multiple effects of guar. *Am. Clin. Nutr.* 48:267-73.

Meyer, J. H., Elashoff, Y. G. J., Reedy, T., Dressman, J., and Amidan, G., 1986. Effects of viscosity and fluid outflow on post cibal gastric emptying of solids. *Am. J. Physiol.* 250:G161-164.

Meyer, J. H., Gu, Y. G., Hehn, D., and Taylor, I.L., 1988. Intragastric vs. intra intestinal viscous polymers and glucose tolerance after liquid meals of glucose. *Am. J. Clin. Nutr.* 48:260-6.

MacFarlane, G. T., Cummings, J. H., and Allison, C., 1986. Protein degradation by human intestinal bacteria. *Gen. Microbiol.* 132:1647-56.

McBurney, M. I., Horvath, P. J., Jeraci, J. L., and Van Soest, P. J., 1985. Effect of in vitro fermentation using fecal inoculum on the water holding capacity of dietary fiber. *Br. J. Nutr.* 53:17-24.

McBurney, M. I., and Thompson, L. U., 1987. Effect of human fecal inoculum on in vitro fermentation variables. *Br. J. Nutr.* 58:233-43.

McBurney, M. I., Thompson, L. U., Cuff, D. J., and Jenkins, D. J. A., 1988. Comparison of ileal effluents, dietary fibers and whole foods in predicting the physiological importance of colonic fermentation. *Am. J. Gastroenterol.* 83:536-540.

McNeil, N. I., Cummings, J. H., and James, W. P. T., 1978. Short chain fatty acid absorption by the human large intestine. Gut 19:819-22.

Narducci, F., Bassotti, G., Gabuni, M., Solinas, A., Fiorucci, S., and Morelli, A., 1985. Distension stimulated motor activity of the human transvene descending and sigmoid colon. Gastroenterology 88:1515.

O'Dea, K., Snow, P., and Nestel, P., 1981. Rate of starch hydrolysis in vitro as a predictor of metabolic responses to complex carbohydrate in vivo. *Am. J. Clin. Nutr.* 34:1991-3.

Read, N. W., Welch, I. M., and Austen, C. J. et al 1986. Swallowing food without chewing: A simple way to reduce postprandial glycaemia. *Br. J. Nutr.* 55:43-7.

Richardson, A., Delbridge, A. T., Brown, N. J., Rumsey, R. D. E., and Read, N. W., 1991. Short chain fatty acids in the terminal ileum ccelerate stomach to cecum transit time in the rat. Gut 32:266-9.

Rowland, I. R., and Mallett, A. K., 1990. The influence of dietary fiber on the microbial enzyme activity in the Gut. *In*: Dietary Fiber—Chemistry, Physiology and Health Effects. eds., D. Kritchevsky, C. Bonfield, J. W. Anderson. Plenum Press, New York: pp. 195-206.

Sakata, T., 1987. Stimulatory effect of short chain fatty acids on epithelial cell proliferation in the rat intestine: a possible explanation for the trophic effects of fermentable fiber, gut microbes and luminal trophic factors. *Br. J. Nutr.* 58:95-103.

Sandberg, A. S., Ahderinne, R., Andersson, H., Hallgreen, B., and Hulten, L., 1983. The effect of citrus pectin on the absorption of nutrients in the small intestine. *Hum. Nutr. Clin. Nutr.* 37:171-83.

Satchithanandam, S., Vargofcak-Apker, M., Calvert, R. J., Leeds, A. R., and Cassidy, M. M., 1990. Alteration of gastrointestinal mucin by fiber feeding in rats. *J. Nutr.* 120:1179-84.

Spiller, R. C., Brown, M. L., and Phillips, S. F., 1986. Decreased fluid tolerance, accelerated transit and abnormal motility of the human colon induced by oleic acid. Gastroenterology 91:100-7.

Spiller, R. C., Brown, M. L., and Phillips, S. F., 1987. Emptying of the terminal ileum in intact humans influence of meal residue and ileal motility. Gastroenterology 92:724-9.

Squires, P., Rumsey, D., Edwards, C. A., and Read, N. W. The effect of short chain fatty acids on the contractile activity and fluid flow in the rat large bowel in vitrol. *Am. J. Physiol.* In press.

Stephen, A. M., and Cummings, J. H., 1980. The microbial contribution to human fecal mass. *J. Med. Microbiol.* 13:45-56.

Tomlin, J., and Read, N. W., 1988a. The effect of inert plastic particles on colonic function in human volunteers. *Br. Med. J.* 297:1175-6.

Tomlin, J., and Read, N. W., 1988. The relation between bacterial degradation of viscous polysaccharides and stool output in human beings. *Br. J. Nutr.* 60:666-75.

Topping, D. L, Mock, S., Trimble, R. P., Storer, G. B., and Illman, R. J., 1988. Effects of varying the content and proportions of gum arabic and cellulose on cecal volatile fatty acid concentrations in the rat. Nutrition Research 8:1013-20.

Traianedes, K., and O'Dea, K., 1986. Commerical canning increases the digestibility of beans in vitro and postprandial metabolic responses to them in vivo. *Am. J. Clin. Nutr.* 44:390-7.

Vince, A. J., McNeil, N. I., Wager, J. D., and Wnoy, O. M., 1990. The effect of lactulose, pectin, arabimogalactan, and cellulose on production of organic acids and metabolism of ammonia by intestinal bacteria in a fecal incubation system. *Br. J. Nutr.* 63:17-26.

Weaver, G. A., Krause, J. A., Miller, T. L., and Wolin, M. J., 1992. Corn starch fermentation by the colonic microbial community yields more butyrate than does cabbage fiber fermentation; corn starch fermentation rates correlate negatively with methanogenesis. *Am. J. Clin. Nutr.* 55:70-7.

Yajima, T., 1985. Contracile effect of short chain fatty acids on the isolated colon of the rat. *J. Physiol.* 368:667-78.

Modulation of Intestinal Development by Dietary Fiber Regimens

Marie M. Cassidy and Leo R. Fitzpatrick

Department of Physiology, The George Washington University Medical Center, Washington, D.C. 20037

1. Introduction

The mucosal lining of the gastrointestinal tract exhibits an extremely rapid turnover rate. Cell proliferation occurs in precursor cells within the intestinal or colonic crypts and differentiation of the major cell types (absorptive, goblet, and enteroendocrine) occurs during escalation of these cells as they migrate to the tip of the intestinal villus or colonic fold. Intestinal cell growth and replenishment appears to be physiologically regulated so that under normal conditions a steady state is maintained.

Dowling[10] has proposed that two types of intestinal adaption can be observed under a variety of conditions. *Physiological adaptation* or Type 1 hypoplasia arises as a consequence of starvation, intestinal bypass or parenteral nutrition. Type 2 or *pathological adaptation* is a repair process in response to mucosal injury. Type 2 hyperplasia occurs following intestinal resection, lactation, and cold adaptation with associated hyperplasia, while Type 2 hypoplasia is seen in the intestine of germ free animals. Intestinal mucosal mass demonstrates adaptive plasticity at the gross, microscopic, and ultrastructural level. Starvation, for example, results in a reduction in intestinal length and microvillar height. At the microscopic level increases in intestinal mass per unit length are at least partially due to variations in the height of the villi and both the number and configuration of villi per unit surface area.[8,10] De-privation of luminal or local nutrition either by starvation or by surgical exclusion leads to progressive structural and functional atrophy.

Relatively few studies have been conducted concerning the effect of dietary fiber on intestinal structure.[12,15,16] It is known that, at birth, rats possess regular finger-shaped small intestinal villi comparable to the morphological appearance of the villi in human small intestine. As these animals mature on a maintained standard laboratory diet the villi become leaf-shaped and then ridged in appearance.[4,5,29] Brown et al[3] observed a significantly increased crypt depth and a greater villus height in the jejunum and ileum of adult animals fed pectin, compared to the normal diet. It has also been suggested that the addition of dietary fiber to low residue diets has a favorable effect on the maintenance of intestinal architecture and function during parenteral feeding.[18] Tasman-Jones[28,29] examined the small intestinal mucosa of developing rats, for the effect of some components of dietary fiber on morphology. Jejunal and colonic mucosal structures were studied in weanling rats fed either regular chow, a fiber-free diet, or one containing either cellulose or pectin. Animals deprived of fiber and those receiving cellulose did not develop the ridged pattern, characteristic of villus maturation. Leaf and ridge-shaped patterns were observed with both the pectin and 'full' fiber laboratory diets. Younoszai et al[30] using young rats found that the presence of mixed fiber of vegetable origin was associated with enhanced growth of the small intestine and more strikingly in the colon. We have previously reported our findings relating to the effects of dietary fiber intake on the histology and surface structure of adult rat jejunum and colon.[4,5] In a series of experiments a detailed morphological and biochemical survey of the effect of dietary manipulation during the neonatal period of ontogeny was carried out.[6] Various parameters of intestinal growth and morphogenesis were examined during the pre-weaning period and post-weaning on to diets of variable composition.

2. Materials and Methods

2.1 Animal Maintenance and Dietary Composition

Lactating female Sprague-Dawley rats with litters of ten male pups were obtained from Zivic-Miller Laboratories (Allison Park, Pennsylvania) or Microbiological Associates (Bethesda, Maryland). At different times postnatally, three rats were removed from the litter for morphological studies. The remainder of the litter was weaned at approximately day 21 after birth, on to one of five different diets. The animals were housed four to a cage and were fed either a control (chow) diet or one of four other diets (see below). Thus, equal numbers of littermates of the same age were subjected to different dietary regimens. The rats were fed for a 4-week period and food and water were provided ad libitum. All animals were maintained at 25°C, with a 12 h light-dark cycle. Individual body weight measurements were done weekly on rats whose tails had been marked for identification purposes. Food consumption measurements were always conducted at approximately the same part of the day to minimize diurnal variation.

Five diets were used during the course of this study. These diets were: (1) Rodent Laboratory Chow 5001 (Ralston Purina Company, St. Louis, Missouri); (2) standard Vivonex, a nutritionally complete elemental liquid diet (Norwich-Eaton Pharmaceauticals, Norwich, New York); (3) a basal diet prepared by Bioserve; (4) the basal diet plus fiber as 10% cellulose; (5) the basal diet plus fiber as 5% guar gum.

2.2 Morphological Measurements

The experiments described in this section were done on pair-fed littermates that were randomly assigned to either a control dietary group (chow) or one of four other test dietary groups. Tissue from the mid-jejunum and the colon from suckling rats and three rats from each dietary group were fixed and processed for light and electron microscopy as previously described.[5] Following the dehydration step, samples for scanning electron microscopy evaluation were critical point-dried with CO_2 and mounted on aluminum stubs (Joel Ltd., Tokyo, Japan).

2.3 Biochemical Markers of Proliferation

Mucosa harvested from the small and large intestines of animals from this study were assayed for RNA, DNA, DNA synthesis, and ornithine decarboxylase activity. Cytokinetic parameters of cell production and migration were also examined. The tissues used in these assays were derived from pair-fed littermates that were randomly assigned to either a control chow group or one of the test dietary groups to permit wider testing of variance. All animals were fasted overnight and all experiments were initiated between 6:00 a.m. and 11:00 a.m. to minimize diurnal variation. Following anesthesia, the mid 10–15 segment of the jejunum and the entire length of the colon were removed and the mucosal tissues scraped with a glass slide and weighed. Tritiated Thymidine incorporation into DNA was measured in vitro and used as an index of DNA synthesis based on the technique of Majumdar and Johnson.[21] The extraction of DNA from the precipitate was performed according to Johnson and Guthrie.[17] RNA was removed by treating the precipitate containing the labeled thymidine in 0.3 N KOH for 90 minutes at 37°.

DNA and protein were then re-precipitated with 2 ml of 10% perchloric acid. Following boiling, denatured protein was removed by centrifugation and filtration. The incorporation of 3H thymidine into DNA was determined by liquid scintillation spectrophotometry at 22% efficiency and expressed as DPM/100 mg wet wt. or DPM/µg DNA. Another aliquot of the final filtrate was assayed for DNA content by the technique of Giles and Myers.[14] Calf thymus DNA (Calbiochem) was used as the standard. The RNA content of the supernatant was determined by the methods of Munro and Fleck[23] and Fleck and Begg.[13] In the fed animals RNA contents was determined at 260 nm. Ornithine decarboxylase activity was assayed by a minor modification of the method described by Russell and Snyder.[25] Protein was determined by the Lowry method.[20]

2.4 Autoradiography and Cell Turnover Measurements

Six rats from each group were anesthetized and injected via the jugular vein with (6-³H) thymidine (NEN, Boston, Mass) at a dose level of 7µ ci$u$/g pf body weight. Animals were sacrificed at 1 and 24 hours following the injection of tritiated thymidine. Jejunal and colonic segments were fixed in 3% buffered glutataraldehyde, post-fixed in osmium tetroxide, and embedded in Araldite resin. 500 nM sections were prepared, coated with Kodak emulsion and developed in Kodak D19 developer. The left sides of the jejunal villi and colonic crypt were used to determine the position of labelled cells at 1 and 24 hours after thymidine injection. The difference obtained by subtracting the time positions (cell#) of the leading edge at these time points permits an estimate of the distance migrated by the fastest labelled cell in a 23 hr. period. Dividing this distance in cell position by 23 provides a value for the migration rate in cell position per hour. It is thus possible to calculate the cell turnover time; ie., the time required for the leading edge of labelled cells, assuming a constant velocity to migrate to the tip of the jejunal villus or colonic crypt from whence it is exfoliated.

3. Results

3.1 Biochemical Parameters

In Table 1 is shown a summary of the biochemical measurements used to assess the effect of the immediate post-weaning diet on small intestinal growth and adaptation. No significant differences for thymidine incorporation into DNA (DNA synthesis) were observed in the jejunum of rats maintained on the various dietary regimens. Animals fed the basal fiber-free diet demonstrated significant increments in DNA and RNA content, as well as in ormithine decarboxylase activity, compared to chow-fed rats. The Vivonex liquid diet resulted in lower tissue contents of RNA and DNA and depressed enzyme activity, with respect to the fiber-free diet. The presence of 5% guar gum (a specific gel type fiber) was associated with the highest level of jejunal RNA content.

3.2 Morphologic Parameters

The typical appearance of jejunal villi in suckling rats at day 12 post-natally is smooth and finger-shaped. Ninety-eight percent of the villi examined showed this type of micro-architecture. At day 19, while still in the pre-weaning period many of the villi have assumed a broader configuration at the base, and the surface has become more convoluted: The normal appearance of adult rat villi is ridged, convoluted, and has an indented structure. This pattern was typical of the neonate rats weaned

Table 1. Summary of the effects of the post-weaning diet on growth/adaptation of the jejunum

Parameter measured	Chow	Vivonex	Fiber free	10% Cellulose	5% Guar Gum
DNA Synthesis (DPM/μgDNA)	76 ″ 12	84 ″ 19	47 ″ 13	72 ″ 19	42 ″ 8
DNA Content (μg/100 mg tissue)	77 ″ 9	74 ″ 18 <	142 ″ 11 *	76 ″ 18 <	106 ″ 14
RNA Content (μg/100 mg tissue)	241 ″ 11	262 ″ 24	351 ″ 38 **	281 ″ 27	325 ″ 48 *
ODC Activity (pmol/mg protein/30 min)	128 ″ 36	66 ″ 13 <<	340 ″ 88 **	348 ″ 127 **	85 ″ 23 <<

* $p < 0.05$ from chow. ** $p < 0.01$ from chow. < $p < 0.05$ from fiber-free. << $p < 0.01$ from fiber-free.

Table 2. Small intestine villus maturation (% finger or leaf/ridged shaped villi)[a]

Dietary condition	Finger-shaped	Leaf/ridge shaped
Suckling (12-day-old)	98	2
Chow	0	100
Vivonex	1	99
Fiber-free	5	95
10% Cellulose	79	21
5% Guar gum	20	80

[a] All of the diets were fed immediately post-weaning for a period of 4 weeks.

on to regulatory chow for a period of 4 weeks (Table 2). Rats weaned directly on to a 10% cellulose diet exhibited little villus maturation. In the remaining diets tested, the majority of the villi were of the mature leaf or ridge-shaped variety. The largest number of jejunal villi per unit area were observed in the suckling animals, and the least number of such structures were seen in the Vivonex-fed rats. In marked contrast, the surface structure of the developing colon does not alter significantly with age or weaning. In the topography of the colon at day 12 post-birth, goblet cells are prominent, as in the adult state, but the microvilli of the colonocytes are more sparse than in the mature state. The colon of suckling and guar gum fed rats had the largest number of colonic folds per unit area while, conversely, the lowest number of folds was found in the large intestine of the rats consuming 10% cellulose.

3.3 Cell Turnover in Jejunum and Colon

Figs. 1 and 2 are a graphic summary of the effect of the post-weaning diet on cell migration and turnover in the mid-jejunum and mid-colon respectively. In the jejunum, at 1 hour following injection of the label

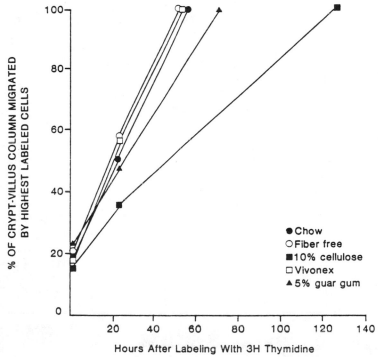

Figure 1. This figure depicts a graphic summary of the effect of the post-weaning diet for 4 weeks on cell migration and turnover in the mid-jejunum.

(3H thymidine) cellular migration had proceeded approximately 20% up the crypt-villus column in all dietary groups with the exception of the 5% guar gum dietary group. Final cell turnover times (the time taken to migrate 100% of the jejunal crypt-villus column) were approximately the same in the fiber-free, chow and Vivonex dietary groups. Conversely they were significantly longer in the small intestine of animals fed a specific form of dietary fiber as either 10% cellulose or guar gum. In the colon (Fig. 2) cellular migrating had proceeded almost 50% of the way up the crypt in guar gum fed animals and only 30% in cellulose fed rats at 1 hour post labelling. Cell turnover times (time taken for 100% crypt migration) were shortest in the chow and Vivonex fed animals, at intermediate levels in the mid-colon of fiber-free and 5% guar gum groups and, as in the jejunum, longest in the 10% cellulose fed rats.

4. Discussion

The results from this study suggest the need for non-gel-forming, insoluble type fiber, like cellulose, or which is likely to be present in a chow diet, to allow normal rates of body growth during the immediate

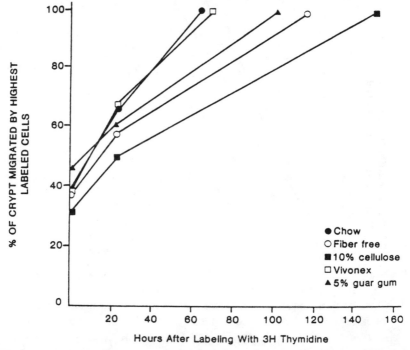

Figure 2. This figure shows the effect of the post-weaning diet for 4 weeks on cell migration and turnover in the mid-colon.

post-weaning period. Newly weaned rats were also able to adapt fairly well to the feeding of a non-fiber containing elemental liquid diet (Vivonex). In contrast, the feeding of a fiber-free pellet diet or a diet containing the gel type fiber, guar gum resulted in significantly decreased body weight gains.[6]

In these experiments we attempted to elucidate possible regulatory mechanisms which may modulate the adaptational response of the intestine to dietary influence. In particular we wished to compare the possible differential effects of the post-weaning diet in terms of the presence or absence of different types of dietary fiber on the growth of the small intestine and colon.

There is good experimental evidence that luminal nutrients are important for the maintenance of normal small and large intestinal mucosal structure and function in addition to redirecting the adaptive changes consequent to surgical manipulation.[11,18] The mechanism whereby local or luminal nutrition exerts its trophic effect is not understood but is believed to involve the release of trophic peptides from intestinal cells. These factors may then stimulate biochemical and cell biological regulators such as the ornithine decarboxylase enzyme system and DNA synthesis. The investigations of Clarke[7] did not support this concept of luminal nutrition as a major controller of epithelial cell replacement. He proposed a mechanism based on the secretory and absorptive workload required of the tissue as a determinant of the replacement rate of the enterocytes and irrespective of the nutrient value of the absorbed material. Creamer[8,9,19] has proposed that villus shape is determined by the number of epithelial cells which are present. When abundant cells are available, a finger-like shape is formed, while with fewer cells, leaf and ridge like villi are present. The results from this study suggest that this hypothesis may have some merit. Animals weaned on to the chow, Vivonex, or fiber free diets maintained a normal pattern of jejunal villus development. In contrast, in the jejunum of rats fed a specific form of dietary fiber as either 10% cellulose or 5% guar gum, 79% and 20% of the villi, respectively, retained the finger-like shape characteristic of early postnatal development. The feeding of these specific forms of dietary fiber also resulted in a larger number of villi, suggesting another adaptational response of the small intestine. Dowling[10] suggested that intestinal adaptation could be classified as either physiological or pathological. He proposed that pathological adaptation was a repair process in response to mucosal injury (hyperplasia) or lack of trauma (hypoplasia). With pathological hyperplasia such as occurs with coeliac disease or tropical sprue, the small intestinal mucosa is characterized by an enlarged crypt area and a corresponding decrease in villus size. The results from this study suggests that rats fed either the fiber free or 5% guar gum diets were exhibiting pathological adaptational hyperplasia, similar to that described by Dowling. In the jejunum of 5% guar gum fed rats, this pathological hyperplasia seems to be occurring without an associated increase in proliferative activity. (Fig. 3) In contrast, the mid-jejunum of 10% cellulose fed animals appears to be in a hypoplastic state. This hypoplasia seems to be a physiological response to the feeding of this insoluble, bulk type fiber and is similar to the physiological hypoplasia.

Ornithine decarboxylase (ODC) has been shown in various mammalian systems, including the GI tract to be one of the earliest biochemical parameters associated with cellular replacement and development.[22,25] Both food and insulin stimulate ODC intestinal activity, while a fast of 72 hours decreases enzyme activity by 41% in the jejunum and by 66% in the colon.[18] Various investigators[18,22] have recently found that ornithine decarboxylase is preferentially associated with the non-dividing cells of the intestinal villus, rather than the proliferating cells of the crypt area. They have suggested a role for ODC in small intestinal cellular differentiation rather than proliferation.[12,18] The results from this cumulative study would seem to offer further support for such a role; particularly under different dietary conditions. In the colon, the presence in the diet of the gel type fiber, guar gum, or the products of its degradation, resulted in a significant trophic influence on the mucosal layer. As was the case in the jejunum, no atrophic effect was found in the colonic

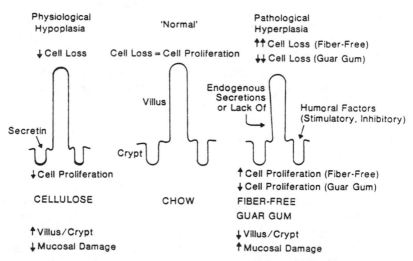

Figure 3. Adaptational response of the neonate rat jejunum to the post-weaning diet.

mucosa of Vivonex fed rats. The feeding of the bulk type fiber, cellulose, at a 10% level, resulted in damage to approximately 50% of the colonic folds.[6] This was in comparison to a disruptive effect of only 5% on the villi of the mid-jejunum. In contrast, the viscous, gel type fiber, guar gum at a 5% level, caused damage to 61% of the jejunal villi and only 13% of the colonic folds[6] (Fig. 4). This suggests differential effects on the mucosal surface architecture, with different types of fibers, in different areas of the intestinal tract, during the immediate post-weaning period.

The mid-colon of 10% cellulose fed rats was characterized by decreased proliferative activity and a corresponding increase in cell turn-over time (Fig. 2). The morphometric, cytokinetic, and biochemical results from the present study, collectively, suggest a colonic hypoplastic state for the cellulose dietary group. Interestingly, this colonic hypoplasia seems to be occurring despite a significant amount of damage to the colonic mucosa. As was the case for the 10% cellulose dietary group, fiber free fed rats also appear to be exhibiting colonic hypoplasia. The *fiber free dietary group* was unique, in that it exhibited *small intestinal hyperplasia* in association with *colonic hypoplasia*.

The results derived from this study relating to the effect of diet on intestinal growth/adaptation are probably due to the influence of a num-

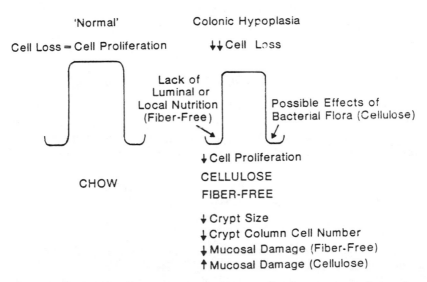

Figure 4. Adaptational response of the neonate rat colon to the post-weaning diet.

ber of extrinsic factors, which are altered by different dietary regimens. These factors include pancreaticobiliary secretions, bacterial flora, and gastrointestinal hormones. In summary, therefore, the intrinsic regulation of intestinal proliferation and growth may be affected directly by dietary manipulation, or indirectly by various luminal and systematic factors brought into play with dietary manipulation. These factors vary in their importance during ontogenic development or with the feeding of specific types of dietary fiber and their effects on intestinal growth/ adaptation appear to differ in various parts of the intestinal tract.

Clinical Significance

Intestinal biopsy samples from asymptomatic healthy persons differ quite marketly when the nature of the diet is taken into consideration. Wide villous structures, exhibiting leaf-like arrays are characteristic of vegetarian diets whether these are examined in the US vegetarian population[1] or in populations within developing countries.[26,27] Both of these groups have a relatively low incidence of Western 'life-style' diseases. In contrast human adult intestine in the U.S. reveals blunt, finger-shaped villi and demonstrates a pattern similar to that of the suckling rat and neonate rats weaned on to a diet containing 10% cellulose. Thus the architectural topography of human small intestine has been correlated with dietary intake. The underlying mechanism has barely been probed and deserves more attention with respect to intestinal pathophysiology. The most obvious hypothesis worthy of pursuit, lies in the area of cell replenishment and the biochemical factors responsible for this remarkable facet of homeostasis.

Summary

1) In the jejunum of animals fed a specific form of dietary fiber, either 10% cellulose or 5% guar gum 79% and 20% of the villi, respectively, retained the finger-like shape characteristic of early postnatal development. Chow fed animals showed uniformly leaf and ridge shaped villi.

2) The feeding of a liquid element diet, post weaning does not appear to adversely affect intestinal mucosal growth.

3) The presence of dietary fiber either bulk type (cellulose) or gel-type (guar gum) does not exert a trophic influence on the rat jejunum.

4) The jejunum of fiber-free and guar-gum fed rats appears to exhibit *pathological adaptational hyperplasia.*

5) The small intestinal mucosa of the cellulose group of animals demonstrated *physiological adaptational hypoplasia.*

6) The presence of the gel fiber, guar gum, appears to *stimulate colonic mucosal growth.*

7) Colonic mucosa from fiber-free and cellulose fed groups exhibits a degree of *hypoplasia*, compared to animals weaned on to a regular chow diet.

8) The fiber-free dietary group was unique among the diets studied in that these animals exhibited *jejunal hyperplasia* in association with *colonic hypoplasia.*

References

1. Baker, S. J.: Geographical variations in the morphology of the small intestinal mucosa in apparently healthy individuals. Patho. Microbiol. 1973, 39:222-237.
2. Banwell J G, Hutt M S T, Tunnicliffe R: Observations on jejunal biopsy in Ugandan Africans. East Afr. Med. J. 41:46-54, 1964.
3. Brown R. C., Kelleher J. K., and Losowsky M. S. The effect of pectin on the structure and function of the rat small intestine. Brit. J. Nutr. 42:351-356, 1979.
4. Cassidy, M. M., Lightfoot, F. G., Grau, L., Story, J. A., Kritchevsky, D., and Vahouny, G. V. Effect of chronic intake of dietary fibers on ultrastructural topography of rat jejunum and colon: a scanning electron microscopy study. Am. J. Clin. Nutr. 34:18-228, 1981.
5. Cassidy, M. M., Lightfoot, F. G. and Vahouny, G. V. Dietary fiber, bile acids and Intestinal morphology. In dietary Fiber in Health and Disease, (eds. by G. V. Vahouny and D. Kritchevsky). Plenum Press, New York, pp. 239-264. 1982.
6. Cassidy, M. M., Fitzpatrick, L., and Vahouny, G. V. Dietary fiber in the post-weaning diet on nutritional and intestinal morphological indices in the rat. In: Basics of Dietary Fiber (eds. G. Vahouny and D. Kritchevsky), Plenum Publishing Co. New York 1985.
7. Clarke, R M: 'Luminal nutrition' versus 'functional work-load' as controllers of mucosal morphology and epithelial replacement in the rat small intestine. Digestion 15:411-424, 1977.
8. Creamer, B: Intestinal structure in relation to absorption. Biomembranes 4A,0:1-42, 1974.
9. Creamer, B: Variations is small intestinal villus shape and mucosal dynamics. Brit. Med. J. 2:1371-1375, 1964.
10. Dowling, R H: Small bowel adaptation and its regulation. Scan J Gastroenterol 17(Suppl.);74:53-74, 1982.
11. Dworkin, L D, Levine, G M, Farber, N J, and Spector, M H: Small intestinal mass is partially determined by indirect effects of intraluminal nutrition. Gastroenterology 7:626-630, 1976.
12. Ecknauer, R, Sircar, B, and Johnson, L R: Effect of dietary bulk on small intestinal morphology and cell renewal in the rat. Gastroenterology 81:781-786, 1981.
13. Fleck, A., and Begg, D. The estimation of ribonucleic acid using ultraviolet ab-

sorption measurements. Biochim. Biophysics. Acta. 108:333-339, 1954.

14. Giles, K. W., and Myers, A. An improved diphenylamine method for the estimation of deoxyribonucleic acid. Nature 206:93, 1965.

15. Jacobs, L R, and Lupton J R: Effect of dietary fibers on rat large bowel mucosal growth and cell proliferation. Am. J. Physiol. G3788-385, 1984.

16. Jacobs, L R: Effects of dietary fiber on mucosal growth and cell proliferation in the small intestine of the rat: A comparison of oat bran, pectin and guar with total fiber deprivation. Am. J. Clin, Nutr. 37L954-960, 1983.

17. Johnson, L. R. and Guthrie, P. D. Mucosal DNA synthesis: a short term index of the trophic action of gastrin. Gastroenterology 67:453-459, 1974.

18. Lipkin, M., Proliferation and differentiation of gastrointestinal cells in normal and disease states, 1981 In Physiology of the Gastrointestinal Tract. Edited by L. R. Johnson Raven Press, 145-168.

19. Loehry, C A, and Creamer, B: Three-dimensional structure of the rat small intestinal mucosa related to mucosal dynamics. Part II: Mucosal structure and dynamics in the lactating rat. Gut 10:116-118, 1969.

20. Lowry, O. H., Rosebrough, N .J., Farr, A. L. et al. Protein measurements with Folin phenol reagent. J. Biol. Chem. 193:265-275, 1951.

21. Majumdar, A. P., and Johnson, L. R. Gastric mucosal cell proliferation during development in rats and effects of pentagastrin. Am. J. Physiol. 242 (Gastrointest. Liver. Physio.): 6135-6139, 1982.

22. Maudsley D. V., Leif, J., and Kobayoshi, Y. Ornithine decarboxylase in rat small intestine: stimulation with food or insulin, Am. J. Physiol. 1976 231:1557-1561

23. Munro, H. N. and Fleck, A. Recent developments in the measurements of nucleic acids in biological materials. Analyst 91:78-88, 1966.

24. Owen, R. L. Brandborg, L. L. Jejunal morphologic consequences of vegetarian diet in humans. Gastroenterology 72:1111, 1977

25. Russell, D. H. and Snyder, S. H. Amine synthesis in rapidly growing tissues: Ornithine decarboxylase activity in regenerating rat liver, chick embryo and various tumors. Proc. Nat. Acad. Sci. U.S.A. 60:1420-1427, 1968.

26. Russell P K, Aziz M A, Ahmad H, Kent T H, Gangerosa E J: Enteritis and gastritis in young asymptomatic Pakistani men. Am J Dig Dis II:296-306, 1966.

27. Sprinz H, Sribhibhadh R, Gangerosa E J, Benyajati C, Kundel K, Halstead S: Biopsy of small bowel of Thai people. 38,7:43-51, 1962.

28. Tasman-Jones C T, Effects of dietary fiber on the structure and function of the small intestine. In Topics in Gastroenterology 67-74, 1981.

28. Tasman-Jones CT, Owen RL, Jones AL: Semipurified dietary fiber and small bowel morphology in rats. Dig. Disc Sci. 27:519-524, 1982.

30. Younoszai M. K., Adedoyun M, and Ranswaw J, Dietary Components and gastrointestinal growth in rats. 1978, J. Nutr. 108: 341-350.

II. Lipids and Nutrient Metabolism

Effect of Dietary Fiber on Alimentary Lipemia

Barbara O. Schneeman

Department of Nutrition
University of California
Davis, CA 95616

Introduction

Most individuals spend 12 hours or more in an alimentary or post-prandial state. After the first meal of the day, the typical pattern of meal eating is likely to sustain a lipemic state throughout the day. During postprandial lipemia, a dynamic remodeling of lipoprotein particles occurs. Thus the metabolism of lipoprotein fractions during the alimentary period is important for understanding the effect of dietary factors on lipoprotein composition and their relationship to risk of cardiovascular disease. The experimental evidence that dietary fiber slows digestion and absorption of lipid and promotes more lipid absorption along a greater length of the intestine has lead several investigators to speculate that consumption of fiber is likely to alter the pattern of postprandial lipemia. To consider the effect of dietary fiber on postprandial lipemia, this paper will first review, briefly, the importance of postprandial lipemia in lipoprotein metabolism and the effect of fiber on lipid digestion and absorption.

Lipoprotein Metabolism During the Alimentary Period

During the consumption of a meal that contains dietary lipid, triglyceride-rich lipoproteins (TRL) appear in the blood (Cohn et al., 1988;

1989). These TRL are derived in part from the intestinal enterocytes, which secrete chylomicron particles into the lymph. The chylomicrons are large, spherical particles (100–1000 nm), and the major lipid components are TG (88%), phospholipid (8%), and cholesterol (4%). Protein is 1–2% of chylomicrons. In studies in which the test meal fed provides at least one-third of the total daily energy and contains at least 40% energy from fat, the peak in alimentary triglyceride concentration typically occurs at 3–4 hours postprandial. The increase in plasma triglycerides after a meal is derived from both intestinal and hepatic sources as indicated by increases in the concentration of both apolipoprotein (apo) B48 and apo B100 in TRL (Cohn et al., 1989; 1991). Apo B48 is derived from secretion of chylomicrons from the small intestine, whereas apo B100 is predominantly associated with TRL made in the liver.

In contrast to the increase in plasma triglycerides postprandially, plasma cholesterol levels are typically unchanged or decrease after a test meal (Cohn et al., 1988; 1989; 1991). However, the movement of cholesterol between lipoprotein fractions appears to be stimulated during the postprandial period. The net transport of cholesterol from cell membranes to plasma, esterification of cholesterol by lecithin cholesterol acyl transferase (LCAT), and transfer by cholesterol ester transfer protein to TRL and LDL fractions is stimulated by postprandial lipemia (Castro and Fielding, 1985; Tall et al., 1986). TRL, including chylomicrons, are effective acceptors of cholesterol esters derived from the LCAT reaction. Normally chylomicrons are cleared rapidly from the plasma (half-time for disappearance is < 1 hour), which provides a route for reverse cholesterol transport, but their rapid clearance may limit the amount of cholesterol ester that can be transferred to these particles and subsequently be cleared by the liver. Fielding et al. (1989) demonstrated that the ability to facilitate reverse cholesterol transfer by this mechanism depends on the level of fat in the diet. Baboons adapted to a low fat diet have enhanced transfer of cholesterol from cells to lipoprotein fractions, whereas those fed a high fat diet have enhanced transfer of cholesterol from lipoproteins to cell membranes. They proposed that chronic high fat and cholesterol consumption overwhelm this system and stimulate cholesterol loading during the postprandial period rather than unloading of cholesterol by cells.

Among individuals, considerable variability in the pattern of postprandial lipemia exists. The degree of increase in triglycerides appears to be lower in premenopausal females than males and in active than sedentary subjects. In females versus males and in active versus sedentary individuals, this blunting of the postprandial response has been associated with an inverse relationship between plasma triglyceride and HDL-cholesterol concentrations and with higher activity of lipoprotein lipase.

Additionally the lipemic response is correlated with fasting triglyceride concentration and is influenced by apo E phenotype (Brown and Roberts, 1991; Weintraub et al., 1987b). The amount and fatty acid composition of the lipid in the test meal has been reported to change the postprandial lipemic response (Weintraub et al., 1987a). However, there is little information on whether altering lipid digestion and absorption will influence the postprandial pattern. Cholestyramine, which binds bile acids and phospholipids and reduces lipid available for absorption in the small intestinal contents (Gallaher and Schneeman, 1986), has been reported to enhance triglyceridemia in type II patients (Weintraub et al., 1987a).

Effect of Fiber on Lipid Digestion and Absorption

The ability of sources of dietary fiber to interfere with rapid digestion and absorption of lipid has been well-documented (Schneeman, 1990; Schneeman and Gallaher, in press). This effect of fiber sources on lipid digestion and absorption has been associated with viscous polysaccharides that can interfere with micelle formation or disrupt mixing within the small intestinal contents and with cereals that contain lipase inhibitor activity (Schneeman, 1990; Schneeman and Gallaher, in press; Lairon et al., 1985). Sources of viscous polysaccharides slow the disappearance of lipids from the digestive tract. Studies with ileostomy patients indicate that lipid in the ileostomy fluid increases by about 50% in patients fed guar gum and by about 36% in patients given pectin (Higham and Read, 1992; Sandgerg et al., 1983). In contrast, wheat bran does not significantly increase fat excretion in ileostomy fluid (Sandberg et al., 1981).

Animal studies have confirmed that consumption of viscous polysaccharides delay the disappearance of lipid from the small intestine.

Table 1. Effect of fiber on the disappearance of cholesterol and triglyceride from the small intestine

	^{3}H-Cholesterol		^{14}C-Triolein	
	small intestine contents	small intestine tissue	small intestine contents	small intestine tissue
	(% of label emptied from the stomach)			
Cellulose	33[a]	57[c]	7[a]	20[c]
Guar gum	43[b]	45[b]	9[b]	11[b]
Glucomannan	58[c]	27[a]	12[c]	1[a]

[a,b,c]Values with different superscripts differ significantly (p < 0.05).
Ebihara and Schneeman 1989.

Ebihara and Schneeman (1989) reported that isotopically labeled triolein and cholesterol is significantly higher in the intestinal contents and significantly lower in the small intestinal tissue at 2.5 hours after a test meal in rats fed glucomannan and guar gum than in rats fed cellulose (Table 1).

Fiber and Postprandial Lipemia

The ability of viscous polysaccharides to slow the disappearance of lipid from the small intestine leads to an alteration in the pattern of alimentary lipemia. However, results of studies conducted on the effect of fiber on alimentary lipemia have not resulted in a clear picture of fiber's effects. Anderson et al (1980) reported that in subjects fed a high carbohydrate, high fiber, low fat meal the increase in alimentary triglyceridemia was significantly less than in subjects fed meals with a higher fat and lower carbohydrate level. However, in this study the difference in fat content undoubtedly accounts for the difference in postprandial lipemia. Jenkins (1978) reported that addition of pectin or guar gum to a Lundh test meal resulted in a higher triglyceride response at 3 h postprandial than a non-fiber supplemented meal. No differences in the postprandial increase in triglycerides were reported if bran or psyllium husk was added to a test meal of cream; however, this study is limited based on the type of meal (bolus of cream) and the apparent limitation in the number of subjects (Miettinen, 1987). Gatti et al. (1984) reported that in normal subjects the rise in postprandial triglycerides was essentially prevented when subjects consumed pasta made with guar gum. The complete lack of increase in triglycerides after the meal is surprising given the fat content (50% of energy) and suggests that the properties of guar gum may change markedly with processing to make pasta.

Table 2. Lymphatic recovery of triglycerides and cholesterol in rats adapted to fiber

Fiber source	Cholesterol		Oleic acid	
	4 hours	24 hours	4 hours	24 hours
	(% of dose infused intestinally)			
None	18.9	49.0	48.5	70.0
Cellulose	8.3*	37.5	37.0	67.0
Pectin	5.0*	18.0*	26.0*	55.0
Guar gum	6.1*	28.0*	32.5*	50.0
Psyllium	3.2*	12.0*	19.0*	27.5*

*Values differ significantly from the fiber-free control (none) $p < 0.05$.
From Vahouny et al. 1988.

Cara et al. (1992) reported that certain cereal fibers blunt the increase in postprandial triglycerides when incorporated into a test meal (Table 3).

Based on these and other data (Lairon et al., 1985), these investigators speculate that the reduction of postprandial lipemia due to cereals is due to the presence of lipase inhibitors that affect the digestion of triglycerides. Although the lipase inhibitors in cereals may blunt the alimentary increase in triglycerides by slowing absorption, it is not clear the inhibiting lipase activity will affect cholesterol absorption. Gallaher and Schneeman (1985) reported the triolein disappearance from the small intestine was slowed due to inhibition of lipase activity by cellulose, but cholesterol disappearance was not affected.

Redard et al. (1990) reported that the percent increase from baseline in triglycerides was significantly higher in subjects who consumed a test meal supplemented with guar gum and oat bran than when they consumed the meal without fiber. These data are consistent with the earlier report of Jenkins (1978) that pectin and guar gum enhanced the triglyceride response to a Lundh test meal. He speculated that the effect of these polysaccharides on triglyceride response could be mediated by a lower insulin release affecting the clearance of TRL.

The differences in postprandial lipemic response to fiber supplemented meals suggest that we currently have a poor understanding of the relationship between the rate and site of lipid digestion and absorption and postprandial lipemia. The studies by Redard et al (1990) and Jenkins (1978) suggest that if a high proportion of viscous polysaccharide is present, postprandial triglyceridemia may be enhanced, while the study of Cara et al. (1992) indicates that postprandial lipemia is likely to be blunted if the diet is rich in insoluble polysaccharides or fiber sources that inhibit lipase activity. These differences imply that some sources of fiber are more likely to affect the secretion of intestinal lipoproteins, whereas other fiber sources are more likely to affect the clearance of TRL postprandially. A significant factor in all of these studies is likely to be the type and amount of fat included in the test meal. Postprandial test meals typically have contained 50% energy from fat or higher. However, it is possible that at lower fat intakes, fiber may be more ef-

Table 3. Serum triglyceride response to fiber-supplemented meals

Oat bran	75*
Rice bran	89
Wheat fiber	66*
Wheat germ	79*

*Differed significantly from control ($p < 0.05$).
From Cara et al. 1992.

fective in modulating the rate of lipid absorption. Likewise, in conjunction with a low fat intake, fiber may be more effective in prolonging the intestinal contribution to alimentary lipemia and thus the opportunity for reverse cholesterol transport.

Conclusions

Lipid digestion and absorption have classically been studied under conditions that favor rapid uptake of lipid from the duodenum and upper jejunum. Studies in gastrointestinal physiology have indicated that the length of intestine exposed to dietary nutrients is an important regulator of gastrointestinal response to diet (Lin et al., 1992a, b; 1989). Fiber, as a normal constituent of the diet, is an important modulator of the rate and site of lipid absorption from the gut, e.g., consumption of viscous polysaccharides can carry lipid into more distal sections of the small intestine and slow disappearance of lipid from the intestine. Our understanding of the relationship between fiber's effects on the rate and site of absorption and postprandial lipemia is currently incomplete, but progress in this area will provide insight on the potential effects of fiber on lipoprotein metabolism.

Acknowledgements

Part of this work has been supported by NIH grant DK20446 and by USDA grant 9000697.

References

Anderson, J. W., Chen, W.-J. L., and Siebling, B., 1980, Hypolipidemic effects of high-carbohydrate, high fiber diets, *Metabolism* 29:551-558.

Brown, A. J., and Roberts, D. C. K. 1991, The effect of fasting triacylglyceride concentration and apolipoprotein E polymorphism on postprandial lipemia, *Arterioscler. Thromb.* 11:1737-1744.

Cara, L., Dubois, C., Borel, P., Armand, M., Senft, M., Portugal, H., Pauli, A.-M., Bernard, P.-M., and Lairon, D., 1992, Effects of oat bran, rice bran, wheat fiber, and wheat germ on postprandial lipemia in healthy adults, *Am. J. Clin. Nutr.* 55:81-88.

Castro, G. R., and Fielding, C. J. 1985, Effects of postprandial lipemia on plasma cholesterol metabolism, *J. Clin. Invest.* 75:874-882.

Cohn, J. S., Lam, C. W. K., Sullivan, D. R., and Hensley, W. J. 1991, Plasma lipoprotein distribution of apolipoprotein (a) in fed and fasted states, *Atherosclerosis* 90:59-66.

Cohn, J. S., McNamara, J. R., Cohn, S. D., Ordovas, J. M., and Schaefer, E. J. 1988, Plasma apolipoprotein changes in the triglyceride-rich lipoprotein fraction of human subjects fed a fat-rich meal, *J. Lipid Res.* 29:925-936.

Cohn, J. S., McNamara, J. R., Krasinski, S. D., Russell, R. M., and Schaefer, E. J. 1989, Role of triglyceride-rich lipoproteins from the liver and intestine in the etiology of postprandial peaks in plasma triglyceride concentration, *Metabolism* 38:484-490.

Ebihara, K., and Schneeman, B. O. 1989, Interaction of bile acids, phospholipids, cholesterol, and triglyceride with dietary fibers in the small intestine of rats. *J. Nutr.* 119:1100-1106.

Fielding, P. E., Jackson, E. M., and Fielding, C. J. 1989, Chronic dietary fat and cholesterol inhibit the normal postprandial stimulation of plasma cholesterol metabolism, *J. Lipid Res.* 30:1211-1217.

Gallaher, D., and Schneeman, B. O., 1985, Effect of dietary cellulose on site of lipid absorption, *Am. J. Physiol.* 249:G184-G191.

Gallaher, D., and Schneeman, B. O. 1986, Intestinal interaction of bile acids, phospholipids, dietary fibers, and cholestyramine, *Am. J. Physiol.* 250:G420-G426.

Gatti, E., Catenazzo, G., Camisasca, E., Torri, A., Denegri, E., and Sitori, C. R., 1984, Effects of guar-enriched pasta in the treatment of diabetes and hyperlipidemia, *Ann. Nutr. Metab.* 28:1-10.

Higham, S. E., and Read, N. W. 1992, The effect of ingestion of guar gum on ileostomy effluent, *Br. J. Nutr.* 67:115-122.

Isaksson, G., Lundquist, I., Akesson, B., and Ihse, I., 1988, Effects of pectin and wheat bran on intraluminal pancreatic enzyme activities and on fat absorption as examined with the triolein breath test in patients with pancreatic insufficiency, *Scan. J. Gastroenterol.* 19:467-472.

Jenkins, D. J. A., 1978, Action of dietary fiber in lowering fasting serum cholesterol and reducing postprandial glycemia: Gastrointestinal mechanisms *in*: International Conference on Atherosclerosis (L. A. Carlson, ed.) Raven Press, New York, pp. 173-182.

Lairon, D., Borel, P., Termine, E., Grataroli, R., Chabert, C. and Hauton, J. C., 1985, Evidence for a proteinic inhibitor of pancreatic lipase in cereals, wheat bran and wheat germ. *Nutr. Rep. Int.* 32:1107-1113

Lin, H. C., Kim, B. H., Elashoff, J. D., Doty, J. E., Gu, Y.-G., and Meyer, J. H., 1992, Gastric emptying of solid food is most potently inhibited by carbohydrate in the canine distal ileum, *Gastroenterology* 102:793-801.

Lin, H. C., Moller, N. A., Wolinsky, M. M., Kim, B. H., Doty, J. E., and Meyer, J. H., 1992, Sustained slowing effect of lentils on gastric emptying of solids in humans and dogs, *Gastroenterology* 102:787-792.

Lin, H. C., Doty, J. E., Reedy, T. J., and Meyer, J. H., 1990, Inhibition of gastric emptying by sodium oleate depends on the length of intestine exposed to nutrient, *Am. J. Physiol.* 259: (Gastrointest. Liver Physiol. 22):G1031-G1036.

Miettinen, T. A., 1987, Dietary fiber and lipids, *Am. J. Clin. Nutr.* 45:1237-1242.

Redard, C. L., Davis, P. A. and Schneeman, B. O., 1990, Dietary fiber and gender: effect on postprandial lipemia, *Am. J. Clin. Nutr.* 52:837-845.

Sandberg, A. S., Ahderinne, R., Andersson, H., Hallgren, B., Hasselblad, K., Isaksson, B., and Hulten, L., 1983, The effects of citrus pectin on the absorption of nutrients in the small intestine. *Human Nutrition: Clinical Nutrition* 37C:171-183.

Sandberg, A. S., Andersson, H., Hallgren, B., Hasselblad, K., Isaksson, B., and

Hulten, L., 1981, Experimental model for in vivo determination of dietary fibre and its effects on the absorption of nutrients in the small intestine, *Br. J. Nutr.*, 45:283-294.

Schneeman, B. O. 1990, Macronutrient absorption, *in* Dietary Fiber (D. Kritchevsky, C. Bonfield, J.W. Anderson, eds.) Plenum Press, New York, pp. 157-166.

Schneeman, B. O., and Gallaher, D., in press, Effects of dietary fiber on digestive enzymes, *in* Handbook of Dietary Fiber in Human Nutrition, 2nd edition, (G. A. Spiller, ed.), CRC Press, Boca Raton, FL.

Tall, A., Sammett, D., and Granot, E. 1986, Mechanisms of enhanced cholesteryl ester transfer from high density lipoproteins to apoB-containing lipoproteins during alimentary lipemia. *J. Clin. Invest.* 77:1163-1172.

Vahouny, G. V., Satchithanandam, S., Chen, I., Tepper, S. A., Kritchevsky, D., Lightfoot, F. G., and Cassidy, M. M., 1988, Dietary fiber and intestinal adaptation: Effect on lipid absorption and lymphatic transport in the rat, *Am. J. Clin. Nutr.* 47:201-206.

Weintraub, M. S., Eisenberg, S., and Breslow, J. L. 1987a, Different patterns of postprandial metabolism in normal, type IIa, type III, and type IV hyperlipoproteinemic individuals, *J. Clin. Invest.* 79:1110-1119.

Weintraub, M. S. Eisenberg, S., and Breslow, J. L. 1987b, Dietary fat clearance in normal subjects is regulated by genetic variation in apolipoprotein E, *J. Clin. Invest.* 80:1571-1577.

Dietary Fiber and Lipid Absorption: Interference of Chitosan and Its Hydrolysates with Cholesterol and Fatty Acid Absorption and Metabolic Consequences in Rats

Ikuo Ikeda,[1] Michihiro Sugano,[2] Katsuko Yoshida,[2] Eiji Sasaki,[1] Yasushi Iwamoto,[3] and Kouta Hatano[3]

[1]Laboratory of Nutrition Chemistry and [2]Laboratory of Food Science, Kyusu University School of Agriculture, Fukuoka 812, Japan, and [3]Biological Engineering Laboratory, Asahi Industries Co., Ltd., Saitama 367-02, Japan.

Introduction

Chitosan, a polymer of glucosamine and a typical animal fiber, has a marked hypocholesterolemic activity, and also decreases hepatic cholesterol and triglyceride in experimental animals (Sugano et al., 1978; Kobayashi et al., 1979; Nagyvary et al., 1979; Sugano et al., 1980; Sugano et al., 1988; Jennings et al., 1988; Hirano et al., 1990). Chitosan interferes with lymphatic absorption of cholesterol and oleic acid (Vahouny et al., 1983), and increases fecal excretion of neutral steroids in rats (Sugano et al., 1978; Sugano et al., 1980). These observations explain the mechanism by which chitosan exerts a hypocholesterolemic effect. The recommendation of chitosan as a hypocholesterolemic agent is reasonable, since its side effect is lower as compared with cholestyramine (Gordon and Besch-Williford, 1984; Jennings et al., 1988).

Chitosan is prepared by deacetylation of chitin, but the degree of deacetylation varies from essentially 100% to approximately 20%. Since the primary base, the amino group, is exposed by deacetylation, chitosan in solution can behave as a weak anion exchange resin. This property may at least in part be responsible for its prominent hypocholesterolemic activity as presumed from the action of cholestyramine, a strong anion exchange resin. Chitosan prepared from naturally occurring chitin is soluble at acidic pH, and the solution is highly viscous. Since viscous fibers such as pectin and guar gum are well known to have a hypocholesterolemic effect (Vahouny, 1982; Edwards, 1988), the viscous property is also thought to be involved in the inhibitory effect of chitosan on cholesterol and fatty acid absorption.

However, the high viscosity of chitosan in solution hinders its use as a food additive as in the case of guar gum. Hence, it is desirable to prepare chitosans with low viscosity without largely influencing a hypocholesterolemic potential. Our previous study showed that various commercially available chitosans which have viscosity between 17 and 1620 cps as 1% solution have an equal hypocholesterolemic activity when fed to rats (Sugano et al., 1988). Thus, the cholesterol-lowering activity of chitosans was independent of their viscosity and hence, molecular weight insofar as the preparations have high viscosity. However, since glucosamine oligomer composed mainly of three to five aminosugar residues did not show a hypocholesterolemic activity, some molecular size should be necessary to exert a desirable effect (Sugano et al., 1988). In the preliminary study in which the effect of partial hydrolysates of chitosan on serum and liver cholesterol levels was examined, we found that chitosan with a molecular weight of approximately 10,000 has still a significant hypocholesterolemic activity (Sugano et al., 1992). Hence, we focused on the effect of chitosan hydrolysates with varying molecular weights on lipid metabolism and lymphatic lipid absorption in rats.

Some Properties of Chitoson Hydrolysates with Different Molecular Weights

Chitosan hydrolysates were prepared from a relatively low molecular weight chitosan (average molecular weight 50,000, Kimitsu Chemical Industries Co., Tokyo, Japan) by using chitosanase from *Verticillium* sp., AF9-V-156 (Iwamoto et al., 1990; Sakamoto et al., 1991).

Table 1 shows some properties of chitosan hydrolysates used in this study. Molecular weight distributions of the hydrolysates as measured by gel-filtration are shown in Figure 1. Average molecular weights of these preparations were 2,000 (LP-2), 5,000 (LP-5), 10,000 (LP-10), and

20,000 (LP-20) as compared with 50,000 in unhydrolyzed chitosan (LP-50). Viscosity, measured as 1% solution in 0.5% acetic acid, of these hydrolysates was apparently the same with that of water. Since the extent of deacetylation was 80% in all preparations, the effect of molecular weight can be compared as a sole variable. Effect of pH on solubility of chitosan preparations was also measured as shown in Table 1. LP-50 precipitated at pH 6.6, whereas LP-5, LP-10, and LP-20 formed precipitation at pH 7.0–8.3. LP-2 did not form precipitation up to pH 10.

Table 1. Characterization of chitosan hydrolysates

Preparations	Average molecular weight	Degree of deacetylation	Viscosity (cps)[1]	pH precipitated
LP-2	2,000	80%	1.1	...[2]
LP-5	5,000	80%	1.3	7.8–8.3
LP-10	10,000	80%	1.6	7.0–7.4
LP-20	20,000	80%	1.9	7.1–7.3
LP-50	50,000	80%	11.0	6.6

[1] Viscosity was measured as 1% solution in 0.5% acetic acid.
[2] No precipitate formed up to pH 10.

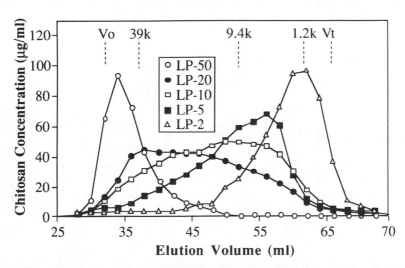

Figure 1. Gel-filtration pattern of the hydrolysates of chitosan. Figures at the top represent molecular weights of the markers. The average molecular weights of LP-50, LP-20, LP-10, LP-5, and LP-2 were 50,000, 20,000, 10,000, 5,000 and 2,000, respectively.

Effects of Chitosan Hydrolysates on Serum and Liver Lipid Levels and on Fecal Steriod Excretion

Male Sprague-Dawley rats, weighing on an average 88g, were fed experimental diets ad libitum for 14 days. The control diet contained 4% cellulose, and 0.25% cholesterol and 0.06% Na-cholate. Testing materials were added to the diet at the 2% level at the expense of cellulose. Rats were killed by decapitation after fasting for 7 hr at 13:00 hours. Feces were collected for 2 days between days 11 and 13.

Food intake and growth of rats fed chitosan preparations were comparable with rats fed cellulose except for the LP-2 group in which these parameters were unexpectedly and significantly lower during the second week than those of rats. Enlargement of liver due to feeding a cholesterol-enriched diet was significantly prevented by all groups of rats fed chitosan preparations.

The concentration of serum cholesterol was comparable among the groups, except for the LP-2 group in which it was significantly higher than the other groups (Figure 2). However, when we measured serum cholesterol one week after feeding experimental diets, it was significantly lower in rats fed LP-5, LP-10, and LP-20 as compared with those fed cellulose, the LP-2 preparation did not show any cholesterol-lowering effect. In a preliminary experiment the partial hydrolysate of guar gum showed a serum cholesterol-lowering activity, but in contrast to the chitosan hydrolysate it did not lower liver cholesterol level. There

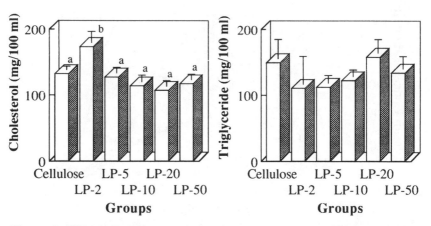

Figure 2. Effects of chitosan hydrolysates on serum cholesterol and triglyceride levels of rats fed cholesterol-enriched diets for 14 days. Mean ± SE of 6 rats. [ab]Values not sharing a common letter are significantly different at $p < 0.05$.

is no significant difference in serum triglyceride concentration among all groups.

In contrast, the concentration of liver cholesterol was significantly reduced by feeding chitosan hydrolysates with molecular weights above 5,000 compared with cellulose and the hydrolysates with a molecular weight of 2,000 (Figure 3). The preparations with molecular weights above 10,000 showed a comparable lowering effect and were more effective than the molecular weight 5,000 preparation. All the hydrolysates reduced liver triglyceride to a comparable extent as compared with cellulose.

Weight of feces was significantly higher in the LP-20 and LP-50 groups, whereas significantly lower in the LP-2 group than in the cellu-

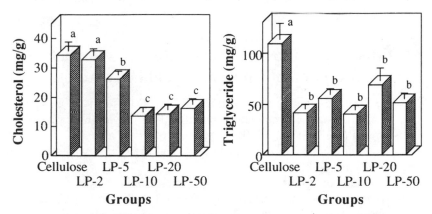

Figure 3. Effects of chitosan hydrolysates on liver cholesterol and triglyceride levels of rats fed cholesterol-enriched diets for 14 days. Mean ± SE of 6 rats. [abc]Values not sharing a common letter are significantly different at p < 0.05.

Table 2. Fecal excretion of neutral and acidic steroids

| Groups | Weight of feces | Neutral steroids | | | Acidic steroids |
		Cholesterol	Coprostanol	Total	
		(mg/day)			
Cellulose	1.40 ± 0.10^a	7.80 ± 0.97^a	1.02 ± 0.72^a	8.81 ± 1.04^a	4.60 ± 0.37^{ab}
LP-2	0.76 ± 0.08^b	7.38 ± 1.19^a	1.30 ± 0.16^{ac}	8.68 ± 1.22^a	$3.96 \pm .80^a$
LP-5	1.49 ± 0.08^{ac}	16.8 ± 2.5^b	1.73 ± 0.53^{ac}	18.6 ± 2.4^b	5.61 ± 0.98^{ab}
LP-10	1.54 ± 0.14^{ac}	19.3 ± 3.7^b	6.65 ± 0.97^b	25.9 ± 3.6^{bc}	6.97 ± 1.56^b
LP-20	1.81 ± 0.11^c	22.9 ± 1.3^b	5.85 ± 1.38^{bd}	28.8 ± 1.5^c	5.04 ± 0.50^{ab}
LP-50	1.77 ± 0.08^c	21.7 ± 4.2^b	3.63 ± 0.57^{cd}	25.3 ± 4.7^{bc}	5.55 ± 0.65^{ab}

Mean ± SE of 6 rats. Feeding periods for 2 weeks.
[a,b,c]Values not sharing a common superscript letter are significantly different at p < 0.05.

lose group as shown in Table 2. Fecal excretion of neutral steroids as cholesterol and coprostanol significantly increased in rats fed chitosan hydrolysates except for LP-2. The hydrolysates with molecular weights above 10,000 were more effective in enhancing fecal neutral steroids, whereas the effect of LP-5 was moderate. Fecal excretion of neutral steroids was inversely correlated with the concentration of liver cholesterol. The neutral steroid excretion observed with LP-10, LP-20, and LP-50 preparations was comparable with that of more viscous chitosans (Sugano et al., 1988). However, the effect of chitosan hydrolysates on the composition of neutral steroids was not necessarily similar depending on the preparations. Excretion of total acidic steroids slightly increased in rats fed chitosan hydrolysates except for LP-2. In particular, the excretion in the LP-10 group was 1.5-fold higher than that in the cellulose group.

Effects of Chitosan Hydrolysates on Lymphatic Absorption of Cholesterol and Fatty Acids

Male Sprague-Dawley rats weighing 260 to 300 g received an operation of a left thoracic lymphatic cannula and an indwelling catheter in the stomach (Ikeda et al., 1989). They were received a freshly prepared test emulsion (Table 3) via stomach tube, and the lymph was collected periodically for 24 hr.

Lymphatic absorption of radioactive cholesterol is shown in Figure 4. Rats given cellulose most effectively absorbed cholesterol during 24 hr. Cholesterol absorption in the LP-2 group was comparable with the cellulose group at 24 hr after administration, but it was lower at 6 and 9 hr. The lowering effect of LP-5, LP-20 and LP-50 on cholesterol absorption was comparable, and was effective for 24 hr. The effect of LP-10 was moderate until 9 hr after administration, but at 24 hr the absorption rate was comparable with the hydrolysates with higher molecular weights.

Thus, the inhibitory effect of chitosan hydrolysates on cholesterol ab-

Table 3. Composition of fat emulsion

Components	Amounts
Sodium taurocholate	200 mg
Albumin (fatty acid free)	50 mg
Cholesterol	10 mg
[^{14}C] Cholesterol	1 μCi
Triolein	200 mg
Test material	50 mg
Distilled water	to 3 ml

sorption was confirmed more directly. Consistent with the results in a feeding experiment, the reduction of cholesterol absorption by chitosan hydrolysates was observed in LP-5, LP-10, LP-20, and LP-50. Although the inhibitory effect of LP-5 on cholesterol absorption was comparable

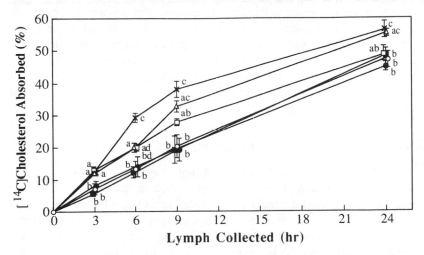

Figure 4. Effects of chitosan hydrolysates on lymphatic absorption of cholesterol in rats. Mean ± SE of 6 rats. [abcd]Values not sharing a common letter are significantly different at p<0.05.

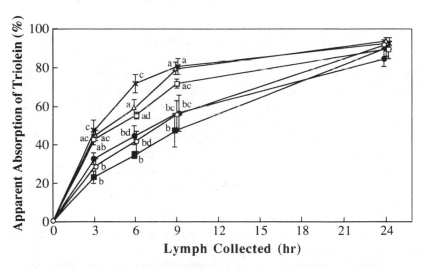

Figure 5. Effects of chitosan hydrolysates on lymphatic absorption of triglyceride (triolein) in rats. Mean ± SE of 6 rats. [abcd]Values not sharing a common letter are significanlty different at p<0.05.

with LP-20 and LP-50, the effect of the former on liver cholesterol and fecal excretion of neutral steroids was less marked than the latter two preparations, suggesting the threshold of the molecular weight required for the cholesterol-lowering activity.

Lymphatic absorption of triolein is shown in Figure 5. Absorption of oleic acid administered as triolein was comparable among the groups at 24 hr after administration, but there was a considerable difference in the absorption pattern. Rats given cellulose most effectively absorbed oleic acid at 3, 6, and 9 hr after administration. Apparent delayed absorption of oleic acid was observed in rats given LP-5, LP-20, and LP-50 until 9 hr after administration. The interfering effect of LP-10 on oleic acid absorption was comparable with that of LP-2.

Discussion

The results presented here showed that low molecular weight chitosan hydrolysates inhibit cholesterol absorption in the intestine and as a result, increase fecal neutral steroid excretion to a similar extent as high viscous chitosan. Moreover, the effect was observed on the hydrolysates with a molecular weight above 5,000. The molecular weight 2,000 preparation appeared to be less effective in this respect. Although the serum cholesterol-lowering effect was not confirmed after 2 weeks of feeding, it was clear after 1 week. There was a marked decrease in liver cholesterol after feeding the hydrolysates with molecular weights above 10,000.

The lymphatic absorption of oleic acid as triolein was delayed, and the concentration of liver triglyceride was decreased by chitosan hydrolysates. However, at 24 hr after administration, oleic acid absorption was comparable among the groups given chitosan hydrolysates and cellulose. In contrast, high molecular weight chitosan reduced absorption of both cholesterol and fatty acids (Vahouny et al., 1983; Ikeda et al., 1990) and liver triglyceride (Sugano et al., 1988). Therefore, the inhibition of fatty acid absorption in the intestine is at least one of the mechanisms of the decrease in liver triglyceride in high molecular weight chitosan, and the mechanism of action on absorption of fatty acid might be different between the hydrolysates and high molecular weight chitosan.

Acidic steroid excretion slightly increased when rats were fed chitosan hydrolysates with molecular weights above 5,000, contrary to the previous observations with high molecular weight chitosans in which acidic steroid excretion did not increase (Sugano et al., 1980). Since chitosan contains primary bases in its molecule and can act as an anion exchanger, the increase in acidic steroid excretion by chitosan is plausible. The discrepancy, therefore, may be explained by the difference in the solubility in the intestine.

Several mechanisms have been proposed to the inhibitory effect of chitosan on lipid absorption. High viscosity of chitosan may be primarily responsible for the inhibition of cholesterol and fatty acid absorption as in the case of guar gum and pectin (Ikeda et al., 1990), and in fact the hypocholesterolemic activity was independent of the viscosity when it is above 17 cps (Sugano et al., 1988). Therefore, it is not obvious whether the mechanism proposed for viscous fiber, the reduction of diffusion of micellar lipids to intestinal walls and the coating effect on inner intestinal wall (Vahouny, 1982), is applicable to chitosan hydrolysates.

Chitosan, as an anion-exchanger, may bind bile acid and fatty acid by ionic bond at pH lower than 6.0 (Furda, 1983) and hence, the binding may occur in the stomach and/or the jejunal lumen. This effect may disturb micellar solubility of cholesterol and fatty acid and inhibits their absorption. Since bile acid and fatty acid are released from chitosan at pH>6.0, these anions will become available for absorption in the middle to lower intestine, and hence, absorption of fatty acids may be delayed. Since chitosan preparations retarded oleic acid absorption, the action as an anion exchanger is plausible. The slowed absorption of fatty acid may be concerned with the reduction of hepatic triglyceride by dietary chitosan (Sugano et al., 1980; Sugano et al., 1988). There is a possibility that the low rate of triglyceride absorption in the intestine alters the composition and the size of lipoproteins synthesized in the mucosal cells, and consequently, influences clearance of triglyceride in the liver and also in peripheral tissues. Moreover, the action as a weak anion exchanger may also explain the observations that fecal excretion of bile acids is not increased (Sugano et al., 1980) or slightly increased as in the present study, since most of bile acids are reabsorbed from the lower intestine.

Nauss et al. (1983) measured lipid binding capacity of chitosan in vitro in micellar solution and artificial mixed microemulsion containing radioactive bile salt, triglyceride, and cholesterol. Chitosan bound all of these compounds, and the binding capacity was 4–5 times of its weight. They suggested that the primary driving force for the binding is determined by ionic interactions, and hydrophobic binding is also involved.

Based on the available data, two major mechanisms have been proposed by Furda (1983), "polar entrapment" of whole micelles containing cholesterol, fatty acid, and bile acid and "disintegration" of mixed micelles. He also suggested another possibility that before micelle is formed in the intestine, negatively charged fatty acid and bile acid are bound to positively charged amino groups of chitosan. Precipitation and aggregation of chitosan at pH 6.0–6.5 has been thought to be concerned with the entrapment of whole micelles. All the chitosan hydrolysates except for LP-2 formed precipitation at pH between 7.0 and 8.3 as shown in Table 1. Since pH in the upper intestinal lumen is around 7.4, it is not clear whether the precipitation of the hydrolysates influences the inhibitory effect on lipid absorption. However, since LP-2 which was not precipitated at any pH did not show an inhibitory effect on cholesterol and triglyceride absorption, the influence of the precipitation process can not be ruled out.

Conclusion

The partial hydrolysates of chitosan interfered with intestinal absorption of cholesterol and increased fecal excretion of neutral steroids in rats. Although feeding study did not necessarily show a significant hypocholesterolemic effects, they markedly reduced the concentration of liver cholesterol and triglyceride. From the results of the two different approaches, chitosan hydrolysates with water-like viscosity and molecular weights of 5,000 to 20,000 were as effective as high-viscous chitosans with molecular weights of 50,000 or above. The effect appeared to be more preferable than the guar gum hydrolysates. From these results, chitosan hydrolysates can be applied as food additives without largely influencing the properties of the products.

References

Edwards, C. A., Physiological effect of fiber, in: "Dietary Fiber," Kritchevsky, D., Bonfield, C., and Anderson, J. W., eds., 1988, Plenum Press, New York.

Gordon, D. T., and Besch-Williford, C., Action of amino polymers on iron status, gut morphology, and cholesterol level in the rat, in: Chitin, Chitosan, and Related Enzymes, Zilahis, J. P., ed., 1984, Academic Press, Orlando.

Furda, I., Aminopolysaccharides-their potential as dietary fiber, in: Unconventional sources of dietary fiber, Furda, I., ed., 1983, American Chemical Society, Washington, D.C.

Hirano, S., Itakura, C., Seino, H., Akiyama, Y., Nonaka, I., Kanbara, N., and Kawakami, T., Chitosan as an ingredient for domestic animal feeds, J. Agric. Food Chem. 38:1214 (1990).

Ikeda, I., Tomari, Y., and Sugano, M., Interrelated effects of dietary fiber and fat on lymphatic cholesterol and triglyceride absorption in rats, J. Nutr. 119:1383 (1990).

Iwamoto, Y., Koga, K., Kaneko, Y., and Hatano, K., Methods for producing low molecular weight chitosans. Japan Patent in application, 90, 214664 (1990).

Jennings, C. D., Boleyn, K., Bridges, S. R., Wood, P. J., and Anderson, J. W., A comparison of the lipid-lowering and intestinal morphological effects of cholestyramine, chitosan, and oat gum in rats, Proc. Soc. Exp. Biol. Med. 189:13 (1988).

Kobayashi, T., Otsuka, S., and Yugari, Y., Effect of chitosan on serum and liver cholesterol levels in cholesterol-fed rats, Nutr. Rep. Int. 19:327 (1979).

Nagyvary, J. J., Falk, J. D., Hill, M. L., Schmidt, M. L., Wilkins, A. K., and Bradbury, E. L., The hypolipidemic activity of chitosan and other polysaccharides in rats, Nutr. Rep. Int. 20:677 (1979).

Nauss, J. L., Thompson, J. L., and Nagyvary, J., The binding of micellar lipids to chitosan, Lipids 18:714 (1983).

Sakamoto, H., Iwamoto, Y., Kaneko, Y., and Hatano, K., Methods for producing chitosanase. Japan Kokai Tokkyo Koho, 91, 280878 (1991).

Sugano, M., Fujikawa, T., Hiratsuji, Y., and Hasegawa, Y., Hypocholesterolemic effects of chitosan in cholesterol-fed rats, Nutr. Rep. Int. 18:531 (1978).

Sugano, M., Fujikawa, T., Hiratsuji, Y., Nakashima, K., Fukuda, N., and Hasegawa, Y., A novel use of chitosan as a hypocholesterolemic agent in rats, Am. J. Clin. Nutr. 33:787 (1980).

Sugano, M., Watanabe, S., Kishi, A., Izume, M., and Ohtakara, A., Hypocholesterolemic action of chitosans with different viscosity in rats, Lipids 23:187 (1988).

Sugano, M., Yoshida, K., Hashimoto, M., Enomoto, K., and Hirano, S., Hypocholesterolemic activity of partially hydrolyzed chitosan in rats, Proceedings of 5th International Conference on Chitin and Chitosan, Elsevier, Barking, (1992) in press.

Vahouny, G. V., Dietary fiber, lipid metabolism and atherosclerosis, Fed. Proc. 41:2801 (1982).

Vahouny, G. V., Satchithanandam, S., Cassidy, M. M., Lightfoot, F. B., and Furda, I., Comparative effects of chitosan and cholestyramine on lymphatic absorption of lipids in the rat, Am. J. Clin. Nutr. 38:278 (1983).

Correspondence should be addressed to Dr. Michihiro Sugano, Laboratory of Food Science, Department of Food Science and Technology, Kyushu University School of Agriculture 46-09, Fukuoka 812, Japan.

The Role of Viscosity in the Cholesterol-Lowering Effect of Dietary Fiber

Daniel D. Gallaher and Craig A. Hassel
Department of Food Science and Nutrition
University of Minnesota
St. Paul, MN 55108

Introduction

The reduction of serum cholesterol by dietary pectin was first demonstrated in rats and humans 30 years ago.[1,2] Since that time many human and animal trials have been carried out testing a variety of dietary fiber types for their ability to reduce serum cholesterol. Guar gum, pectin, and psyllium seed hydrocolloid have repeatedly been demonstrated to reduce serum cholesterol. The majority of studies investigating various forms of oats (e.g., rolled oats, oat bran, or oatmeal) have also shown this capacity. In contrast, cellulose and wheat bran have consistently failed to reduce serum cholesterol. Many other fiber sources have been studied, generally with inconsistent results.

The mechanism by which certain fibers elicit their cholesterol-lowering effect remains to be established. For example, the demonstration that certain fibers bind bile acids *in vitro* raised the possibility that such fibers lowered serum cholesterol by increasing bile acid excretion. In order to maintain the bile acid pool, more cholesterol would be diverted to bile acid synthesis. Alternatively, binding of bile acids within the small intestine could disrupt micellar structure and lead to decreased absorption of cholesterol.[4] Yet another hypothesis states that propionate derived from large intestinal fermentation of fibers reduces hepatic cholesterol synthesis.[5] Numerous hypotheses have been put forth, but no one hypothesis satisfactorily explains all the experimental data.

When the fiber types with serum cholesterol-lowering abilities are examined, most share attributes of viscosity and fermentability within the large intestine. If the attribute of dietary fiber responsible for cholesterol-lowering could be identified, this would provide a focus for further mechanistic studies. For example, if a high viscosity could be established as the responsible attribute, this would suggest that a reduced efficiency of bile acids and/or cholesterol absorption may be responsible for cholesterol lowering. If fermentation is the key attribute, this would lend weight to other hypotheses.

Fermentation versus Viscosity

We have recently conducted a series of studies designed to determine which attribute of dietary fiber, fermentability or viscosity, is the primary determinant of the serum cholesterol-lowering effect of dieatry fibers. In these studies we have employed hamsters as the animal model, as hamsters appear to have certain advantages over rats in studies of cholesterol metabolism. These include greater similarity to humans with regard to hepatic cholesterol synthesis rates, lipoprotein profiles, LDL metabolism, and greater sensitivity to dietary factors known to influence plasma cholesterol in humans. We have also found that the hamster fecal bile acid profile is somewhat more similar to the human than is that of the rat (unpublished results).

In our first experiment, we choose guar gum and hydroxypropyl methylcellulose (HPMC) as our fiber sources. Native guar gum is highly viscous, highly fermentable, and reproducibly reduces serum cholesterol in both animals and humans. HPMC is a synthetic cellulosic ether that is available in a wide range of viscosities. HPMC is essentially unfermentable in rats.[6] In designing this experiment, we took advantage of the ability to reduce the viscosity of guar gum by limited acid hydrolysis. We were thus able to design a 2 × 2 factorial experiment, where the factors were fermentability and viscosity. The high viscosity HPMC and native guar gum had an *in vitro* viscosity of 100,000 cP and the low viscosity HPMC and acid-hydrolyzed guar gum had a viscosity of 100 cP (as 2% solutions, at 20°C). The experimental diets were modified AIN-76A diets, which contained 10% palm oil and 0.12% cholesterol. The final fiber concentration in each diet was 5%.

Three feeding trials were carried out using this experimental design. In one, animals were fed their respective diets for 3 weeks, fasted overnight, and presented with a 2 g meal of their respective diet the following morning. Two hours after presentation of the meal, the animals were anesthetized, blood was collected for plasma cholesterol determination, and the small intestine removed and the contents collected. The intestinal contents were centrifuged at 30,000 × g for 1 hour and the viscosity of the supernatants measured using a cone/plate viscometer. In a second trial, animals were fed their respective diets for 6 weeks, fasted overnight, anesthetized, blood collected for analysis of plasma lipoproteins and liver taken for determination of cholesterol and cholesteryl esters. In a third trial, animals were fed their respective diets for 11 weeks. After an overnight fast, each animal was given an intraperitoneal injection of ^3H_2O to determine *in vivo* sterol synthesis.

The *in vitro* viscosities and the intestinal contents (*ex vivo*) viscosities are shown in Table 1. Unexpectedly, there was a lack of correlation between these two viscosity measures. The high viscosity HPMC showed a much higher *ex vivo* viscosity than did the native guar gum, in spite of their similar *in vitro* viscosity. Likewise, the low viscosity HPMC had a higher *ex vivo* viscosity than the hydrolyzed guar gum. We believe the unexpectedly low viscosities of the contents of the guar-fed animals may be due fermentation in the hamster stomach. In the hamster, unlike the rat, the stomach is separated into a pregastric pouch and a gastric pouch. The pregastric pouch has a higher pH than the gastric pouch. In addition, the presence of short chain fatty acids in the pregastric pouch contents and the keratinized epithelial lining (similar to a cecum) of the pouch all point to the pregastric pouch as a site of active fermentation.[7] Thus, we believe the guar gum was fermented in the pregastric pouch sufficiently to reduce its *ex vivo* viscosity.

Given the unexpected *ex vivo* results, the appropriate comparison for examining the role of viscosity is the high viscosity HPMC group with the low viscosity HPMC group. For examining the role of fermentation, the comparison of interest would be the low viscosity HPMC group with the native guar group, as both these fibers had similar *ex vivo* viscosities.

Table 1. *In vitro* and intestinal contents supernatants *ex vivo* viscosity in hamsters fed hydroxypropylmethylcellulose (HPMC) or guar gum (GG) of different viscosities

Diet group	Dietary fiber 2% solution (in vitro)	Intestinal contents (ex vivo)
	cP	
High viscosity GG	100,000	230 ± 89
Low viscosity GG	100	56 ± 19
High viscosity HPMC	100,000	2,665 ± 648
Low viscosity HPMC	100	274 ± 63

Figure 1 shows plasma cholesterol concentrations of each group at 3 weeks, 6 weeks, and 11 weeks. By 11 weeks, plasma cholesterol concentrations had still not reached a plateau. Regardless of the time point chosen, the high viscosity HPMC group had lower plasma cholesterol concentrations than the low viscosity HPMC group.

These results provide clear evidence that the increased viscosity has a role in plasma cholesterol reduction. Plasma cholesterol concentrations were lower in animals fed native guar compared to low viscosity HPMC; however, this difference was statistically significant only at the 6 week time period. These results suggest the possibility that fermentation may be involved in plasma cholesterol lowering.

Plasma lipoproteins were examined at the 6 week period. Table 2 shows lipoprotein cholesterol concentrations. Low density lipoprotein (LDL) cholesterol concentrations were approximately 0.7 mmol/L and were unaffected by the dietary treatments. Very low density lipoprotein (VLDL) cholesterol concentrations were approximately the same as LDL cholesterol concentrations. However, the high viscosity HPMC group had a significantly lower concentration than did the low viscosity

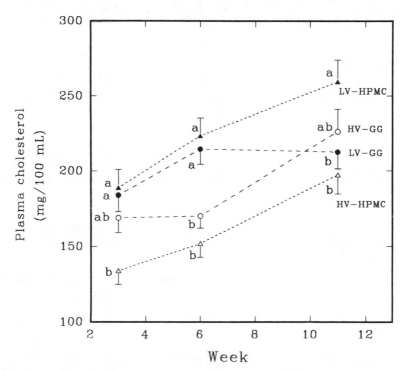

Figure 1. Plasma cholesterol concentrations in hamsters fed either hydroxy-propylmethycellulose guar gum of different viscosities.

HPMC. The highest concentrations of plasma cholesterol were found in the high density lipoprotein (HDL) fraction. This is also where the greatest dietary effects were seen. Again, the high viscosity group had a significantly lower cholesterol concentration compared to the low viscosity HPMC group.

We also examined hepatic cholesterol concentrations (Table 3). Cholesterol ester concentrations were dramatically lower in the high viscosity HPMC group compared to all other groups, but particularly to the low viscosity HPMC group. However, the cholesterol ester concentration of the native guar gum group was significantly lower than the low viscosity HPMC group. Unesterified (free) cholesterol concentration was also influenced by the diet treatments; a significantly lower concentration was found in the high viscosity HPMC group compared to the

Table 2. Lipoprotein cholesterol concentrations in hamsters fed diets containing hydroxypropyl methylcellulose (HPMC) or guar gum (GG) of different viscosities for six weeks[1]

Diet group	Cholesterol (mmol/L)		
	VLDL	LDL	HDL
High viscosity GG	0.60[ab]	0.69	2.54[a]
	±0.05	±0.05	±0.16
Low viscosity GG	0.72[a]	0.68	3.20[b]
	±0.09	±0.04	±0.22
High viscosity HPMC	0.43[b]	0.68	2.08[a]
	±0.05	±0.03	±0.14
Low viscosity HPMC	0.64[a]	0.74	3.34[b]
	±0.06	±0.06	±0.24

[1]Values represent mean ± SEM of pools of plasma from 2 animals; n = 8. Means within the same column not sharing a common superscript are significantly different ($p < 0.05$).

Table 3. Hepatic cholesterol concentrations in hamsters fed diets containing hydroxypropyl methylcellulose (HPMC) or guar gum (GG) of different viscosities for six weeks[1]

Diet group	Cholesterol esters	Free cholesterol
	(μmol/g liver)	
High viscosity GG	19.8 ± 2.1[a]	6.2 ± 0.3[a]
Low viscosity GG	30.3 ± 3.3[b]	7.3 ± 0.5[ab]
High viscosity HPMC	7.2 ± 0.9[c]	6.2 ± 0.3[a]
Low viscosity HPMC	31.2 ± 2.7[b]	8.3 ± 0.8[b]

[1]Values represent mean ± SEM from 16 animals. Means within the same column not sharing a common superscript are significantly different ($p < 0.05$).

low viscosity HPMC group.

Differences in plasma and hepatic cholesterol concentrations induced by the dietary treatment could be the result of changes in the rate of cholesterol synthesis. Table 4 shows hepatic and small intestinal rates of synthesis, measured using tritiated water incorporation into digitonin-precipitable sterols, at the 11 week period.

Synthesis rates are expressed on a per organ basis. There were no differences in hepatic cholesterol synthesis rates among the dietary treatments. There were differences among the groups in small intestinal synthesis rates; the lowest rate was found in the low viscosity HPMC group, the group with the highest plasma cholesterol concentration.

Increased bile acid excretion is another possible mechanism by which dietary fibers may mediate cholesterol reduction. Table 5 shows the to-

Table 4. Hepatic and small intestinal sterol synthesis rates in hamsters fed diets containing hydroxypropylmethylcellulose (HPMC) or guar gum (GG) of different viscosities for eleven weeks[1]

Diet group	Liver	Small intestine
	(nmol DPS/h•organ^{-1})	
High viscosity GG	29.7 ± 6.9^a	48.5 ± 6.1^a
Low viscosity GG	23.6 ± 2.7^a	39.6 ± 2.7^{ab}
High viscosity HPMC	21.8 ± 3.8^a	41.8 ± 3.4^{ab}
Low viscosity HPMC	23.4 ± 1.8^a	32.9 ± 3.3^b

[1]Values represent mean $\pm$ SEM from 9-10 animals. Means within the same column not sharing a common superscript are significantly different ($p < 0.05$). DPS, digitonin-precipitablesterols.

Table 5. Fecal bile acid excretion in hamsters fed diets containing hydroxypropylmethylcellulose (HPMC) or guar gum (GG) of different viscosities for six weeks[1]

	Diet group (μmoles/d)			
	HV-GG	LV-GG	HV-HPMC	LV-HPMC
3a, 7a-Diol-12-one-5β-cholanic acid	1.42 ± 0.47^a	0.68 ± 0.17^b	0.37 ± 0.10^b	0.29 ± 0.10^b
Cholic acid	0.29 ± 0.12^a	0.06 ± 0.02^b	0.03 ± 0.01^b	0.03 ± 0.01^b
Chenodeoxycholic acid	0.18 ± 0.04^{ab}	0.26 ± 0.05^a	0.16 ± 0.03^{ab}	0.12 ± 0.02^b
Deoxycholic acid	0.55 ± 0.10^a	0.39 ± 0.07^a	0.45 ± 0.08^a	0.37 ± 0.06^a
Lithocholic acid	0.35 ± 0.07^a	0.63 ± 0.11^b	1.17 ± 0.10^c	0.71 ± 0.12^b
Total bile acids[2]	2.97 ± 0.48^a	2.24 ± 0.36^{ab}	2.35 ± 0.13^{ab}	1.63 ± 0.19^b

[1]Values represent mean $\pm$ SEM from 16 animals. Means within the same column not sharing a common superscript are significantly different ($p < 0.05$). Abbreviations are HV-GG, high viscosity GG; LV-GG, low viscosity GG; HV-HPMC, high viscosity HPMC; LV-HPMC, low viscosity HPMC.

tal and major individual fecal bile acids excreted per day in the four dietary treatments at the 6 week time period. Total fecal bile acid excretion was highest in the high viscosity guar gum-fed group, and significantly higher than the total excreted by the low viscosity HPMC group. Thus, consumption of a fermentable fiber was associated with a higher bile acid excretion than a non-fermentable fiber of similar *ex vivo* viscosity. The higher excretion rate in the high viscosity guar gum group was largely due to a higher excretion rate of two relatively polar bile acids, 3-alpha, 7-alpha-diol-12-one-5β-cholanic acid and cholic acid.

In summary, these experiments strongly indicate a role for viscosity in plasma and liver cholesterol reduction. We suggest that dietary treatments that increase the viscosity of the small intestinal contents are likely to produce reductions, regardless of whether they are fermented. However, the lower plasma cholesterol concentrations in the native guar gum group compared to the low viscosity HPMC group (signficant only at 6 weeks) as well as the lower hepatic cholesterol ester concentrations suggest that fermentation may have a role in plasma cholesterol lowering independently of viscosity. It is not clear how these cholesterol reductions are mediated. It is apparently not due to reductions in hepatic cholesterol synthesis, as these rates were unchanged by the dietary treatments.

Degree of Viscosity

One of several questions raised by these studies is the question of dose response. That is, how viscous must the fiber fed be to produce a cholesterol-lowering effect to answer this question, HPMC preparations with a wide range of *in vitro* viscosities were fed to cholesterol-fed hamsters for three weeks. In addition, one group was fed cellulose only. The diets used were the same as described above, except that the fiber sources (HPMC or cellulose) were incorporated into the diets to a final concentration of 4%.

Figure 2 shows the plasma cholesterol response of the different groups based on the *ex vivo* viscosities resulting from feeding the different diets. Animals fed the HPMC preparation that produced an *ex vivo* viscosity of about 100 cP had a plasma cholesterol concentration almost as low as those with an *ex vivo* viscosity of 480 cP. When *ex vivo* viscosity is plotted on a logarithmic scale, the relationship between plasma cholesterol and viscosity is highly linear ($r^2 = 0.99$). Thus, using HPMC as the dietary fiber source, there is a strong association between viscosity and plasma cholesterol lowering in the hamster.

Discussion

There have been few studies addressing the dose-response relationship between the viscosity of the fiber and a hypcholesterolemic effect. Topping et al.[8] fed rats methylcellulose of low, medium and high *in vitro* viscosity (range 25–1500 cP, using a 2% solution). These investigators found no changes in plasma or liver cholesterol concentrations among the groups fed the different viscositiesof methylcellulose preparations compare to those used in the hamster studies described above. However, the lack of agreement between our results and those of Topping et al. may also be due to differences in the animal model or experimental diets. In their experiment, rats were fed cholesterol-free diets, whereas in the present experiment cholesterol-fed hamsters were used. Sugano et al.[9], using chitosan as a fiber source, also failed to find a dose-response relationship between apparent *in vitro* viscosity of the fiber and a hypocholesterolemic efffect. In their study, plasma cholesterol was lowered to an equal extent by all the chitosan preparations.

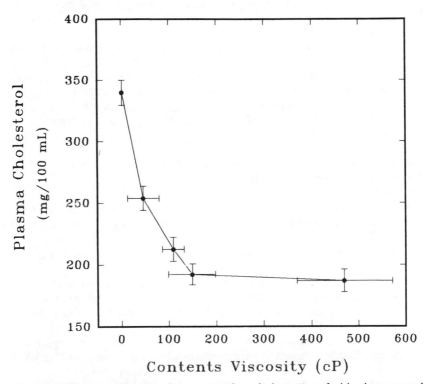

Figure 2. Plasma cholesterol concentrations in hamsters fed hydroxypropyl methycellulose of different viscosities.

Although this could suggest that a viscosity dose-dependent relationship is dependent on the type of fiber, it should be noted that chitosans are insoluble at pH > 6[10]. Thus, it is not clear that the chitosans produced an increase in intestinal contents viscosity (no *ex vivo* viscosity data were reported). Consequently, the ability of chitosans to reduce plasma cholesterol could be unrelated to changes in intestinal viscosity.

Our results suggest that dietary fibers that increase the viscosity of the small intestinal contents will exert a hypocholesterolemic effect. Further, our results from the dose response study suggest that extremely high intestinal contents viscosities are not necessary to achieve a significant reduction in plasma cholesterol. How an increase in viscosity influences plasma cholesterol remains unclear, although a likely explanation may be a viscosity-related interference with cholesterol absorption or reabsorption within the small intestine.

References

1. A. F. Wells and B. H. Ershoff, Beneficial effects of pection in prevention of hypercholesterolemia and increase in liver cholesterol in cholesterol-fed rats, *J. Nutr.* 11:433 (1963).
2. A. Keys, F. Grande, and J. T. Anderson, Fiber and pection in the diet and serum cholesterol concentration in man. *Proc. Soc. Exp. Biol. Med.* 106:555 (1961).
3. J. A. Story and D. Kritchevsky, Comparison of the binding of various bile acids and bile salts in vitro by several types of fiber, *J. Nutr.* 106:292 (1976).
4. G. V. Vahouny, R. Tombes, M. M. Cassidy, D. Kritchevsky, and L. L. Gallo, Dietary fibers. V. Binding of bile salts, phospholipids and cholesterol from mixed micells by bile acid sequestrants and dietary fibers. *Lipds* 15:1012 (1980).
5. J. W. Anderson W-J. L. Chen, Plant fiber. Carbohydrate and lipid metbolism. *Am. J. Clin. Nutr.* 32:346 (1979).
6. W. H. Braun, J. C. Ramsey, and P. J. Gehring, The lack of significant absorption of methylcellulose, viscosity, 3300 CP, from the gastrointestinal tract following single and multiple oral doses to the rat, *Fd. Cosmet. Toxicol.* 12:373 (1974).
7. W. H. Hoover, C. L. Mannings, and H. E. Sheerin, Observations digestion in the golden hamster. *J. Anim. Sci.* 28:349 (1969).
8. D. L. Topping, D. Oakenfull, R. P. Trimble, and R. Illman, A viscous fibre (methylcellulose) lowers blood glucose and plasma triacylglycerols and increases liver glycogen independently of volatile fatty acid production in the rat. *Br. J. Nutr.* 59:21 (1988).
9. M. Sugano, S. Watanabe, A. Kishi, M. Izume, and A. Ohtakara, Hypocholestermicaction of chitosans with different viscosity in rats, *Lipids* 23:187 (1988).
10. I. Furda, Aminopolysaccharides—their potential as dietary fiber, *in* "Unconventional Sources of Dietary Fiber," I. Furda, ed., American Chemical Society, Washington, DC (1983).

Fat/Fiber Interactions: Effect on Colon Physiology and Colonic Cytokinetics

Joanne R. Lupton

Human Nutrition
218 Kleberg
Texas A&M University
College Station, TX 77843

Introduction

Fat is thought to be promotive, and fiber protective of colon cancer (Shankar and Lanza 1991), yet epidemiological studies and experimental data do not always support this hypothesis (Klurfeld and Kritchevsky 1986; Lewin 1991; Roberfroid 1991). Kritchevsky (1990) and others have suggested that the effects of fat and fiber must be considered in the context of the total diet and interactions of dietary components. This paper discusses three possible explanations for inconsistencies in the fat/fiber/colon carcinogenesis literature: different types of fats and fibers have different effects; effects are site specific; effects are interactive. Data are presented in support of each of these three possible explanations.

Different Types of Fats and Fibers Have Different Effects

Although the general statement is made that *fat* is promotive and *fiber* is protective against colon carcinogenesis, it is clear that not all fats behave the same, nor do all fibers.

Effects of Different Fats

Ninety five percent of ingested lipids are in the form of triglycerides, which may differ from each other in their fatty acid composition. Chain length and degree of saturation are properties of fatty acids which produce differential physiological effects. For example, shorter chain lengths and greater degrees of unsaturation result in preferential absorption from the small intestine, with a smaller proportion of these fatty acids reaching the large intestine (Hofmann and Borgstrom 1963). Unsaturated fatty acids are more fluid than their saturated counterparts, and thus their incorporation into cell membranes would produce a membrane with different physicochemical properties than a membrane composed of a greater proportion of saturated fatty acids. Studies have shown that colonic mucosal phospholipids do change in response to the fatty acid composition of the diet (Lindner 1991; Minoura et al. 1988; Robblee et al. 1988). Specific fatty acids, such as arachidonic acid, are precursors for prostaglandins which in turn modulate colonic carcinogenesis (Metz et al. 1981), whereas other fatty acids, such as omega 3 fatty acids (found predominantly in fish oils) may inhibit prostaglandin synthesis by inhibiting the conversion of C18:2n-6 to C20:4n-6 (Brenner and Peluffo 1967).

Most epidemiological studies do not discriminate between the effects of specific fatty acids on colon cancer incidence. Instead, broad classifications, such as fats from animal sources vs fats from vegetables or fish have been tested. The epidemiological studies generally show that animal sources of fat are promotive (Graham et al. 1988; Willett et al.

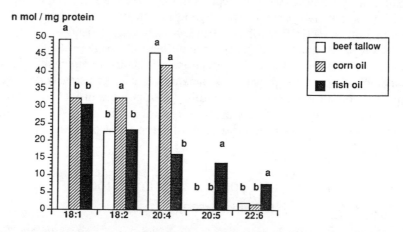

Figure 1. Modification of fatty acid composition of colonic phospholipids by dietary fat. For each fatty acid, bars not having the same letter are significantly different at P < 0.05. Data are from Lee et al. 1992.

1990) and fats from fish are protective (Lanier 1976). In a recent prospective study of 88,751 women, the relative risk of colon cancer for the highest quintile for animal fat was 1.89 times that of the lowest quintile (Willett et al. 1990). The role of polyunsaturates from vegetable sources in less clear. The same study which showed a positive association of animal fat with the risk of colon cancer, showed no association for vegetable fat (Willett et al 1990).

In studies designed to test the effect of specific fatty acids on experimentally induced colon cancer, saturated fatty acids and omega-6 fatty acids are generally promotive, whereas omega-3 fatty acids are generally protective (Minoura et al. 1988; Deschner et al. 1990; Reddy et al. 1991; Linder 1991). The issue of whether saturated fatty acids or omega-6 fatty acids are more promotive has not been resolved. Nicholson et al. (1990) found a more promotive effect of beef suet on colon cancer as compared to corn oil (suggesting a more promotive role for saturated fatty acids), whereas Sakaguchi et al. (1986) found a more promotive effect of unsaturated fat diets made by adding linoleic acid to basal diet compared to saturated fat diets made by adding stearic acid to the basal diet. It should be noted that oleic acid, not stearic acid, is the major fatty acid in beef fat, and Lindner (1991) has demonstrated a strong positive correlation between oleic acid and tumors in the colon.

In a study using equlvalent amounts of corn oil, fish oil or beef tallow, we found that fish oil feeding resulted in higher levels of n-3 fatty acids in colonic mucosal phospholipids than beef tallow or corn oil feeding, and lower levels of n-6 fatty acids (Lee et al. 1992) (Figure 1).

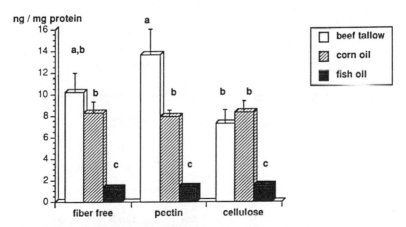

Figure 2. Effect of dietary fiber and fat on PGE_2 synthesis of proximal colon. For each fiber, bars not having the same letter are significantly different at $P < 0.05$. Data are from Lee et al. 1992.

The increased levels of fish oil derived n-3 fatty acids in mucosal phospholipids were associated with decreased cell proliferation ($r = -0.73$, $P < 0.05$). There was a concomitant dramatic reduction of the production of prostaglandin E_2 by fish oil feeding ($P < 0.001$) (Figure 2). Since increases in cell proliferation are considered tumor promoting (Cohen and Ellwein 1990) these data would suggest a protective role for fish oils against colon carcinogensis.

Effects of Different Fibers

The primary way in which fiber affects the colonic luminal environment is through its fermentation, as illustrated in Figure 3. Both the degree to which fiber is fermented and the specific fermentative products produced are important. Approximately three times as much total short chain fatty acids (SCFA) are produced from a highly fermentable fiber such as pectin as from the fermentation of the less fermentable cellulose (Table 1). This is important because SCFA have been shown to stimulate cell proliferation (Sakata 1984, 1987; Sakata and Engelhardt 1983).

An important consequence of the fermentation of fiber and the production of SCFA is that these acids acidify colonic pH, as shown in Figure 4. The significance of this acidification is discussed in detail by Newmark and Lupton (1990). Epidemiologic studies have generally supported a reduced incidence of colon cancer with lower fecal pH

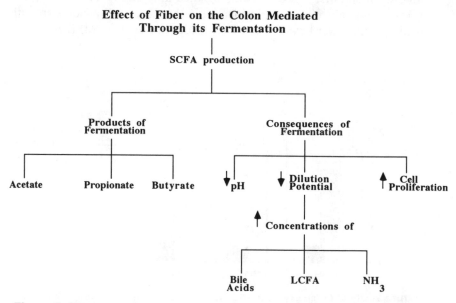

Figure 3. Diagrammatic representation of the effect of fiber on the colon, as mediated through its fermentation.

(Malhotra 1982) but experimental studies are equivocal, with one showing significant tumor inhibition with lower fecal pH (Samelson et al. 1985) and the other showing the opposite effect (Jacobs and Lupton 1986).

Another very important consequence of the fermentation of fiber to SCFA is that once the fiber is fermented, it is no longer available to contribute to fecal bulk. Figure 5 is the result of a 4 week feeding study in which the in vivo diluting ability of dietary fiber was tested by providing 90 male Sprague-Dawley rats with a fiber-free control diet, or that diet diluted by 8% dietary fiber from pectin, guar, cellulose, wheat bran or oat bran (Gazzaniga and Lupton 1987). Chromic oxide, a non-

Table 1. Ratio of total SCFA from pectin/cellulose

	Ratio*	Significance†
Humans	3.0	$P < 0.01$
Baboons	2.2	$P < 0.05$
Pigs	1.3	NS
Rats	3.0	$P < 0.01$

*The ratio is the amount of total SCFA produced from the fermentation of pectin divided by the total SCFA produced from the fermentation of cellulose for that particular species.
†P values are for a comparison of the total SCFA produced from the fermentation of cellulose to the total SCFA produced from the fermentation of pectin, within a series. These data are from Lupton, 1991.

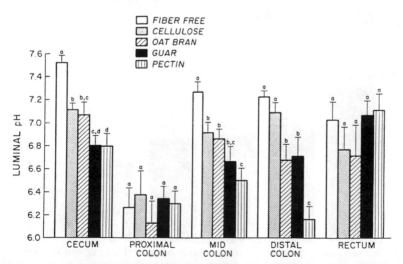

Figure 4. Long-term effects of dietary fiber supplements on large-bowel luminal pH. Small vertical bars indicate SEM. At each anatomic site, means with a different letter are significantly different (P < 0.05). For complete details, see Lupton et al., 1988.

absorbable marker, was incorporated into all diets at 0.4% by weight. In vivo samples of colonic contents from the cecum, proximal and distal colon were analyzed for chromium concentration using atomic absorption spectrophotometry. At all sites, the best in vivo diluters were the least fermentable fibers, cellulose and wheat bran.

Dilution potential of the fiber, although important, is not the only way in which fibers affect the luminal concentration of cancer promoters such as secondary bile acids. A recent report by Reddy et al. (1992) in which subjects consumed 13–15 g of wheat, oat or corn bran daily showed that wheat bran reduced the concentrations of most bile acids, neutral sterols and the activities of all bacterial enzymes measured. Oat bran had no effect on secondary bile acids and the bacterial enzymes measured. Oat bran had no effect on secondary bile acids and the bacterial 7 alpha-dehydroxylase but decreased other bacterial enzymes. Corn bran increased the levels of some bile acids and decreased those of others. This study reinforces the concept that dilution is not the only way in which concentration of bile acids is decreased, since wheat bran and corn bran should be equivalent in vivo dilutors. An interesting study by Calvert et al. tested the theory that wheat bran is protective of colon cancer due to its dilution of fecal bile acids (Calvert et al. 1987). They added bile salts to the diets of wheat bran supplemented animals to equal the concentration of fecal bile acids seen with animals receiving no fiber supplement. Wheat bran was still protective against 1,2-di-

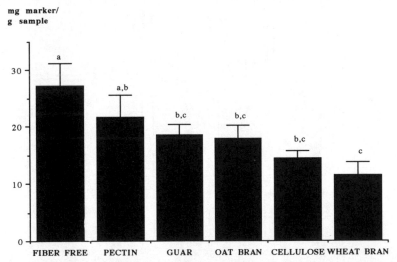

Figure 5. In vivo diluting ability of dietary fiber in the proximal colon (mg marker/g sample). Data are from Gazzaniga and Lupton, 1987. Results are expressed as means ± SEM on a sample size of 15 rats/group Means not sharing the same superscript are significantly different (P < 0.05).

methylhydrazine induced colon carcinogenesis, despite fecal bile acid concentrations equilvalent to the fiber-free controls.

In summary, the effect of fiber on the colonic luminal environment is mediated, in large part, through its fermentation to short chain fatty acids. The degree to which a particular fiber is fermented in turn affects pH and dilution potential. The greater the production of SCFA the lower the pH. Also, the greater the degree to which the fiber is fermented the lower its dilutions potential. Mitogenic factors such as bile acids, long chain fatty acids and ammonia are in lower concentrations in stools from animals supplemented with insoluble fiber sources. Thus, fermentable fibers, such as pectin, or guar, may actually enhance colon carcinogenesis by stimulating cell proliferation (Jacobs and Lupton 1984; Jacobs and Lupton 1986; Lupton et al. 1988), whereas the less fermentable fibers such as cellulose and wheat bran may be protective by diluting carcinogens (Gazzaniga and Lupton 1987).

Effects of Fats and Fibers Are Site Specific

Previous studies have shown that the main effects of fiber fermentation on cell proliferation are seen in the proximal colon (Jacobs and Lupton 1984; Jacobs and Lupton 1986; Lupton et al. 1988). This effect appears to be mediated through the fermentation of fiber, resulting in the production of short chain fatty acids and a lower luminal pH. Both short chain fatty acids (Sakata and Yajima 1984) and an acidic luminal pH (Lupton et al. 1985) have been demonstrated to stimulate colonic cell proliferation.

In a 3 × 3 factorial experiment conducted to examine how dietary fiber and fat interactively affect cell proliferation of the colon in rats, the main effect of dietary fiber on cell proliferation was found in the proximal colon where the pectin diet stimulated cell proliferation compared to the cellulose and fiber-free diets (Lee et al. 1992). In contrast, the main effect of fat was seen in the distal colon where the beef tallow diet stimulated cell proliferation to a greater degree than did the fish oil diet ($P < 0.05$) (Lee et al. 1992). Most epidemiological studies on diet and colon cancer do not discriminate between proximal and distal colon. However, in one that does (West et al. 1989) fats (odds ratio = 2.7–8.8) increased the risk of cancer of the ascending, or proximal colon, while protein (OR = 3.8) was a risk factor for cancer of the distal colon.

Effects of Fats and Fibers Are Interactive

In a recent study, McGarrity et al. (1991) evaluated the effects of fat and fiber on the growth of human colon cancers xenografted to athymic nude mice. The high fat/no fiber group resulted in a greater tumor burden than the normal fat/no fiber group. High fat/high fiber produced an attenuating effect for fiber. Sinkeldam et al. (1990) used three levels of fiber (wheat bran) and three levels of fat (lard) to test their interactive effects on colon cancer in rats treated with N-methyl-N′-nitro-N-nitrosoguanidine. The highest colon cancer incidence was observed in the animals fed the medium-fat/medium-fiber diet. An enhancing effect of fat on both tumor incidence and tumor multiplicity was present for the low-fiber diets, whereas fat had no effect when the fiber content of the diet was high. The authors conclude that both dietary fiber and fat affect colon carcinogenesis in a complex, interactive manner (Sinkeldam et al. 1990). An epidemiological study involving 8,006 American-Japanese men also examined the relationship between amount of fat and fiber and colon carcinogenesis (Heilbrun et al. 1989). The authors found a significant negative association between fiber intake and colon cancer incidence) (P = 0.042), but only in men consuming less than 61 g/d of fat.

Little information is available on interactive effects of types of fibers and fats. In a recent study (Lee et al. 1992) the effects of dietary fibers on rat proximal colonic crypt size were highly dependent on the source of fat in the diet. Fiber supplementation only resulted in larger crypt sizes than fiber-free diets when the dietary fat source was corn oil. This is important because corn oil is traditionally used in nutrition and cancer studies since it is the lipid component of the AIN 76 diet (A.I.N., 1977). Effects of dietary fat were also significantly influenced by the type of fiber in the diet. For example, the corn oil diet resulted in a significantly higher labeling index than the beef tallow diet only when pectin was the fiber source (Lee et al. 1992).

In conclusion, the effects of fats and fibers on colonic cell proliferation and colon carcinogenesis are complex. Part of the explanation as to why fat is not always shown to be promotive, and fiber protective of colon cancer may be that different fats and fibers have different effects; the effects are site specific; and the effects are interactive. The recommendation is made that a broader perspective be used for diet/colon cancer studies which is not limited to single nutrients or isolated dietary components.

Acknowledgments

The contribution of Dong-Yeon K. Lee for the fat/fiber interactive study and Robert S. Chapkin for the collaboration on mucosal lipids and prostaglandins is gratefully acknowledged. Support for this research was provided, in part, by the American Institute for Cancer Research.

References

American Institute of Nutrition. Report of the AIN Ad Hoc Committee on standards for nutritional studies. J. Nutr. 107:1340-1348, 1977.

Brenner, R. R., and Peluffo, R. O. Inhibitory effect of docosa-4,7,10,13,16,19-hexaenoic acid upon the oxidative desaturation of linoleic into gamma-linolenic acid and of alpha linolenic acid into octadeca-6,9,12,15-tetraenoic acid. Biochim. Biophys. Acta 137:184-186, 1967.

Cohen, S. M. and Ellwein, L. B. Cell proliferation in carcinogenesis. Science 249:1007-1011, 1990.

Deschner, E. E., Lytle, J. S., Wong, G., Ruperto, J. F., and Newmark, H. L. The effect of dietary omega-3 fatty acids (fish oil) on Axosymethanol-induced focal areas of dysplasia and colon tumor incidence. Cancer 66:2350-2356, 1990.

Gallaher, D. D., Locket, P. L., and Gallaher, C. M. Bile acid metabolism in rats fed two levels of corn oil and brans of oat, rye and barley and sugar beet fiber. J. Nutr. 122:473-81, 1992.

Gazzaniga, J. M., and Lupton, J. R. Dilution effect of dietary fiber sources: an in vivo study in the rat. Nutr. Res. 7:1261-1268, 1987.

Graham, S., Marshall, J., Haughey, B., Mittelman, A., Swanson, M., Zielezny, M., Byers, T., Wilkinson, G., and West, D. Dietary epidemiology of cancer of the colon in Western New York. Am. J. Epidemiol. 128:490-503, 1988.

Heilbrun, L. K., Nomura, A., Hankin, J. H., and Stemmermann, G. N. Diet and colorectal cancer with special reference to fiber intake. Int. J. Cancer 44:1-6, 1989.

Hofmann, A. F. and Borgstrom, B. Hydrolysis of long chain monoglycerides in micellar solution by pancreatic lipase. Biochim. Biophys. Acta 70:317-331, 1963.

I.A.C.R. Intestinal Microecology Group. Dietary fiber, transit time, fecal bacteria and steroids in two scandinavian populations. Lancet II:207-211, 1977.

Jacobs, L. R., and Lupton, J. R. Effect of dietary fibers on rat large bowel mucosal growth and cell proliferation. Am. J. Physiol., 346 (Gastrointest. Liver Physiol. 9):G378-G385, 1984.

Jacobs, L. R., and Lupton, J. R. Relationship between colonic luminal pH, cell proliferation, and colon carcinogenesis in 1,2 Dimethylhydrazine treated rats fed high fiber diets. Cancer Res. 46:1727-1734, 1986.

Klurfeld, D. M., Kritchevsky, D. Dietary fiber and human cancer: critique of the literature. Adv. Exp. Med. Biol. 206:119-35, 1986.

Kritchevsky, D. Fiber and cancer. Med. Oncol. Tumor Pharmacother. 7:137-41, 1990.

Lanier, A. P., Bender, T. R., Blot, W. J., Fraumeni, Jr., J. F., and Hurlburt, W. B. Cancer incidence in Alaska natives. Int. J. Cancer 18:409-412, 1976.

Lee, D-Y. K., Chapkin, R. S. and Lupton, J. R. Modulation of markers of colon carcinogenesis by dietary fiber and fat: I. Interactive effect of different types of fiber and fat on cell proliferation. Cancer Res. (Submitted for publication), 1992.

Lewin, M. R. Is there a fibre-depleted aetiology for colorectal cancer? Experimental evidence. Rev. Environ. Health 9:17-30, 1991.

Linder, M. A. A fish oil diet inhibits colon cancer in mice. Nutr. Cancer 15:1-11, 1991.

Lupton, J. R., Coder, D. M., and Jacobs, L. R. Influence of luminal pH on rat large bowel epithelial cell cycle. Am. J. Physiol. 249 (Gastrointest. Liver Physiol. 12):G382-G388, 1985.

Lupton, J. R., Coder, D. M., and Jacobs, L. R. Long-term effects of fermentable fibers on rat colonic pH and epithelial cell cycle. J. Nutr., 118:840-845, 1988.

Malhotra, S. L. Faecal urobilinogen levels and pH of stools in population groups with different incidence of cancer of the colon, and their possible role in aetiology. J R Soc Med 75:709-714, 1982.

McGarrity, T. J., Peiffer, L. P., Kramer, S. T. and Smith, J. P. Effects of fat and fiber on human colon cancer xenografted to athymic nude mice. Dig. Dis. Sci. 36:1606-10, 1991.

Metz, S. A., McRae, J. R., and Robertson, R. P. Prostaglandins as mediators of paraneoplastic syndromes: review and update. Metabolism 30:299-316, 1981.

Minoura, T., Takata, T., Sakaguchi, M., Takata, H., Yamamura, M., Hioki, K., and Yamamoto, M. Effect of dietary eicosapentaenoic acid on azoxymethane-induced colon carcinogenesis in rats. Cancer Res. 48:4790-4794, 1988.

Newmark, H. L. and Lupton, J. R. Determinants and consequences of colonic luminal pH: implications for colon cancer. Nutr. Cancer 14:161-73, 1990.

Nicholson, M. L., Neoptolemos, J. P., Clayton, H. A., Talbot, I. C., and Bell, P. R. F. Inhibition of experimental colorectal carcinogenesis by dietary n-6 polyunsaturated fats. Carcinogenesis 11:2191-2197, 1990.

Nigro, N. D. Animal studies implicating fat and fecal steroids in intestinal cancer. Cancer Res. 41:3769-3770, 1981.

Reddy, B. S. Nutrition and colon cancer. Adv Nutr Res 2:199-218, 1979.

Reddy, B. S., Burill, C., and Rigotty, J. Effect of diets high in w-3 and w-6 fatty acids on initiation and postinitiation stages of colon carcinogenesis. Cancer Res. 51:487-491, 1991.

Reddy, B. S., Engle, A., Simi, B. and Goldman, M. Effect of dietary fiber on colonic bacterial enzymes and bile acids in relation to colon cancer. Gastroenterology 102:1475-82, 1992.

Reddy, B. S., Hedges, A. R., Laakso K., and Wynder, E. L. Metabolic epidemiology of large bowel cancer: fecal bulk and constituents of high risk North American and low risk Finnish population. Cancer 42:2832-2838, 1978.

Roberfroid, M. B. Dietary modulation of experimental neoplastic development: role of fat and fiber content and calorie intake. Mutat. Res. 259:351-62, 1991.

Robblee, N. M., Farnworth, E. R., and Bird, R. P. Phospholipid profile and production of prostanoids by murine colonic epithelium: effect of dietary fat. Lipids 23:334-339, 1988.

Sakaguchi, M., Minoura, T., Hiramatsu, Y., Takada, H., Yamamura, M., Hioki, K., and Yamamoto, M. Effects of dietary saturated and unsaturated fatty acids on fecal bile acids and colon carcinogenesis induced by azoxymethane in rats. Cancer Res. 46:61-65, 1986.

Sakata, T. Short chain fatty acids as the luminal trophic factor. Can. J. Anim. Sci. 64(Suppl.):189-190, 1984.

Sakata, T. Stimulatory effect of short-chain fatty acids on epithelial cell prolifertion in the rat intestine: a possible explanation for trophic effets of fermentable fibre, gut microbes and luminal trophic factors. Br J Nutr 58:95-103, 1987.

Sakata, T. and Engelhardt, W. V. Stimulatory effect of short chain fatty acids on the epithelial cell proliferation in rat large intestine. Comp Biochem and Phys A74:459-462, 1983.

Sakata, T., and Yajima, T. Influence of short chain fatty acids on the epithelial cell division of digestive tract. Q. J. Exp. Physiol. 69:639-648, 1984.

Samelson, S. L. Nelson, R. L. and Nyhus, L.M. Protective role of faecal pH in experimental colon carcinogenesis. J R Soc Med 78:230-233, 1985.

Shankar, S. and Lanza, E. Dietary fiber and cancer prevention. Hematol. Oncol. Clin. North Am. 5:25-41, 1991.

Sinkeldam, E. J., Kuper, C. F., Bosland, M. C., Hollanders, V. M. and Vedder, D. M. Interactive effects of dietary wheat bran and lard on N-methyl-N'-nitro-N-nitrosoguanidine-induced colon carcinogenesis in rats. Cancer Res. 50:1092-6, 1990.

Willett, W. C., Stampfer, M. J., Colditz, G. A., Rosner, B. A. and Speizer, F. E. Relation of meat, fat, and fiber intake to the risk of colon cancer in a prospective study among women. N. Engl. J. Med. 323:1664-72, 1990.

Wynder, E. L. and Hirayama, T. Comparative epidemiology of cancers in the United States and Japan. Prev Med 6:567-594, 1977.

Cholesterol-Lowering Effects of Soluble Fiber in Humans

James W. Anderson, M.D.

Metabolic Research Group
VA Medical Center and University of Kentucky
Lexington, KY 40511

Introduction

Foods rich in soluble fiber, such as oat and bean products, and purified fibers, such as gums, pectins, and psyllium, have important hypocholesterolemic effects in humans and experimental animals. Insoluble fibers, such as cellulose and wheat bran, usually do not affect serum cholesterol concentrations (1,2). The mechanisms responsible for these hypocholesterolemic effects are still under investigation but it seems likely that several mechanisms are operating concurrently (1).

The effects of foods such as oat and bean products on serum cholesterol are of particular interest. In addition to their hypocholesterolemic effects, these foods have been used for millennia, are safe and well accepted, and bring important macronutrients and micronutrients into the diet. Over the past 30 years many studies document the significant hypocholesterolemic effects of oat products (3–7). The early studies of Groen et al (8) and Luyken et al (9) identifying the important hypocholesterolemic effects of beans have been well confirmed (6,10–13). Thus these two types of foods exert significant hypocholesterolemic effects in humans and have important implications for coronary heart disease.

This review will focus on the cholesterol-lowering effects of oat bran and beans, two widely available food sources of soluble fiber, and examine current considerations regarding the mechanisms for hypocholesterolemia.

Metabolic Ward Studies

Oat bran studies

Since 1977 our metabolic research group has studied the cholesterol-lowering effects of oat bran and beans at the Special Diagnostic and Treatment Unit in the VA Medical Center. Because the research participants ate only the food served from the metabolic kitchen while living on the metabolic ward for periods of two to four weeks, we were able to precisely control the diet and obtain weights of all food consumed. These studies thus reflect the maximal effects of these foods on serum lipoproteins. Issues of the practical implications of these observations for free-living individuals must be determined from studies of free-living individuals. The outcomes of ambulatory studies, however, are highly related to diet adherence, which probably varies widely from center to center.

Preliminary studies using oat bran in animals (14) and humans (15) stimulated us to perform carefully controlled metabolic ward studies of hypercholesterolemic men. Using a random-allocation, cross-over design, we studied the effects of response of eight hypercholesterolemic men to 94 grams of oat bran daily for two weeks (4). Table 1 summarizes the responses. The control responses during three metabolic ward studies (4,16,17) are averaged in Table 1 for ease of comparison; serum lipid values did not change significantly with control diets. However, during the oat bran period (OB 1) serum cholesterol and LDL-cholesterol decreased significantly by 13.0% and 13.6%, respectively.

Subsequently, we examined the effects of oat bran or bean intake on serum cholesterol values of 20 hypercholesterolemic men (11). While

Table 1. Response of hypercholesterolemic men on a metabolic research ward to control and test diets with oat bran or beans

Study	g/d	Chol.	LDL-Chol.	HDL-Chol.	Trigly-cerides	Body wgt. (% change)
OB1	94	−13.0	−13.6	−2.0	−9.3	−1.9
OB2	98	−19.3	−21.6	−5.6	−18.7	−1.2
OB3	106	−12.8	−12.1	−7.4	−10.2	−1.4
OB avg	98	−15.0	−15.8	−5.0	−12.7	−1.5
Bean 1	101	−18.7	−23.1	−12.7	−3.0	−1.3
Bean 2	67	−11.6	−10.0	−11.7	−14.5	−1.7
BN avg	83	−15.2	−16.7	−12.2	−8.8	−1.5
CTL avg		−0.9	−0.6	−2.3	−11.7	−0.8

Abbreviations: Chol, cholesterol; OB, oat bran; BN, bean; CTL, control.

these men were on a control diet for one week, control values from a cross-over or a parallel group are not available. The oat bran diet (OB 2) decreased serum total and LDL-cholesterol significantly by 19.3% and 21.6%. Dietary total fat, saturated fat, and cholesterol intakes were essentially identical on the control and oat bran diets.

To rigorously compare the effects of oat bran and wheat bran we recruited 20 hypercholesterolemic men and randomly allocated them to diets containing either 100 grams oat bran per day or 40 grams wheat bran per day (17). These diets were virtually identical in nutrient and total fiber content and differed primarily in the soluble fiber content, which was 13.4 grams per day with oat bran and 7.8 grams per day with wheat bran. Figure 1 and Table 1 compare the responses of serum total and LDL-cholesterol to oat-bran and wheat-bran diets. With wheat-bran diets serum total and LDL-cholesterol decreased nonsignificantly by 4.4% and 5.5%, respectively. In contrast, with oat-bran diets serum total and LDL-cholesterol decreased significantly by 12.8% and 12.1%, respectively (OB 3).

In these three studies between 94 and 106 grams of oat bran was fed daily. Average changes in serum values were: cholesterol −15%; LDL-cholesterol −15.8%; HDL-cholesterol −5%; and triglycerides −12.7%. The average changes with these control diets were: cholesterol −0.9%; LDL-cholesterol −0.6%; HDL-cholesterol −2.3%; and triglycerides −11.7%. By subtracting the control values from the oat bran values, the net effect of oat bran administration can be estimated. Feeding approximately 98 grams of oat bran daily to hypercholesterolemic men on a metabolic ward for two to three weeks produces these net changes in serum lipids: cholesterol −14.1%; LDL-cholesterol −15.2%, HDL-

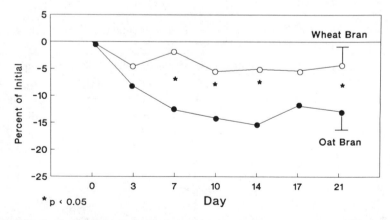

Figure 1. Percent reduction of serum cholesterol in oat-bran (OB 3) and wheat-bran treated hypercholesterolemic men.

cholesterol −2.7%; and triglycerides −1.0%. These observations suggest that oat bran intake significantly reduces serum total cholesterol and LDL-cholesterol concentrations and does not significantly affect serum HDL-cholesterol or triglyceride concentrations. While greater reductions in body weight were seen with oat-bran diets than control diets, no significant correlations were observed between weight changes and serum cholesterol (11).

Bean studies

In two metabolic ward studies (11,12) the cholesterol lowering effects of dried beans or canned beans were assessed. The first bean study, see Table 1 (Bean 1), was conducted in parallel to the second oat bran study. Twenty hypercholesterolemic men were randomly allocated to oat-bran or bean diets after one week on a control diet. The control and bean diets were virtually identical in energy and nutrient content and varied only in the fiber content of the bean diet. When 101 grams (dry weight) of beans were prepared and served in the metabolic research ward, significant reductions in serum total and LDL-cholesterol resulted. Serum total and LDL-cholesterol decreased 18.7% and 23.1% respectively.

The second bean study (Bean 2) compared the effects of canned beans on serum cholesterol of hypercholesterolemic men. The control and bean diets were virtually identical in energy and nutrient content but the bean diet, providing 83 grams (dry weight) of beans per day, had more total and soluble fiber. The bean diet significantly decreased total and LDL-cholesterol by 11.6% and 10.0%, respectively.

Bean intake on a metabolic research ward had these average effects on serum values: cholesterol −15.2%, LDL-cholesterol −16.7%, HDL-cholesterol −12.2%, and triglycerides −8.8%. The net effect of bean intake can be estimated by using the control values obtained during the oat bran studies. Using these calculations, intake of 83 grams of beans per day for hypercholesterolemic men has these net effects on serum values: cholesterol −14.3%, LDL-cholesterol −16.1%, HDL-cholesterol −9.9%, and triglycerides −2.8%.

Ambulatory Studies

Ambulatory studies of free-living subjects are difficult to evaluate because of wide variability in adherence of subjects to the prescribed diet. Of course, differences in study design also confound analysis and comparison of studies. One highly publicized study (18), for example, was widely criticized for a number of flaws in its design (19–21). Furthermore, oat bran products manufactured in the United States (22) and in New Zealand (23), for example, appear to differ significantly in composition. Even if subjects consume the foods under investigation, it is unclear how variations in day-to-day intake of saturated fat, cholesterol and energy affect results. Two studies we performed point to the limitations of ambulatory studies as currently conducted. We will present our own experience and summarize ambulatory studies from other investigators.

Oat bran studies

The 10 hypercholesterolemic men who participated in the oat bran versus wheat bran metabolic ward study also received 100 g oat bran per day for an additional 10 weeks after discharge from the hospital. Table 2 shows their serum lipid responses over this 13 week period.

In response to this regimen, hypercholesterolemic men had a 13% reduction in serum cholesterol on the metabolic ward. However, when they resumed their home diet but included 100 g/d of oat bran, their serum cholesterol increased. By 9 weeks, serum cholesterol values were similar to control values. LDL-cholesterol followed a similar pattern. Serum HDL-cholesterol decreased initially and then increased to values higher than initial. Because of the increase in HDL-cholesterol, the LDL/HDL ratio was lower throughout the ambulatory period. This study demonstrates different response patterns of hypercholesterolemic men to metabolic ward and ambulatory protocols. However, it does not document whether there was poor adherence to product, poor adherence to diet, or whether the day-to-day variation in diet produced these responses.

The effects of oat bran intake on serum cholesterol has been examined in several carefully controlled ambulatory studies (5,7,24,25). These studies indicate that oat bran intake decreases total and LDL-

Table 2. Response of 10 hypercholesterolemic men to metabolic ward (MW) and ambulatory (A) incorporation of 100 g/d oat bran into diet

Week	Serum lipid values, mg/dl			
	Total Chol.	LDL-Chol.	HDL-Chol.	LDL/HDL
0 (MW)	266 ± 15	193 ± 13	36 ± 2	5.36
3 (MW)	230 ± 9	165 ± 13	33 ± 1	5.00
5 (A)	257 ± 13	176 ± 10	38 ± 2	4.63
7 (A)	261 ± 11	183 ± 9	37 ± 1	4.94
9 (A)	265 ± 14	192 ± 11	37 ± 2	5.05
11 (A)	258 ± 11	175 ± 8	38 ± 1	4.52
13 (A)	251 ± 10	175 ± 8	37 ± 2	4.72

cholesterol by 2.2% to 9.5% and 3.9% to 15.9%, respectively. In a careful meta-analysis of 12 ambulatory studies, Ripsin et al (26) documented that oat bran intake produced a small, but statistically significant reduction in serum total and LDL-cholesterol when compared to responses to the control diet.

Bean studies

The effects of canned beans for 24 healthy ambulatory male and female subjects aged 30 to 60 years were evaluated using a random-allocation, cross-over design. Subjects received 8 ounces of canned ravioli daily during the control diet and 8 ounces of canned beans during the bean diet. In this controlled study for the first six weeks 12 subjects received canned beans while 12 subjects received canned ravioli. After a four-week washout period, the subjects crossed over and 12 received canned ravioli while 12 received canned beans for the next six weeks. Four blood samples were obtained during the control, ravioli and bean periods. Table 3 demonstrates the serum lipid values during these three periods.

Despite similar intakes of nutrients with the ravioli and bean diets, serum cholesterol levels were significantly higher on ravioli than control while values on beans were not changed. Serum total and LDL-cholesterol values were lower, but not significantly so, on bean than ravioli diets. The LDL/HDL ratio was distinctly lower on bean than ravioli diets. Although subjects reported good compliance to bean intake, the cholesterol reduction was much less than observed for hypercholesterolemic men consuming similar amounts of canned beans on a metabolic research ward (see Table 1, Bean 2).

This ambulatory study using canned beans follows the same trend seen with the ambulatory oat bran study. Using the same product in the ambulatory setting produces substantially smaller changes in serum total and LDL-cholesterol than using the same product on a metabolic research ward. Further study is required to explain these differences.

Table 3. Serum lipid responses of 24 healthy subjects to control diet and diets containing either canned ravioli or canned beans

Measurement mg/dl	Period		
	Control	Ravioli	Bean
Cholesterol	203 ± 8	213 ± 10*	211 ± 9
LDL-cholesterol	120 ± 8	125 ± 10	116 ± 7
HDL-cholesterol	56 ± 4	58 ± 3	59 ± 3
LDL/HDL ratio	2.37	2.33	2.13*

*P vs. control <0.025.

Proposed Mechanisms for Hypocholesterolemic Effects of Fiber

Proposed mechanisms for the hypocholesterolemic effects of dietary fiber are reviewed elsewhere (1,2). While most prior investigation has focused on the fiber effects on fasting serum lipoproteins, recent studies have examined postprandial lipid responses. (27,28). Thus, when considering the cholesterol-lowering effects of dietary fiber, the effects on postprandial events must be considered.

Different dietary fibers have different effects on gastrointestinal physiology (29), and preliminary evidence indicates that they have different effects on rates of fat absorption (30). Dietary fibers may affect fasting lipoproteins and postprandial lipid metabolism by these and other mechanisms (30): *altering gastric emptying*—soluble fibers such as gums slow gastric emptying which would delay lipid absorption (29,31–34); *influencing intestinal transit time*—wheat bran and other insoluble fibers hasten intestinal transit while soluble fibers may slow the process in manners which might affect the timing and quantity of lipid hydrolysis, absorption, and secretion as chylomicrons (29,33,34); *modifying pancreatic secretion or pancreatic enzyme activity*—fiber may bind, inactivate, or physically separate enzymes from lipids and thus affect their hydrolysis (34,35); *acting upon micelle formation*—binding of bile acids or decreased mixing may decrease micelle formation and slow or decrease lipid hydrolysis and absorption (32–34); *varying intestinal motility*—soluble fiber may decrease while insoluble fibers may increase mixing of intestinal contents in such a way as to affect micelle formation and exposure of lipids to hydrolytic enzymes and absorptive surfaces (31); *changing transport barriers such as the unstirred layer*—soluble fibers may decrease lipid absorption by affecting transport barriers (32–34); *altering lymphatic flow rates* to affect rate of entry of lipids into the peripheral circulation (30,33); *fermentation in the colon* to produce short chain fatty acids which may inhibit hepatic cholesterol synthesis (36); and *influencing secretion of insulin or other hormones*—which could affect hepatic lipid and lipoprotein synthesis and secretion rates (29,33,34,37,38).

Discussion

Careful studies on the metabolic research ward indicate that incorporation of 100 grams of either oat bran or dried beans into a typical Western diet leads to a significant reduction in serum total and LDL-cholesterol for hypercholesterolemic men (Table 1). Under these conditions, serum total and LDL-cholesterol decrease 15% and 16%, respectively. Since reductions of serum cholesterol of 1% are estimated to reduce risk for coronary heart disease by 2% (2), these hypocholesterolemic effects should have a major impact on risk for coronary heart disease.

The mechanisms responsible for the hypocholesterolemic effects of soluble fiber are still under investigation. Our research with oat bran indicates that this specific soluble fiber has these actions: increased fecal excretion of bile acids (4,11); increased serum acetate concentrations in humans (39); increased portal vein concentrations of propionate in rats (1); propionate at physiologic concentrations inhibiting hepatic cholesterol synthesis in rat (36); and decreased postprandial serum insulin concentrations (40). Probably several or all of these changes plus additional factors interact to produce the observed serum lipoprotein changes.

Conclusions

Foods rich in soluble fiber have significant hypocholesterolemic effects. Oat and bean products, in amounts commonly consumed by some populations and in amounts easily consumed by Western people, can decrease serum cholesterol by 10% to 15%. Soluble fiber supplements, such as psyllium, can reduce serum cholesterol to a similar degree (41, 42). Using soluble fibers to enhance the hypocholesterolemic effects of fat-restricted diets can decrease serum cholesterol by 20% to 30%. This degree of reduction enables most individuals with elevated serum cholesterol values to satisfactorily manage their hypercholesterolemia without drugs. Since these dietary measures have far fewer side effects than cholesterol-lowering drugs, this approach is preferred by many individuals (2). For soluble dietary fiber to have this important effect on risk for coronary heart disease, both in primary and secondary prevention, health professionals and consumers will need much more education and awareness about these benefits.

Acknowledgments

This research was supported, in part, by grants from the National Institutes of Health (HL-37902 and HL-36552) and from the HCF Nutrition Foundation.

References

1. J. W. Anderson, D. A. Deakins, and S. R. Bridges, Hypocholesterolemic effects of soluble fibers: mechanisms, in: "Dietary Fiber: Chemistry, Physiology, and Health Effects," D. Kritchevsky, C. Bonfield, J. W. Anderson, eds., Plenum

Press, New York (1990).

2. J. W. Anderson, D. A. Deakins, T. L. Floore, B. M. Smith and S. E. Whitis, Dietary fiber and coronary heart disease, Critical Reviews in Food Science and Nutrition 29:95 (1990).

3. A. P. de Groot, R. Luyken and N. A. Pikaar, Cholesterol-lowering effect of rolled oats, Lancet 2:303(1963). (letter).

4. R. W. Kirby, J. W. Anderson, B. Sieling, et al., Oat-bran intake selectively lowers serum low-density lipoprotein cholesterol concentrations of hyper-cholesterolemic men, Am. J. Clin. Nutr. 34:824 (1981).

5. L. V. Van Horn, K. Liu, D. Parker, et al., Serum lipid response to oat product intake with a fat-restricted diet, J. Am. Dietet. Assoc. 86:759 (1986).

6. J. W. Anderson and N. J. Gustafson, Hypocholesterolemic effects of oat and bean products, Am. J. Clin. Nutr. 48:749 (1988).

7. M. H. Davidson, L. D. Dugan, J. H. Burns, J. Bova, K. Story, and K. B. Drennan. The hypocholesterolemic effects of beta-glucan in oatmeal and oat bran, JAMA 265:1833 (1991).

8. J. J. Groen, K. B. Tijong, M. Koster, A. F. Willebrands, G. Verdonck, and M. Pierloot, The influence of nutrition and ways of life on blood cholesterol and the prevalence of hypertension and coronary heart disease among Trappist and Benedictine monks, Am. J. Clin. Nutr. 10:456 (1962).

9. R. Luyken, N. A. Pikaar, H. Polman, and F. A. Schippers, The influence of legumes on the serum cholesterol level, Voeding 23:447 (1962).

10. D. J. A. Jenkins, G. W. Wong, and R. Patten, Leguminous seeds in the dietary management of hyperlipidemia, Am. J. Clin. Nutr. 38:567 (1983).

11. J. W. Anderson, L. Story, B. Sieling, W-J. L. Chen, M. S. Petro, and J. Story, Hypocholesterolemic effects of oat bran or bean intake for hypercholes-terolemic men, Am. J. Clin. Nutr. 40:1146 (1984).

12. J. W. Anderson, N. J. Gustafson, D. B. Spencer, J. Tietyen and C. A. Bryant, Serum lipid response of hypercholesterolemic men to single and divided doses of canned beans, Am. J. Clin. Nutr. 51:1013 (1990).

13. S. M. Shutler, G. M. Bircher, J. A. Tredger, et al., The effects of daily baked beans (*Phaseolus vulgaris*) consumption on the plasma lipid levels of young, normo-cholesterolemic men, Br. J. Nutr. 61:257 (1989).

14. W-J. L. Chen and J. W. Anderson, Effects of plant fiber in decreasing plasma total cholesterol and increasing high density lipoprotein cholesterol, Proc. Soc. Exp. Biol. Med. 162:310 (1979).

15. M. R. Gould, J. W. Anderson and S. O'Mahony, Biofunctional properties of oats, in: "Cereals for Food and Beverages," G. E. Inglett and L. Munch, eds., Academic Press, New York (1980).

16. J. W. Anderson, D. B. Spencer, C. C. Hamilton, et al., Oat-bran cereal lowers serum total and LDL-cholesterol in hypercholesterolemic men, Am. J. Clin. Nutr. 52:495 (1990).

17. J. W. Anderson, N. H. Gilinsky, D. A. Deakins, et al., Lipid responses of hypercholesterolemic men to oat bran and wheat bran intake, Am. J. Clin. Nutr. 54:678 (1991).

18. J. F. Swain, I. L. Rouse, C. B. Curley and F. M. Sacks, Comparison of the effects of oat bran and low-fiber wheat on serum lipoprotein levels and blood

pressure, N. Engl. J. Med. 322:147 (1990).

19. R. A. Roubenoff and R. Roubenoff, Oat bran and serum cholesterol, N. Engl. J. Med. 322:1746 (1990). (letter).

20. B. S. Kanders, N. Istfan and G. L. Blackburn, Oat bran and serum cholesterol, N. Engl. J. Med. 322:1747 (199). (letter).

21. J. W. Anderson and C. L. Wood, Oat bran and serum cholesterol. N. Engl. J. Med. 322:1747 (1990) (letter).

22. J. W. Anderson and S. R. Bridges, Dietary fiber content of selected foods, Am. J. Clin. Nutr. 47:440 (1988).

23. J. Leadbetter, M. J. Ball and J. I. Mann, Effects of increasing quantities of oat bran in hypercholesterolemic people, Am. J. Clin. Nutr. 54:841 (1991).

24. M. Kestin, R. Moss, P. M. Clifton and P. J. Nestel, Comparative effects of three cereal brans on plasma lipids, blood pressure, and glucose metabolism in mildly hypercholesterolemic men, Am. J. Clin. Nutr. 52:661 (1990).

25. J. M. Keenan, J. B. Wenz, S. Myers, C. Ripsin and Z. Huang, Randomized, controlled, crossover trial of oat bran in hypercholesterolemic subjects, J. Fam. Fract. 33:600 (1991).

26. C. M. Ripsin, J. M. Keenan, D. R. Jacobs, Jr., et al. Oat products and lipid lowering: a meta-analysis, J. Am. Med. Assoc. 267:3317 (1992).

27. C. L. Redard, P. A. Davis and B. O. Schneeman, Dietary fiber and gender: effect on postprandial lipemia, Am. J. Clin. Nutr. 92:837 (1990).

28. L. Cara, C. Dubois, P. Borel, et al., Effects of oat bran, rice bran, wheat fiber, and wheat germ on postprandial lipemia in healthy adults, Am. J. Clin. Nutr. 55:81 (1992).

29. J. W. Anderson, Physiologic and metabolic effects of dietary fiber, Fed. Proc. 44:2902 (1985).

30. I. Ikeda, Y. Tomari and M. Sugano, Interrelated effects of dietary fiber and fat on lymphatic cholesterol and triglyceride absorption in rats. J. Nutr. 119:1383 (1989).

31. J. M. Gee, N. A. Blackburn and I. T. Johnson, The influence of guar gum on intestinal cholesterol transport in the rat, Br. J. Nutr. 50:215 (1983).

32. K. Ebihara and B. O. Schneeman, Interaction of bile acids, phospholipids, cholesterol and triglyceride with dietary fibers in the small intestine of rats, J. Nutr. 119:1100 (1989).

33. G. V. Vahouny, Dietary fiber, lipid metabolism, and atherosclerosis, Fed. Proc. 41:2801 (1982).

34. G. V. Vahouny and M. M. Cassidy, Dietary fibers and absorption of nutrients, Proc. Soc. Exper. Biol. Med. 180:432 (1985).

35. B. O. Schneeman and D. Gallaher D. Effects of dietary fiber on digestive enzyme activity and bile acids in the small intestine. Proc. Soc. Exper. Biol. Med. 180:409 (1985).

36. R. W. Wright, J. W. Anderson and S. R. Bridges, Propionate inhibits hepatic lipid synthesis, Proc. Soc. Exper. Biol. Med. 190:26 (1990).

37. Y. Deshaies, F. Begin, L. Savoie, and C. Vachon, Attenuation of the meal-induced increase in plasma lipids and adipose tissue lipoprotein lipase by guar gum, J. Nutr. 120:64 (1989).

38. D. J. A. Jenkins, T. M. S. Wolever, V. Vuksan, et al., Nibbling versus gorging:

metabolic advantages of increased meal frequency, N. Engl. J. Med. 321:929 (1989).

39. S. R. Bridges, J. W. Anderson, D. A. Deakins and C. A. Wood, Oat bran increases serum acetate of hypercholesterolemic men, Am. J. Clin. Nutr. In press. 1992.

40. J. W. Anderson and A. E. Seisel, Hypocholesterolemic effects of oat products, in: "New Developments in Dietary Fiber, Physiologic, Physicochemical, and Analytical Aspects" I. Furda and C. J. Brine, eds., Plenum Press, New York, (1990).

41. J. W. Anderson, N. Zettwoch, T. Feldman, et al., Cholesterol-lowering effects of psyllium hydrophilic mucilloid for hypercholesterolemic men, Arch. Intern. Med. 148:292 (1988).

42. J. W. Anderson, T. L. Floore, P. B. Geil, et al., Hypocholesterolemic effects of different bulk-forming hydrophilic fibers as adjuncts to dietary therapy in mild to moderate hypercholesterolemia, Arch. Intern. Med. 151:1597 (1991).

Dietary Fiber, Carbohydrate Metabolism and Diabetes

David J. A. Jenkins,[1,2] Alexandra L. Jenkins,[1,2]
Thomas M. S. Wolever,[1,2] Vladimir Vuksan,[1,2]
A. Venket Rao,[1] Lilian U. Thompson,[1] and
Robert G. Josse[1,2]

[1]*Department of Nutritional Sciences, Faculty of Medicine;* [2]*Clinical Nutrition and Risk Factor Modification Center and Division of Endocrinology and Metabolism, St Michael's Hospital, University of Toronto*

By the mid 1970's, experimental evidence was accumulating to support the original claim that increased fiber consumption might have a beneficial effect on diabetes and its cardiovascular complications (1–3). Despite the weight of positive evidence, there is still considerable doubt about the validity of these claims (4). Much of this doubt has focused on the fact that a clear demonstration of mechanism has been lacking (4) and that any benefits observed may therefore be related to other factors such as weight loss or reduction of saturated fat intake. Since this debate continues, it seems appropriate to discuss the mechanisms by which fiber may alter carbohydrate and lipid metabolism which may be relevant to diabetes.

Dietary Fiber and Carbohydrate Metabolism

The action of dietary fiber in reducing postprandial glycemia acutely and its suggested action in improving carbohydrate metabolism in the long term may be dependent on both the small intestinal and colonic effects of fiber. In the small intestine fiber may slow the rate of absorption. This is most readily demonstrated with purified viscous fibers given with glucose or incorporated into test meals. In general the more viscous the fiber the greater the effect (5). By analogy, any other aspect of food which reduces absorption rate will have a similar effect. In the colon there are theoretical reasons why carbohydrate metabolism may be influenced by the products of bacterial fermentation of fiber and carbohydrate which is not absorbed in the small intestine. These products of bacterial metabolism, the short chain fatty acids, may influence both hepatic cholesterol synthesis, the production of glucose and its utilization by peripheral tissues.

Lente Carbohydrate: Nibbling Versus Gorging

There is a growing body of evidence that many of the apparent health benefits related to dietary fiber consumption may be due to the ability of certain types of fiber to slow absorption. The idea of low glycemic index foods which was an offshoot of interest in dietary fiber supported this concept by showing that there was a good correlation between the rate at which a carbohydrate food was digested in vitro and the glycemic response in vivo (6,7). A decade ago when enzyme inhibitors were first being developed to reduce the rate of absorption, it was suggested that slowing the rate of absorption should be regarded as a new therapeutic principle (8). However, these ideas are not new. Possibly the earliest experimental evidence favouring prolongation of the absorption time came from studies of the so called "nibbling versus gorging" paradigm which was an area of active investigation over a quarter of a century ago (8–17). Even further back in time, based on his own experiments, Sanctorius in the 16th century recommended the consumption of frequent small meals rather than one large meal: *"He who eats but one meal a day destroys himself slowly if he eats but a little or a lot."*

It therefore seems appropriate to review what has been learnt from food frequency studies. These studies provide a means of assessing the effect of prolonging absorption time isolated from alterations in the nature of the food or the use of enzyme inhibitors.

Diabetes and carbohydrate metabolism

Early studies by Ellis suggested that insulin requirements in diabetes could be reduced considerably by increasing meal frequency (15). In 1933 he published a series of case reports where patients on high insulin doses with poor control had both control improved and insulin requirements cut when glucose was sipped at *hourly* intervals throughout the day (15). In the 1960's and 70's there was broad interest in the effects of increased food frequency. Studies indicated that when normal volunteers and diabetics were placed on diets of differing food frequency, there was an improvement in glucose tolerance and reduction in postprandial insulin levels (9). Not all studies noted this phenomenon (18) and in one study it appeared that the dietary P:S ratio was a determinant of the effect on the glucose and insulin response (18). There is still debate as to whether the effect is seen only at the time when meal frequency is increased or whether there are longer-term adaptations which can be demonstrated by glucose tolerance testing. More recent acute studies have confirmed that when 50g of glucose in solution was taken over a period of 180 min (sipping) as opposed to being drunk in 5 min (bolus) there was a dramatic reduction in the insulin response area (19). Sipping was also reflected in flatter C-peptide, gastric inhibitory polypeptide, glucagon and enteroglucagon responses. At the same time despite reduced insulin secretion, FFA levels were suppressed similarly by both treatments. However, whereas the FFA levels 180 mins after the bolus drink rose and by 240 mins had overshot baseline values, after sipping the FFA levels remained suppressed for the full 240 mins (19). This suggests that the post bolus undershot in blood glucose level at 180 mins triggered a counteregulatory response which mobilized FFA. In support of this were the significantly higher growth hormone levels seen at 180 mins and the increased urinary catecholamine secretion seen in the first 4 hrs after the glucose bolus. A further feature of interest was the response to intravenous glucose administered at 4 hrs (IVGTT). The IVGTT administered at 4 hrs after the bolus had a KG which was significantly greater than that seen after sipping. This related to a significantly higher FFA level over the course of the IVGTT after the bolus. There was no difference between treatments in insulin, c-peptide, or GIP (19).

This effect may be a reflection of the Staub-Traugott effect, where the closeness of one meal to the next determines the glycemic response to the second meal, the closer the better the glucose tolerance. A similar explanation has been used for the second meal phenomenon observed with viscous fiber. In this situation fiber in one meal, presumably by spreading the nutrient load from the first meal improved carbohydrate tolerance and reduced the insulin response to the second meal (20). Studies in non-diabetic volunteers have been extended to diabetic volunteers. The same insulin economy was seen in NIDDM when over a 12 hour period 240g glucose in solution was either sipped or given as an 80g glucose bolus on three occasions (21). Using foods rather than glucose in NIDDM the economy in insulin secretion was again seen. In these studies three meals taken over 10 hours were compared with hourly feedings of the same food. In this situation mean glucose levels were also significantly reduced together with plasma levels of GIP and 24 hour urinary excretion of C-peptide (22).

In normal volunteers studies were carried out where meals were taken hourly for 16 hours of the day over a two week period (23). These were compared to a two week control period taking the same food as three meals per day. In this longer term comparison the serum insulin and c-peptide responses were moderately reduced. However when a 50g GTT and an IVGTT were performed at the end of each two week period no difference was seen between treatments (23). It can be concluded that the time was too short to produce a chronic change in glucose tolerance or that only at the time when food frequency is increased is the effect seen. Therefore these studies only indicate an acute insulin economy while food frequency is actually increased. Nevertheless if this paradigm as acceptable as a model for slow absorption, then the findings may go some way to explain the effect of fiber acutely in improving glucose tolerance without involving specific attributes of fiber other than its ability to slow small intestinal absorption of nutrients.

Lipid metabolism

Beneficial effects of fiber on lipid metabolism would be of obvious relevance to diabetes and its macrovascular complications. Patients with type II diabetes tend to have low HDL levels and high total:HDL cholesterol ratios. They may also suffer from raised total cholesterol and triglyceride levels. Some of the earliest studies to be conducted on the nibbling versus gorging paradigm involved the effects of food frequency on lipid metabolism. Early studies indicated that hyperlipidemic and normal volunteers showed reductions in total cholesterol (2,3,5,10,16) with some studies showing falls also in plasma phospholipids and triglyceride levels (10). The effects varied with the nature of the fat, the more saturated the greater and more significant the effect (18). The metabolically controlled studies were usually of comparatively short duration, 2–3 weeks but data were also presented which indicated that the effects could be sustained in hyperlipidemic volunteers over study periods lasting for months and in one instance for two years (16). The minimum meal frequency which appeared effective in lowering serum cholesterol was 8 or more when compared to three meals per day. However, the greater difference was between volunteers who consumed only one major meal a day compared to those who consumed three meals daily. Some studies indicated that nibbling induced longer term metabolic changes in terms of post prandial responses following fat challenge with reduced triglyceride rises in response to a fatty test meal after nibbling (18). As with the glucose effect this was only seen after the corn oil as apposed to the butter fat diet (25).

More recently, detailed studies of the blood lipid and lipoprotein changes with increasing meal frequency confirmed the cholesterol lowering effect of increased food frequency (23). Studies using liquid formula diets have indicated that falls in serum cholesterol can be seen during the course of a single day using increased food frequency (24). Two week studies of 17 very small meals per day demonstrated that the fall after two weeks was in the LDL cholesterol fraction with a reduction also in the level of apolipoprotein B (23). No treatment differences were observed in apo AI, HDL cholesterol or serum triglyceride. Furthermore an additional effect of increased food frequency was also seen even when diets were high in carbohydrate (23). The effect was not as pronounced on 20% fat diets as on 30% fat diets, but the absolute level serum cholesterol reached was nevertheless lower (23). The mechanism by which increased food frequency lowers serum lipids is not clear. Only two of the mechanisms suggested for dietary fiber are likely to apply to the nibbling paradigm. The first is the reduction in insulin secretion and post prandial nutrient rises after nibbling. HMGCoA reductase, a rate limiting step in cholesterol synthesis, is stimulated in amount and activity by circulating insulin levels (25). Reduction in insulin levels over the day may result in a reduction of HMGCoA reductase activity and a decrease in the rate of hepatic cholesterol synthesis over the day (25). The second mechanism may relate to an increased rate of bile salt cycling during the day due to the presence of food in the gut for a longer period of time on nibbling. This would result in prolonged exposure of the liver to the recycled bile acids and the inhibitory effect of chenodeoxycholic acid on cholesterol synthesis (26). Although both these mechanisms may operate, neither has yet been demonstrated to be responsible for the often dramatic cholesterol falls observed with increased meal frequency.

Products of colonic fermentation, carbohydrate metabolism

Slow absorption may increase carbohydrate losses to the colon. Although the carbohydrate losses are in general too small to reduce postprandial glycemia by themselves, sufficient fermentable substrates may enter the colon to cause major changes in the amount and possibly the type of short chain fatty acids (SCFA) produced by their bacterial fermentation. The fatty acids commonly reported include acetate, propionate, and butyrate in the approximate proportion of 60:20:20.

Since small intestinal transit times for mixed meals are of the order of 6 hours, colonic fermentation is unlikely to explain the acute effects of slowing small intestinal absorption which follows consumption of test meals containing viscous fiber, low glycemic index foods or enzyme inhibitors. They may, however, influence the metabolism of carbohydrate loads taken later in the day. Acetate which appears in the peripheral circulation may reduce serum FFA levels. This finding is in common with other short chain acids including the ketone bodies acetoacetate and β-hydroxybutyrate (27). The effect appears to be a direct inhibitory effect on adipose tissue lipolysis. Propionate, which is largely extracted by the liver and in consequence does not reach the peripheral circulation, is gluconeogenic in the liver and may increase blood glucose levels.

Despite these theoretical considerations SCFAs taken either by mouth or by rectal infusion do not appear to alter postprandial glycemia following consumption of carbohydrate. Certainly increased colonic fermentation with acetate generated from lactulose, both acutely (28) and in chronic feeding studies (29) or acetate fed (30) or infused per rectum (31) have all been shown to reduce serum FFA levels. However, none of these acetate studies have demonstrated improved carbohydrate tolerance. Propionate, on the other hand, given by rectal infusion has been shown to raise blood glucose levels (31) and when given in bread to reduce glycemia acutely and in the longer term to reduce the glycemic response to a propionate free bread test meal (32). This latter study also demonstrated that propionate incorporated into bread reduced its digestibility and it is therefore difficult to dissociate the effects observed from those of the acute and chronic effects of slowly digested foods. From the perspective of carbohydrate tolerance it appears that the beneficial effects are likely to be due to a reduced rate of small intestinal absorption which can be increased simply by reducing the size of meals and reducing their frequency. The colonic events do not appear to play an essential role in the reduced glycemia seen with fiber, low glycemic index foods or enzyme inhibitors.

Colonic fermentation: lipid metabolism

Early studies indicated that propionate was hypocholesterolemic in pigs (33). Subsequently this explanation was offered to account for the hypocholesterolemic effect of fiber and was supported by evidence in rats that propionate feeding reduced serum cholesterol levels and inhibited cholesterol synthesis in rat liver studies in vitro (34). It was also suggested that acetate may be hypocholesterolemic and it was demonstrated that raised acetate levels were seen over the day when high fiber diets were fed which lowered serum cholesterol levels (35). Furthermore human feeding studies using propionate at a level of 7g/day indicated that total cholesterol levels were reduced (38). On the other hand rectal infusion studies demonstrated that over a 2–3 hour period infusion of 800–1600 ml of 90–180 mmol acetate resulted in measurable rises in serum total and LDL cholesterol (31). Addition of propionate to the perfusate blocked the rise in serum cholesterol. In support of this finding, administration of lactulose over a two week period increased peripheral blood glutamine levels as an indicator of increased SCFA generation but at the same time raised LDL cholesterol and apolipoprotein B levels (29). Since acetate is the major SCFA generated during colonic fermentation these studies suggest that simple fermentation per se with increased acetate production is unlikely to be the major reason for the lipid lowering effects of fiber. It may be that fibers or carbohydrate foods which produce larger amounts of propionate may be of benefit. However, propionate incorporated into bread had a greater effect in lowering HDL cholesterol than in reducing the LDL cholesterol (32). This effect may be very relevant to diabetes, where HDL levels may already be low. Thus, as with the effect of fiber on carbohydrate metabolism, it is likely that the dominant beneficial action of fiber on lipid metabolism takes place in the small intestine. Selection of fiber simply on the basis that it increases colonic fermentation is an issue which requires further investigation.

Conclusion

We conclude that the value of high fiber foods lies principally in their ability to prolong absorption in the small intestine. The effects on carbohydrate and lipid metabolism can be mimicked by reducing meal size and increasing meal frequency over an extended period of time. The inevitable increase in colonic fermentation which accompanies slowing small intestinal absorption by the use of fiber does not appear to be essential for the metabolic benefits. Indeed it may be counterproductive in certain cases where increased acetate is produced if, for example, cholesterol reduction is the objective. On the other hand, although increasing food frequency may not be a practical approach to many therapeutic problems which may benefit from reducing the rate of absorption it appears to be a useful model to explore what has proved to be an elusive mechanism of action.

References

1. Kiehm, T. G., Anderson, J. W., Ward, K. Beneficial effects of a high carbohydrate high fiber diet in hyperglycemic men. Am J Clin Nutr 1976;29:895-9.
2. Jenkins, D. J. A., Leeds, A. R., Gassull, M. A., Wolever, T. M. S., Goff, D. V., Alberti, K. G. M. M., Hockaday, T. D. R. Unabsorbable carbohdyrates and diabetes: decreased postprandial hyperglycemia. Lancet 1976;2:172-4.
3. Jenkins D. J. A, Wolever, T. M. S., Hockaday, T. D. R., Leeds, A. R., Haworth, R., Bacon, S., Apling, E. C., Dilawari, J. Treatment of diabetes with guar gum. Lancet 1977;2:779-80.
4. NIH Consensus Development Conference Statement on Diet and Exercise. US Department of Health and Human Services. Diabetes Care 1987;10:6.
5. Jenkins, D. J. A., Wolever, T. M. S. , Leeds, A. R., Gassull, M. A., Dilawari, J. B., Goff, D. V., Metz, G. L., Alberti, K. G. M. M. Dietary fibres, fibre

analogues and glucose tolerance: importance of viscosity. Brith Med J 1978; 1:1392-4.

6. Jenkins, D. J. A., Taylor, R. H., Wolever, T. M. S. The diabetic diet, dietary carbohdyrate and differences in digestibility. Diabetologia 1982;23:477-84.

7. Jenkins, D. J. A., Wolever, T. M. S., Thorne, M.J., Jenkins, A. L., Wong, G. S., Josse, R. G., Csima A. The relationship between glycemia response, digestibility, and factors influencing the dietary habits of diabetics. Am J Clin Nutr 1984;40:1175-91.

8. Creutzfeldt, W. Introduction. In: Delaying absorption as a therapeutic principle in metabolic diseases. Eds: Creutzfeldt W, Folsch UR. Thiem-stratton, New York, 1983, p 1.

9. Gwinup, G, Byron, R. C., Roush, W. H., Kruger, F. A., Hamwi, G. J. Effect on nibbling versus gorging on glucose tolerance. Lancet 1963;2:165-7.

10. Gwinup, G., Byron, R. C., Roush, W. H., Kruger, F. A., Hamwi, G. J. Effect on nibbling versus gorging on serum lipids in man. Am J Clin Nutr 1963;13:209-13.

11. Irwin, M. R., Feeley, R. M. Frequency and size of meals and serum lipids,nitrogen and mineral retention, fat digestibility and urinary thiamine and riboflavin in young women. Am J Clin Nutr 1967;2:816-24.

12. Fabry, P., Tepperman, J. Meal frequency—a possible factor in human pathology. Am J Clin Nutr 1970;23:1059-68.

13. Young, C. M., Scanlan, S. S., Topping, C. M., Simko, V., Lutwak, L. Frequency of feeding, weight reduction and nutrient utilization. J Am Dietet Assoc 1971;59:473-80.

14. Bray, G. A. Lipogenesis in human adipose tissue: some efefcts of nibbling and gorging. J Clin Invest 1972;51:537-48.

15. Ellis, A. Increased carbohdyrate tolerance in diabetes following hourly administration of glucose and insulin over long periods. Quart J Med 1934;27:137-53.

16. Cohn, C. Feeding patterns and some aspects of cholesterol metabolism. Fed Proc 1964;23:76-81.

17. Special Report Committee: Guidelines for the nutritional management of diabetes mellitus: A special report from the Canadian Diabetes Association. J Can Dietet Assoc 1981;42:110-8.

18. Jagannathan SN, Connel WF, Beveridge JMR. Effect of gormandizing and semicontinous eating of equicaloric amounts of formula type high fat diets on plasma cholesterol and triglyceride levels in human volunteers subjects. Am J Clin Nutr 1964;15:90-3.

19. Jenkins, D. J. A., Wolever, T. M. S., Ocana, A. M., Vuksan, V., Cunnane, S.C., Jenkins, M., Wong, G. S., Singer, W., Bloom, S.R., Blendis, L.M., Josse, R. G. Metabolic effects of reducing rate of glucose ingestion by single bolus versus continous sipping. Diabetes 1990;39:775-81.

20. Jenkins, D. J. A., Wolever, T. M. S., Nineham, R., Sarson, D. L., Bloom, S. R., Ahern, J., Alberti, K. G. M. M, Hockaday, T. D. R. Improved glucose tolerance four hours after taking guar with glucose. Diabetologia 1980;19:21-4.

21. Jenkins, D. J. A., Wolever, T. M. S., Taylor, R. H., Kannan, W., Sarson, D., Bloom, S. R. Reply to letter by Abraira and Lawrence. Am J Clin Nutr 1983;37:153-4.

22. Jenkins, D. J. A, Ocana, A. M., Jenkins, A. L., Wolever, T. M. S., Vuksan, V., Katzman, L, Hollands, M., Greenberg, G., Corey, P., Patten, R., Wong, G. S., Josse, R. G. Metabolic advantages of spreading the nutrient load: effects of increased meal frequency in non-insulin dependent diabetics. Am J Clin Nutr 1992;55:461-7.

23. Jenkins, D. J. A., Wolever, T. M. S., Vuksan, V., Brighenti, F., Cunnane, S. C., Rao, A. V., Jenkins, A. L., Buckley, G., Patten, R., Singer, W., Corey, P., Josse, R. G. "Nibbling versus gorging": Metabolic advantages of increased meal frequency. New Eng J Med 1989;321:929-93.

24. Wolever, T. M. S. Metabolic effects of continous feeding. Metab 1990;39:947-51.

25. Lakshmanan, M. R., Nepokroeff, C. M., Ness, G. C., Dugan, R. E., Porter, J. W. Stimulation by insulin of rat liver beta-hydroxy-beta-methylglutaryl conenzyme A reductase and cholesterol-synthesizing activities. Biochem Biophys Res Commun 1973;50:704-10.

26. Coyne, M. J., Bonoris, G. G., Goldstein, L., Schoenfield, L. J. Effect of chenodeoxycholic acid and phenobarbital on the rate of limiting enzymes of hepatic cholesterol synthesis in patients with gallstones. J Lab Clin Med 1976;87:281-91.

27. Jenkins, D. J. A. Ketone bodies and the inhibition of free-fatty-acid release. Lancet 1967;2:338-40.

28. Scheppach, W., Cummings, J. H., Branch, W. J., Schrezenmeir, J. Effect of gut-derived acetate on oral glucose tolerance in man. Clin Sci 198?;75:355-61.

29. Jenkins, D. J. A., Wolever, T. M. S., Jenkins, A. L., Brighenti, F., Vuksan, V, Rao, A. V., Cunnane, S. C., Ocana, A. M., Corey, P., Versina, C., Connelly, P., Buckley, G., Patten, R. Specific types of colonic fermentation may raise low-density-lipoprotein-cholesterol concentrations. Am J Clin Nutr 1991;54:141-7.

30. Wolever, T. M. S., Brighenti, F., Royall, D., Jenkins, A. L., Jenkins, D. J. A. Effect of rectal infusion of short chain fatty acids in human subjects. Am J Gastroenterol 1989;84:1027-33.

31. Wolever, T. M. S., Spadafora P., Eshuis H. Interaction between colonic acetate and propionate in man. Am J Clin Nutr 1991. In press.

32. Todesco, T., Rao, A. V., Bosello, O., Jenkins, D. J. A. Propionate lowers blood glucose and alters lipid metabolism in healthy subjects. Am J Clin Nutr 1991; 54:860-5.

33. Thacker, P. A., Salomons, M. O., Aherne, F. X., Milligan, L. P., Bowland, J. P. Influence of propionic acid on the cholesterol metabolism of pigs fed hyper-cholesterolemic diets. Can J Anim Sci 1981;61:969-75.

34. Chen, W.-J. L., Anderson, J. W., Jennings, D. Propionate may mediate the hypocholesterolemic effects of certain soluble plant fibers in cholesterol fed rats. Proc Soc Exp Biol Med 1984;175:215-8.

35. Bridges, S. R., Anderson, J. W., Deakins, D. A., Dillon D. W., Wood, C. A. Oat bran increases serum acetate of hypercholesterolemic men. Am J Clin Nutr 1992;56:455-9.

36. Venter, C. S., Vorster, H. H, Cummings, J. H. Effects of dietary propionate on carbohydrate and lipid metabolism in healthy volunteers. Am J Gastroenterol 1990;85:549-53.

Dietary Fiber and Protein Digestion and Utilization

Bjørn O. Eggum

National Institute of Animal Science
Animal Physiology and Biochemistry
Research Center Foulum
P.O. Box 39, 8830 Tjele
Denmark

Introduction

Dietary fiber (DF) affects many processes along the entire gastro-intestinal (GI) tract from ingestion to excretion (Heaton 1980). In the small intestine, however, the effect of DF depends on the chemical and structural composition of the cell wall materials (CWM). In general, purified viscous substances reduce the rate of nutrient absorption, whereas insoluble DF sources will have only little effect on nutrient absorption in the small intestine. Consequently, DF may modify and usually decrease digestibility of proteins, along with lipids and certain minerals (Kritchevsky 1988).

In the hind-gut DF profoundly alters the metabolism of the bacteria and as a consequence nitrogen metabolism is changed (Mason 1984). The effect of fiber on N balance and N excretory patterns is influenced by many factors, including its chemical composition and degradability (Eggum et al. 1984). The influence of fiber on the apparent digestibility of N depends on the nature of the DF, digestibility of dietary carbohydrates and the digestibility and level of dietary protein (Beames and Eggum 1981). Furthermore, fiber reduces the transit time significantly (Raczynski et al. 1982), and thus leaves less time for microbial fermentation.

The proteins (or rather amino acids) not absorbed from the small intestine, including those of endogenous origin, will sustain the microbial population in the hind-gut with nitrogen (e.g., Beames and Eggum 1981; Mason 1984; Macfarlane et al. 1986). Together with the undigested carbohydrates that act as energy sources, nitrogen will stimulate microbial activity leading to substantial increases of bacterial nitrogen in the faecal matter.

Numerous studies have been carried out to study the effect of fiber on protein utilization (as was reviewed by, e.g., Eggum 1973; Gallaher and Schneeman 1986). Results obtained by different groups have been contradictory in that some found a decrease in protein utilization with increasing fiber levels, and others found no differences. Some of the contradictions may have been due to the type of fiber source that was included in the diets. For example, Eggum (1973) in work with rats found no effect of including cellulose powder up to a level of 30% in the diet on true protein digestibility, biological value, and net protein utilization of casein. On the other hand, Breite (1973) and Meier and Poppe (1977) found a decrease in protein digestibility as well as amino acid availabilities when including increasing amounts of natural DF sources to rats.

However, the validity of the faecal analysis method for determination of the apparent digestibility of protein and amino acids is often questioned partly because of endogenous protein secretions into the digestive tract and partly because of the effects of microorganisms in the hindgut. The microorganisms may influence protein metabolism and thereby confound the determination of protein and amino acid digestibilities. Bacterial enzymes in the large intestine could bring about hydrolyses of undigested protein through peptides of decreasing length to free amino acids. These free amino acids may either be absorbed as such or broken down further to yield ammonia and carbon skeletons. The latter compounds, in turn, may be absorbed by the individual or be used for de novo bacterial protein synthesis (Mason 1984).

It is also demonstrated that amino acids infused into the caecum of pigs rather than fed orally led to almost complete and rapid excretion of their N into the urine and no improvement in N balance (Zebrowska 1973; Just et al. 1981).

An additional problem would be to separate the influence of antinutritional factors associated to the fibers (Liener and Kakade 1980; Bach Knudsen and Eggum 1984; Vandergrift et al. 1983). It is also difficult to separate the nitrogen associated to the fiber having a low availability (Donangelo and Eggum 1985) from other nitrogen containing material in faeces.

It appears from the discussion above that many factors can be of great importance when determining the influence of DF on protein digestion and utilization in vivo. The present work will be discussing several of these aspects based on experiments with rats, pigs and man.

Experiments with Rats

In balance studies with natural protein foods and feeds Eggum (1973) showed that there exists a strict negative relationship (P<0.001) between true protein digestibility (TD) and the fiber level in various protein sources. However, when replacing starch with pure cellulose powder in the diets from 0 to 30% of dry matter (DM) no relationship between the fiber level and TD or protein utilization was found. These two studies indicate that fiber in natural food sources affects protein utilization differently compared to purified fiber sources. However, in the review of Gallaher and Schneeman (1986) it could be seen that also purified fibers could have a negative effect on protein digestibility in studies on rats while the two human studies reported showed no effect of purified fiber on protein digestibility. In studies with 15 natural food sources Mongeau et al. (1989) showed that several food fiber fractions and possibly associated substances, influenced protein digestibility. Purified cellulose did not have the same physiological behavior as food cellulose from the viewpoint of protein digestibility and fiber fermentability which is in agreement with the studies of Agarwal and Chauhan (1989) who found in experiments with Indian plant foods, high in dietary fiber, that the various food sources affected TD significantly and more than pure cellulose. Radha and Geervani (1985) found that TD of bengal gram decreased with maturity and the authors assumed that this probably was due to an increase in the NDF content.

In work with cereals Heger et al. (1990) found in balance experiments with rats a strict negative relationship between TD, SDF and IDF, respectively, while BV was positively correlated with both fiber fractions. This indicates that fiber can affect the excretory patterns in rats significantly.

Bach Knudsen et al. (1984) showed that the microbial activity in the hind-gut was strongly influenced by the amount and type of nutrients reaching the lower gut. It could be seen that of different botanical fractions of barley the aleurone fractions having a low digestibility in the small intestine, contributed significant amounts of easily fermentable energy and protein to the microflora in the hind-gut.

Increased loss of endogenous faecal nitrogen when fiber is added to the diet may be due to a number of factors. Increased secretion of digestive enzymes (trypsin, chymotrypsin, lipase and amylase) has been shown to occur when pectin is added to diets of rats (Foreman and Schneeman 1980). The possibility that fiber might increase the sloughing of intestinal mucosal cells has been suggested (Bergner et al. 1975; Sheard and Schneeman 1980). A lowering of intestinal reabsorption of endogenous amino acids secreted into the gut has been observed with a fiber-supplemented diet (Bergner et al. 1975). Any reduction in intestinal transit time associated with fiber-containing diets could also leave less time for digestion and absorption of dietary protein. Rémesey and Demigné (1989) measured the specific effects of fermentable carbohydrate on blood urea flux and ammonia absorption in the rat caecum. This study suggests that fermentable NSP will affect protein metabolism in the rat significantly.

Conclusion of Experiments with Rats

From experiments with rats it can be concluded that fiber in general has a negative influence on protein digestibility and utilization. However, several purified fiber sources seem to have a less and often insignificant negative effect, while fiber in natural food sources has a much more pronounced effect. The reason for this is certainly that nitrogen/protein associated with CWM is less digestible than regular storage plant proteins. Furthermore, antinutritional factors are often associated to the fiber-rich parts of plant foods, and this has a negative effect on protein utilization. The influence of fiber is strongly determined by the chemical composition of the DF fraction. Fermentable fiber in the digestive tract will be a better energy source for the micro flora than less fermentable DF—and thus more nitrogen will be built into microbial protein and thus escape absorption.

Experiments with Pigs

The fistulated pig is a frequently used animal model when studying the significance of the micro flora in the digestive tract on the utilization of various nutrients. Since the fistulation technique on pigs has become routine more detailed information can be obtained as sampling of digesta can be performed at various sites of the digestive tract (Low and Zebrowska 1989). As the microbial activity primarily is located to the hind-gut (Bach Knudsen et al. 1990) it is convenient to be able to sample digesta prior to this organ. By comparing values obtained on digesta collected at the terminal ileum with values obtained on faecal material, a good estimate of the influence of the microbial activity on various nutrients can be obtained since dietary fiber can be metabolized only through microbial fermentation, under the use of nitrogen, this model will give detailed information concerning the influence of dietary fiber on protein digestion and utilization.

The catabolic activities of the bacteria in the large intestine are closely related to the inflow of nitrogenous compounds which leave the ileum. These consist partly of undigested dietary residues but also substantial amounts of endogenous proteins from epithelial cells mucus, as well as urea and bacteria (Zebrowska et al. 1977; Low 1979).

The anabolic processes of the microflora are as dependent on available substrates as are the catabolic processes. The bacterial requirements for their own cell components and secretions are largely met by urea, ammonia, amino acids, and peptides, together with a suitable energy source—usually carbohydrate and mostly in the form of non-starch polysaccharides. The quantitative importance of this activity is indicated by the observation that 60–80 percent of faecal N in pigs appears to be bacterial (Mason et al. 1976; Low et al. 1978; Meinl and Kreienbring 1985). More recently, Mason et al. (1982) found that substitution of one third of the cereal in a high-barley diet with grass meal increased faecal and bacterial N output by 60 and 63 percent, respectively, resulting in a low protein digestibility.

Infusion of starch into the caecum of pigs given a barley-meat and bone meal diet (Zebrowska et al. 1980) depressed faecal apparent digestibility of nitrogen by 3–4 percentage units, and of amino acids by 4–7 units, compared with the control group. N excretion in the urine was reduced, and N balance was unaffected, indicating that the route of nitrogen excretion was modified by starch and that microbial growth and metabolism was limited by the available energy supply. When cellulose rather than starch was infused into the caecum of pigs, however, little effect on digestibility of N was observed (Zebrowska et al. 1978) because of its low fermentability.

Den Hartog et al. (1988) compared the effects of different carbohydrate sources on amino acid digestibility. They substituted 50 g/kg of a basal diet containing corn, barley, soybean meal, and meat meal with either pectin, cellulose, or ground straw (as a lignin-rich source). All amino acids (except arginine) were digested to a lower extent when straw meal was incorporated in the diet. There was no statistically significant effect of either pectin or cellulose inclusion on ileal amino acid digestibility. However, Dierick et al. (1983) found that the addition of pectin and sugar beet pulp had a much larger effect on ileal digestibility of essential and nonessential amino acids than addition of cellulose. There was a considerable reduction in digestion of the nutrients at the ileal level dependent on source and level of fiber. The influence of pectin and dried sugar beet pulp was much more pronounced than cellulose. The significant reduction in digestion of dry matter, protein and amino acids amounted to 10 to 15 units at the ileal level. The effect in the faeces was greatly reduced, illustrating the importance of hind-gut fermentation.

The referred works with fistulated pigs demonstrate an excellent model for studying the fate of undigested protein in the large bowl of monogastric animal and man and the importance of NSP in this respect.

Conclusion of Experiments with Pigs

The referred experiments with pigs demonstrate a similar negative influence of dietary fiber on protein digestibility and utilization as in rats. Purified fiber sources of low fermentability have a much lower negative effect than more fermentable fibers in natural foods. This is probably due to associated factors as antinutritional components in common feed and foodstuffs.

Experiments with Man

In most studies of the effects of fiber on humans, cereal fibers were given (Gallaher and Schneeman 1986). However, Stephen and Cummings (1980) showed that cabbage fiber, which is extensively broken down, provides a readily usable substrate for the stimulation of microbial growth, whereas wheat fiber remains largely undigested and retains water in the gut lumen. These authors compared the effect of 18 g fiber given as wheat bran or as cabbage to a control diet. The changes seen with cabbage fiber were quite different. Among other changes nitrogen excretion increased from 1.5 g to 2.1 per day.

Cabbage fiber influences colonic function through its stimulation of microbial growth. Analysis of the bacterial fraction for nitrogen in the study of Stephen and Cummings (1980) showed that 0.42 g of the 0.67 g per day (63%) increase in nitrogen excretion is associated with this fraction, whereas with wheat fiber only 0.18 g of the 0.53 g (34%) increase is in the bacteria. Two distinct mechanisms thus emerge whereby fiber affects the human colon. Stephen and Cummings (1980) assume that the stimulation of microbial growth is the more usual one in man because very little fiber survives digestion by the bacteria when sources such as apple, carrot, guar, pectin or mixed diets are fed. Wheat fiber and most cereals in general, may prove to be the exception as they have small cells with highly lignified cell walls which resist digestion. The rest of the nitrogen is presumably present in the undigested cell wall material.

Kelsay et al. (1981) studied the effects of diets containing fruits and vegetables as sources of DF. A low DF diet was compared to three diets containing increasing levels of fiber in fruits and vegetables. Nitrogen digestibilities decreased from 89.9% on the low fiber diet (1.9 g/d) to 81.2% on the high fiber diet (25.6 g/d) containing the highest amount of fruits and vegetables. Apparent digestibility of NDF was in the range of 30 to 40% for all diets and did not differ significantly. This indicates an active microbial protein fermentation which can explain the decreasing nitrogen digestibility with increasing fiber in the diets.

Legumes in general have a low protein digestibility (Beames and Eggum 1981). This was also confirmed in studies on man by Radha and Geervani (1984). They gave three cereal legume diets differing in NDF content to women in a balance study. Three groups were given a low fiber diet, a normal diet or a high fiber diet. In this study the mean faecal excretion of nitrogen on the low fiber diet was 2.13 g/d, while it was 2.50 g/d on the normal diet and 4.21 g/d on the high fiber diet. The results indicate strict adverse influence of fiber on nitrogen utilization. The study of Radha and Geervani (1984) demonstrates that dietary fiber might adversely affect the protein situation of a population when protein supply is marginal. Kaneko et al. (1986) thus demonstrated that the negative effect of fiber on apparent protein digestibility was more pronounced on a low protein diet (27 g/d) compared to a high protein diet (67 g/d).

The fate of undigested protein in the colon of man is not so intensively studied as in pigs, although this topic has attracted special interest. Only few data are available concerning the physiological mechanisms which control protein breakdown or amino acid fermentation in vivo. About 50% of normal adults harbour methanogenic bacteria in their large intestine (Miller et al. 1984). The presence of methane producing bacteria would probably alter the end-products formed during protein breakdown.

Protease activities in human ileal effluent are approximately 20-fold greater than in normal faeces of man (Macfarlane et al. 1988). Substantial quantities of proteinaceous material enter the human large intestine (ca. 12 g/d) in the form of a complex mixture of proteins and peptides, that are of both endogenous and dietary origin. In the large gut, these substances are metabolized by the micro flora to produce organic acids, toxic metabolites such as ammonia, phenols and indoles, and the gases hydrogen, carbon dioxide and methane (Macfarlane and Allison 1986). The initial step in protein degradation by bacteria involves hydrolysis of polypeptides and amino acids that are produced and then become available for assimilation.

Conclusion of Experiments with Man

Although less detailed information is available from studies on man compared to rats and pigs concerning the influence of fiber on protein digestion and utilization, very similar conclusions can be drawn. Fiber, especially fiber associated with natural food sources, has a negative influence on protein utilization. The influence depends greatly on the structure and composition of the DF. Soluble DF found primarily in fruits and vegetables is more fermentable than insoluble DF, mainly found in cereals, and will as such stimulate microbial growth resulting in a relatively high excretion of microbial proteins together with undigested protein.

General Conclusion

In the present study the current knowledge of the effects of dietary fiber and associated components on protein digestibility and utilization are discussed. Results from rats, pigs and humans are included. Although it is not fully understood how DF affects the utilization of various nutrients, it can be concluded that the implications and the mechanisms behind the effect of soluble and insoluble DF on protein digestibility and utilization are quite different. Hence, insoluble DF, because of its low degradability by the microflora will effect increased faecal bulk and faecal nitrogen excretion primarily due to an increased excretion of cell wall bound protein. Contrary to this, soluble DF increases faecal bulk and faecal nitrogen due to an increased excretion of microbial nitrogen. The overall effect of both mechanisms is a decrease in apparent protein digestibility. Furthermore, antinutritional factors are often associated to the fibrous parts of plant foods, which can have additional negative effect on protein digestibility and utilization.

A matter of controversy is the influence of DF on endogenous nitrogen excretion and factors affecting the losses of nitrogen in this way. Although it is now widely recognized that very substantial amounts of protein are secreted into the digestive tract, it is not known if fiber as a dietary component acts as a secretogogue. Such information could lead to methods of reducing endogenous losses with consequent improved metabolic efficiency of dietary protein. It is still extremely hazardous to distinguish with confidence between dietary and endogenous proteins within the digestive tract, although knowledge of such partition would be helpful in interpreting data on digestibility of dietary proteins. Fundamental studies on the hormonal regulation of endogenous secretions are clearly worthwhile from both fundamental and practical viewpoints.

References

Agarwal, V., Chauhan, B. M., 1989, Effect of feeding some plant foods as source of dietary fibre on biological utilization of diet in rats. *Plant Foods Hum Nutr.* 39:161-167.

Bach Knudsen, K. E., Eggum, B. O., 1984, The nutritive value of botanically mill fractions of barley. 3. The protein and energy value of pericarp, testa, germ, aleuron, and endosperm rich decortication fractions of the variety Bomi. *Z Tierphysiol Tierernährg u Futtermittelkde* 51:130-148.

Bach Knudsen, K. E., Wolstrup, J., Eggum, B. O., 1984, The nutritive value of botanically defined mill fractions of barley. 4. The influence of hindgut microflora in rats on digestibility of protein and energy of pericarp, testa, germ, aleuron and endosperm rich decortication fractions of the variety Bomi. *Z Tierphysiol Tierernährg u Futtermittelkde* 52:182-193.

Bach Knudsen, K. E., Borg Jensen, B., Andersen, J. O., Hansen, I., 1991, Gastrointestinal implications in pigs of wheat and oat fractions. 2. Microbial activity in the gastrointestinal tract. *Br J Nutr* 65:233-248.

Beames, R. M., Eggum, B. O., 1981, The effect of type and level of protein, fibre and starch on nitrogen excretion patterns in rats. *Br J Nutr* 46:301-313.

Bergner, H., Simon, O., Zimmer, M., 1975, Contents of crude fiber in the diet as affecting the process of amino acid resorption in rats. *Arch Tierernährg* 25:95-104.

Breite. S., 1973, Modeluntersuchungen zum Einfluss exogener Faktoren auf die Aminosäuren resorbierbarkeit. Diss (Promotion A), Univ Rostock.

Den Hartog, L. A., Huisman, J., Thielen, W. J. G., Van Schayk, G. H. A., Boer, H., Van Weerden, E. J., 1988, The effect of including various structural polysaccharides in pig diets on ileal and faecal digestibility of amino acids and minerals. *Livestock Prod Sci* 18:157-170.

Dierick, N., Vervaeke, I., Decuypere, J., Henderickx, H.K., 1983, Influence de la nature et du niveau des fibres brutes sur la digestibilité ileale et fécale apparente de la matiére séche, des proteines et des acides aminée et sur la rétention azotée chez les porcs. *Revue de l'agriculture* 36:1691-1712.

Donangelo, C. M., Eggum, B. O., 1985, Comparative effects of wheat bran and barley husk on nutrient utilization in rats 1. Protein and energy. *Br J Nutr* 54:741-751.

Eggum, B. O., 1973, A study of certain factors influencing protein utilization in rats and pigs. *Rep. No 406, Nat Inst Anim Sci, Copenhagen*, pp 1-173.

Eggum, B. O., Beames, R. M., Wolstrup, J., Bach Knudsen, K. E., 1984, The effect of protein quality and fibre level in the diet and microbial activity in the digestive tract on protein utilization and energy digestibility in rats. *Br J Nutr* 51:305-314.

Foreman, L. P., Schneeman, B. O., 1980, Effects of dietary pectin and fat on the small intestinal contents and exocrine pancreas of rats. *J Nutr* 110:1992-1999.

Gallaher, D., Schneeman, B. O., 1986, Effect of dietary fiber on protein digestibility and utilization. In: Spiller, GA (ed) Handbook of Dietary Fiber in Human Nutrition. CRC Press, Boca Raton, Florida, pp. 143-164.

Heaton, K. W., 1980, Dietary fibre in perspective. *Hum Nutr Clin Nutr* 37C:151-170.

Heger, J., Salek, M., Eggum, B. O., 1990, Nutritional value of some Czechoslovak varieties of wheat, triticale and rye. *Anim Feed Sci and Technol* 29:89-100.

Just, A., Jørgensen, H., Fernandez, J. A., 1981, The digestive capacity of the caecum-colon and the value of the nitrogen absorbed from the hind gut for protein synthesis in pigs. *Br J Nutr* 46:209-219.

Kaneko, K., Nishida, K., Yatsuda, J., Osa, S., Koike, G., 1986, Effect of fiber on protein, fat and calcium digestibilities and fecal cholesterol excretion. *J Nutr Sci* 32:317-325.

Kelsay, J. L., Clark, W. M., Herbst, B. J., Prather, E. S., 1981, Nutrient utilization by human subjects concerning fruits and vegetables as sources of fiber. *J Agric Food Chem* 29:461-465

Kritchevsky, D., 1988, Dietary fiber. *Ann Rev Nutr* 8:301-328.

Liener, I. E., Kakade, M. L., 1980, Protease inhibitors. In: Liener, GE (ed) Toxic constituents of plant foods. Academic Press, New York, pp. 7-71.

Low, A. G., 1979, Studies on digestion and absorption in the intestines of growing pigs. 6. Measurements of the flow of amino acids. *Br J Nutr* 41:147-156.

Low, A. G., Sambrook, I. E., Yoshimoto, J. T., 1978, Studies on the true digestibility of nitrogen (N) and amino acids in growing pigs. EAAP 29th Ann Meeting. Stockholm.

Low, A. G., Zebrowska, T., 1989, Digestion in pigs. In: Bock, H-D., Eggum, B. O., Low, A. G., Simon, O., Zebrowska, T., (eds) Protein Metabolism in Farm Animals. Oxford University Press, VEB Deutscher Landwirtschaftsverlag Berlin, pp. 53-121.

Macfarlane, G. T., Allison, C., 1986, Utilisation of protein by human gut bacteria. *FEMS Microbiol Ecology* 38:19-24.

Macfarlane, G. T., Cummings, J. H., Allison, C., 1986, Protein degradation by human intestinal bacteria. *J of General Microbiol* 132:1647-1656.

Macfarlane, G. T., Allison, C., Gibson, S. A. W., Cummings, J. H., 1988, Contribution of the microflora to proteolysis in the human large intestine. *J of Applied Bacteriol* 64:37-46.

Mason, V. C., 1984, Metabolism of nitrogenous compounds in the large gut. *Proc Nutr Soc* 43:45-53.

Mason, V. C., Just, A., Bech-Andersen, S., 1976, Bacterial activity in the hind-gut of pigs. 2. Its influence on the apparent digestibility of nitrogen and amino acids. *Z Tierphysiol Tierernähr u Futtermittelkde* 36:310-324.

Mason, V. C., Kragelund, Z., Eggum, B. O., 1982, Influence of fibre and Nebacetin on microbial activity and amino acid digestibility in the pig and rat. *Z Tierphysiol Tierernährg u Futtermittelkde* 48:241-252.

Meier, H., Poppe, S., 1977, Zum Einfluss der Rohfaser auf die wahre Verdaulichkeit der Aminosäuren. Vth International Symposium on Amino Acids. Budapest.

Meinl, M., Kreienbring, F., 1985, Investigations into the bacterial contribution in pig faeces. *Archiv f Tierernährg* 35:33-44.

Miller, T. L., Weaver, G. A., Wolin, M. J., 1984, Methanogens and anaerobs in a colon segment isolated from the normal fecal stream. *Apppl Environ Microbiol* 48:449-450.

Mongeau, R., Sarwar, G., Peace, R. W., Brassard, R., 1989, Relationship between dietary fiber levels and protein digestibility in selected foods as determined in rats. *Plant Foods Hum Nutr* 39:45-51.

Radha, V., Geervani, P., 1984, Utilisation of protein and calcium in adult women on cereal legume diets containing varying amounts of fibre. *Nutr Rep Intr* 30:859-864.

Radha, V., Geervani, P., 1985, Influence of neutral detergent fibre and protein in Bengal Gram (Cicer arietinum) on the utilization of proteins by albino rats. *J Sci Food Agric* 36:1212-1218.

Raczynski, G., Eggum, B. O., Chwalibog, A., 1982, The effect of dietary composition on transit time in rats. *Z Tierphysiol Tiernährg u Futtermittelkde* 47:160-167.

Rémesy, C., Demigné, C., 1989, Specific effects of fermentable carbohydrates on blood urea flux and ammonia absorption in the rat cecum. *J Nutr* 119:560-565.

Sheard, N. F., Schneeman, B. O., 1980, Wheat bran's effect on digestive enzyme activity and bile acid levels in rats. *J Food Sci* 45:1645-1648.

Stephen, A. M., Cummings, J. H., 1980, Mechanism of action of dietary fibre in the human colon. *Nature* 284:283-284.

Vandergrift, W. L., Knabe, D. A., Thanksley, T. D., Anderson, J., 1983, Digestibility of nutrients in raw and heated soyaflakes for pigs. *J Anim Sci* 57:1215-1224.

Zebrowska, T., 1973, Digestion and absorption of nitrogenous compounds in the large intestine of pigs. *Rocznik Nauk Rolniczych* 95B (3):85-90.

Zebrowska, T., Buraczewska, L., Buraczewski, S., 1977, The apparent digestibility of amino acids in the small intestine and the whole digestive tract of pigs fed diets containing different sources of protein. *Roczniki Nank Rolniczych* 99B, 1:87-98.

Zebrowska, T., Buraczewska, L., Horaczynski, H., 1978, Apparent digestibility of nitrogen and amino acids and utilization of protein given orally or introduced into the large intestine of pigs. *Roczniki Nauk Rolniczych* 99B:99-105.

Zebrowska, T., Zebrowska, H., Buraczewska, L., 1980, The relationship between amount and type of carbohydrates entering the large intestine and nitrogen excretion in faeces and urine of pigs. Proceedings 3rd EAAP Symposium on protein metabolism and nutrition, pp. 222-226. EAAP Publication No 27.

III. Fiber and Cancer

Fiber and Cancer: Prevention Research

Peter Greenwald, M.D., Dr. P.H.,
and Carolyn Clifford, Ph.D.

Introduction

Cancer is the second leading cause of death in the United States; incidence rates for colon and breast cancer are particularly high, with an annual estimate in 1991 of 160,000 new colon cancer cases and 175,000 new breast cancer cases (National Cancer Institute *et al.* 1991). Epidemiologic and carcinogenesis research over the past 20 years strongly suggests a major role for dietary factors in cancer risk. The NCI believes there is substantial evidence that fiber-rich foods and diets high in fiber-containing foods (fruits, vegetables, and cereal grains) are associated with reduced risk of some types of cancers, particularly colorectal cancer and possibly breast cancer. Dietary objectives include increasing the per capita consumption of fiber from grains, fruits, and vegetables from its current level of about 8–12 grams to 20–30 grams daily (U.S. Department of Health and Human Services, 1986).

Tracking the trends in fiber consumption is difficult; however, observations of fiber intake over time are reported through food disappearance and food supply availability data. From 1909 to 1980, food disappearance data showed a decline in intake of grains, while vegetables and fruits remained stable (Welsh *et al.* 1982). From 1909–13 to 1980 availability of total dietary fiber in the food supply fell from 40 to 26.7 g/day per capita from decreased use of cereal grains and potatoes. Crude fiber in the food supply fell from 6.1 g/day per capita during 1909–13 to 4.1 g/day per capita in 1982 (National Academy of Sciences *et al.* 1989). More recent assessments, using data from the Second National Health and Nutrition Examination Survey (NHANES II), estimate that the average American consumes only 0.7 servings of vegetables (1.5 servings when potatoes and salads are included), 0.7 servings of fruit, and 0.3 servings of legumes and nuts per day (Lanza *et al.* 1987). According to the United States Department of Agriculture, the annual per capita consumption of vegetables and fruits increased 23 percent between 1970 and 1985 (Steinmetz *et al.* 1991).

Over the past decade, progress has been documented in awareness that fiber may reduce cancer risk (U.S. Department of Health and Human Services, 1986). A two-part telephone survey of public knowledge, attitudes, and practices related to cancer prevention and risk was conducted by NCI and FDA as part of a long-term effort to help NCI achieve its year 2000 goal of decreasing cancer mortality. Results indicated that significantly more respondents in Wave II of the survey (0.6% in February–April, 1985) than in Wave I (<0.1% in June 1983) believed not eating enough bran or fiber possibly increased their risk of disease. Also, the proportion of the general population who believed that more fiber in the diet can reduce the risk of developing cancer increased significantly from 2.2 percent in Wave I to 5.4 percent in Wave II.

The scientific evidence outlined below is a basis for assessing whether increased fiber consumption can decrease the risk of several cancers and for the recommendations disseminated to the public as the research continues. The direction of the research agenda includes epidemiologic studies that investigate the associations between dietary fiber and cancer and clinical studies between dietary fiber intake and physiological effects and the underlying mechanisms of action.

Research Evidence as the the Basis for Current Recommendations

Fiber Types

Fiber is defined as the components of dietary plant material that cannot be digested by human enzymes (Pilch, 1987) and consist of a heterogenous mixture of complex polysaccharides and nonpolysaccharide polymers. Categorized by differences in chemical structure, major fiber types are celluloses, hemicelluloses, pectins, gums, mucilages, algal polysaccharides, and lignin. Dietary fiber also can be classified according to water solubility. The structural fibers—cellulose, lignin, and some hemicelluloses—are generally insoluble in water and are nonfermentable, while the natural gel-forming fibers—pectins, gums, mucilages, and the remaining hemicelluloses—are water soluble and fermentable. The nonfermentable, insoluble fiber fractions affect intestinal function by retaining water in the stool, thereby increasing fecal bulk and decreasing gastrointestinal transit time. The fermentable, soluble fiber fractions also contribute to the decrease in transit time by stimulating microbial growth in the intestine, which increases the fecal bacterial mass. Additionally, soluble fiber slows glucose absorption and lowers serum cholesterol (Shankar *et al.* 1991).

The major food sources of fiber are fruits, vegetables, and whole grain cereals (U.S. Department of Health and Human Services, 1988). Although food sources of fiber are complex, they may be rich in specific types of fiber. For example, oat bran is rich in water-soluble gums and is a good source of viscous fiber, while wheat bran contains more insoluble fiber. Vegetables and grain products contain large amounts of cellulose; bran cereals and other whole grain products are the most concentrated sources of hemicellulose; and apples and citrus fruits contain a large amount of pectin (Council on Scientific Affairs, 1989). A summary of the major benefits and sources of the various soluble and insoluble fiber components is presented in Table 1.

Fiber and Colorectal Cancer

Epidemiology. Burkitt in the early 1970's observed that the incidence of colon cancer is rare in most African populations, where a high fiber diet is consumed, and widespread in Western populations, where fiber consumption is relatively low (Burkitt, 1971). The observations made by Burkitt led to numerous epidemiologic studies, as well as experimental and clinical studies that generally demonstrate that the risk of colon cancer and possibly other cancers may be lowered by increasing consumption of foods high in dietary fiber. More recent evidence indicates that fiber may modulate the risk-enhancing effects of fat and/or hormonal influences (Rose *et al.* 1991; Shankar *et al.* 1991; Rose, 1992).

Table 1. The benefits and examples of good sources of both soluble and insoluble fiber

	Soluble fiber	Insoluble fiber
Natural fiber components	Gums, mucilages, pectins, some hemicelluloses	Cellulose, lignins, some hemicelluloses
Benefits	May help in reducing blood cholesterol and controlling blood glucose levels	May help prevent colon cancer. Helps prevent constipation.
Good sources	Oat bran, beans (navy, kidney, pinto, or lima), barley, vegetables, and fruits	Whole-wheat bread, beans (navy, kidney, pinto, or lima), cereals, and the skins of vegetables and fruits

The hypothesis that dietary fiber is protective against colon cancer is generally corroborated by time-trend correlational studies and international comparisons of dietary fiber intake and colon cancer incidence and mortality rates (U.S. Department of Health and Human Services, 1988; Greenwald et al. 1987). An inverse relationship between dietary fiber, fiber-rich diets, or other measures of fiber consumption and colon cancer was seen in 6 of 7 international correlational studies, with the remaining study not showing any relationship. However, the relationships often disappear or are reduced when other dietary factors, such as dietary fat or cholesterol, are controlled. Conversely, when fiber intake was included in a correlational analysis between total fat consumption and colon cancer incidence, the magnitude of the fat-colon cancer relation was reduced (Hursting et al. 1990). One of the 6 studies that found a protective effect of total dietary fiber also showed a protective effect specifically for cereal fiber, even after adjusting for intake of total fat and animal fat and red meats (McKeown-Eyssen et al. 1984).

An analysis of 37 observational epidemiologic studies published between 1970 and 1988 found that the majority of the studies (21 studies, or 57%) supported a strong-to-moderate protective effect for high-fiber intake against colon cancer. A meta-analysis of data from 16 of the 23 case-control studies further supported a protective effect from the consumption of fiber-rich diets, with an estimated combined odds ratio of 0.57 [95% confidence interval = (0.50, 0.64)] when highest and lowest quartiles of fiber intake were compared. Risk estimates based on vegetable consumption were only slightly more protective (O.R. = 0.48) than those based on an estimate of fiber intake (O.R. = 0.58). However, these data do not differentiate between the protective effects of fiber and non-fiber constituents found in vegetables (Trock et al. 1990).

A review of the epidemiologic studies conducted since 1980 showed that of 17 case-control studies on fiber and colon cancer, 12 showed an inverse association, 3 showed no association, and 2 showed a positive association. The protective effect of fiber was enhanced when adjusting for fat or calories in five studies; three studies showed no change; the adjustment was not performed in the remainder of the studies. This evidence suggests that the protective effect of fiber represents more than confounding with fat or calories (Shankar et al. 1991).

Some case-control studies have found inverse associations between intake of grain fiber and colon cancer (Freudenheim et al. 1990), while others have found a protective effect for colon cancer only from a high intake of vegetables and fruits and crude fiber, but not grains (Slattery et al. 1988). The recent prospective study by Willett found a dose-response decrease in risk of colon cancer incidence with increased intake of fruit fiber. In this study total dietary fiber, total crude fiber, vegetable fiber, and cereal fiber were not as clearly associated with risk (Willett *et al.* 1990). In contrast, a recent prospective study of nearly 7,300 men from the Health Professional Followup Study found that fiber from three sources—vegetables, fruits, and grains—was associated with decreased risk for colorectal adenomas, frequently precursors of cancer (Giovannucci *et al.* 1992). Increases in colon cancer risk with high intake of dietary fiber and association between colon cancer and crude fiber intake have also been reported (Jain *et al.* 1980; Potter *et al.* 1986).

Biases inherent in the conduct of epidemiologic studies may partially account for inconsistent results. These biases include difficulties in measuring and estimating the fiber content in food, the availability and accuracy of food composition data, correlations among nutrients within food, and selection bias (Trock *et al.* 1990). Early epidemiologic studies focused on foods and food groups high in fiber rather than fiber per se (Welsh *et al.* 1982) or have used measures of crude fiber content of foods rather than total dietary fiber to estimate fiber intakes—crude fiber represents only about one-fourth to one-third of the total fiber in foods. Further difficulties include lack of a standard chemical definition of fiber and differing methods of food intake assessment (Bingham, 1987). The NCI is completing the development and improvement of analytical methods for the detection and quantification of significant dietary fiber sources in the American diet to refine the reliability across studies of these types of data.

Animal Studies. Animal studies examining the role of various dietary fibers as colon cancer inhibitors have provided mixed results. However, this may mainly be due to methodological variations across studies, such as differences in the nature and amount of carcinogens used to induce tumors, differences in the susceptibilities of rodent strains to carcinogens, and differences in experimental diet compositions (Nigro *et al.* 1987; Reddy, 1986). In a review of these animal models, Reddy concluded that, overall, the results suggest that the inhibitory effect on colon tumors depends on the type of fiber, and that wheat bran inhibits colon tumor development more consistently than any other type of fiber in animal models (Reddy, 1986). However, the relevance of animal models to human cancer cannot be assumed.

Mechanisms. Several mechanistic hypotheses whereby dietary fiber may be protective against colon cancer appear biologically plausible—increasing fecal bulk, which can both dilute fecal mutagen concentration and increase the transit time of fecal material through the colon so that carcinogens have a shorter duration of contact with colonic mucosa; altering the metabolic activities and composition of gut microflora, which can affect the production of initiators and promoters of colon tumors; influencing cell proliferation rates; altering bile acid metabolism;

or reducing fecal pH (Reddy, 1986; Reddy, 1987).

The effects of supplemental fiber on fecal mutagens and bile acids were studied in 19 volunteers, who consumed a high-fat, moderately low-fiber diet, and who were found to secrete high levels of mutagens, which are thought to be important in the pathogenesis of colon cancer. Their normal (control) diet was supplemented with 10 g of dietary fiber from, alternately, wheat bran, oat fiber, or cellulose for 5-week periods, followed by the control diet was consumed after each fiber supplementation period. The concentrations of fecal secondary bile acids and fecal mutagenic activity were significantly lower during the wheat bran and cellulose supplementation periods, but no effect was detected with oat bran supplementation (Reddy *et al.* 1989).

Recent clinical metabolic studies have examined fecal bulk, fecal mutagenic activity, and concentrations of secondary bile acids (deoxycholic acid and lithocholic acid) in various populations in a range of fiber intakes. A study comparing a New York population at high risk for colon cancer with rural Kuopio, Finland, which has one of the lowest colon cancer incidence rates in Europe and a high-fiber and high-fat intake, suggested that of high dietary fiber consumption increases fecal bulk, thereby diluting bile acids, which have tumor-promoting activity (Reddy *et al.* 1978). The possible protective role of fiber also was supported in a study of adult men in Copenhagen, Denmark, and rural Kuopio, Finland, where dietary fat intake levels is similar, but the fiber intake in Copenhagen is half that consumed in Kuopio, and the colon cancer incidence rate is four times greater in Copenhagen than in Kuopio. This study demonstrated that stool weights were higher in the low colon cancer incidence group (MacLennan *et al.* 1978). A further study, consisting of 30 randomly selected men from four areas in Denmark and Finland indicated that a population may have a low colon cancer risk despite a high intake of dietary fat, protein, and meat, and that high carbohydrate and fiber intake may be protective (Jensen *et al.* 1982).

Clinical Trials. Human intervention trials are expected to resolve many of the questions concerning the protective effect of dietary fiber for reducing the risk of colon cancer. Several fiber intervention studies are using protocols that include adenomas, precursor lesions of large bowel cancer. A successful 4-year, randomized, double-blind, placebo-controlled trial demonstrated the inhibition of benign polyps in 58 patients with Familial Adenomatous Polyposis (FAP), a heritable disease that progresses to cancer in almost all cases if left untreated. The results showed that the number and size of the polyps decreased in patients whose diets were supplemented with more than 11 g fiber/day (for a total of 22.5 g fiber/day). Vitamin E and C supplements also were administered, alone or with the fiber supplement; however, no significant effect was observed for the vitamins alone (Decosse et al. 1989). More recently, Alberts and his group have examined the effects of dietary fiber supplementation on rectal epithelial cell proliferation, a marker of carcinogenesis for colorectal cancer. In this small pilot study, [$_3$H]-thymidine labeling index data suggest that 13.5 g/day of a wheat bran fiber dietary supplement inhibited rectal mucosa cell proliferation in a high-risk study group (Alberts et al. 1990).

Results from experimental and clinical research form the basis for the NCI Polyp Prevention Trial, a multi-institute randomized controlled study designed to determine whether a low-fat, high-fiber, and vegetable- and fruit-enriched eating plan will prevent the recurrence of large bowel adenomatous polyps in subjects who have undergone polypectomy but are otherwise healthy individuals. The protocol for this clinical trial is based on the fact that large bowel adenomas are highly prevalent, occurring in 30 percent of middle-aged and older adults; the polyp recurrence rate is high in those individuals who have undergone surgical polyp removal; and the strong association between colon polyps and the development of colon cancer. The subjects in this trial will be followed for 4 years, and the recurrence of polyps will be assessed in both the intervention and control groups at year 1 and year 4 to determine the effects of this dietary intervention on the polyp recurrence rate.

Fiber and Breast Cancer

Experimental Studies. Several studies have investigated the role of fiber-rich foods in protecting against breast cancer. A meta-analysis of the original data of 12 case-control studies was conducted in populations with very different breast cancer risks and dietary habits. After adjusting for total fat intake, there was a significant decrease in breast cancer risk among women in the highest quintile of dietary fiber intake compared to women in the lowest quintile of fiber intake. When the analysis was stratified by menopausal status, similar decreases in risk were observed, although the decrease was statistically significant only among post-menopausal women. However, when fiber, beta-carotene, and vitamin C were analyzed together in the same model in order to estimate the independent effects of each, only vitamin C remained statistically significant in its association with decreased breast cancer risk (Howe et al. 1990).

In a review of individual case-control studies (four of these studies were included in the meta-analysis previously described) that examined the association between breast cancer risk and intake of fiber or fiber-rich foods, six out of seven studies reported inverse relationships. Three of these studies indicated that diets high in fiber and/or cereal reduced the risk of breast cancer, and an additional study suggested a weak protective effect of fiber constituents in vegetables. In five of these seven studies, the relationship between fiber and/or vegetable consumption and breast cancer was stronger than the association with dietary fat intake (Shankar *et al.* 1991). A recent case-control study not included in this review found an inverse association between breast cancer and intake of fiber, even after adjusting for potential confounders. Women in the lowest quartile for consumption of cereal products, beta-carotene, fruits, vegetables, or all vegetable products combined, were at greatest risk of developing breast cancer (Van't-Veer *et al.* 1990).

Very few animal studies examining the effect of fiber on mammary carcinogenesis have been conducted. An early study suggested that a high-fiber diet reduces the incidence of mammary tumors in rats (Carroll *et al.* 1971). Recently a study assessed this possibility directly and demonstrated that supplemental fiber inhibits the promotional phase of MNU-induced mammary carcinogenesis in rats fed a high-fat diet, but not in those fed a low-fat diet (Cohen *et al.* 1991).

Mechanisms. Fiber is thought to modify the biologic actions of hormones, such as lowering circulating levels of estrogen, and may therefore reduce the risk of breast cancer, a hormone-related cancer (Adlercreutz, 1990). The mechanism through which fiber lowers circulating levels of estrogens is not fully understood, although it most likely involves estrogen metabolism and bioactivity, both possibly affecting on the enterohepatic circulation of estrogens and the actions of fiber-associated phytoestrogens (Rose *et al.,* 1990; Rose, 1990).

A review of studies examining the connection between diet and systemic sex hormones reported that a high total fiber intake, and high intakes of vegetable fiber, grain fiber, and fiber from fruits and berries were associated with low levels of testosterone, estrone, androstenedione and plasma percent free estradiol and free testosterone. These high fiber intakes also are associated with high levels of sex hormone-binding globulin (SHBG), the protein to which estradiol is bound (Adlercreutz, 1990).

Two small clinical studies compared healthy omnivorous and vegetarian women and women with breast cancer. One study examined only the postmenopausal women in these study groups and found that the postmenopausal women with breast cancer consumed significantly less total fiber, nongrain fiber, and grain calories than women in the other two groups, and had higher plasma levels of androstenedione, testosterone, and free testosterone, and lower plasma concentrations of SHBG than women in either of the two control groups (Adlercreutz *et al.* 1989). The second study examined only premenopausal women in these groups and found the main dietary difference to be a low intake of grain products and grain fiber among the breast cancer patients compared with the omnivorous and vegetarian control women. Estrogen production and urinary estrogen profiles did not differ among the three groups, with the exception of a lower 4-hydroxyestrone (4-OH-E1) excretion and higher urinary 2-OH-E1 to 4-OH-E1 ratio, a ratio which appears to depend on diet, among the premenopausal breast cancer women when compared with the control women (Adlercreutz *et al.* 1989).

High dietary fat intake associated with high circulating estrogen concentrations, a possible risk factor for breast cancer, was shown to be favorably modified by a high fiber intake. The daily diets of 62 premenopausal women were supplemented with 15 g wheat, corn, or oat bran to increase their daily fiber consumption from 15 g to 30 g/day, with no significant decrease in daily dietary fat consumption. The wheat-bran supplemented group demonstrated significant reductions at two months in serum estrone and estradiol, but no change in serum progesterone or SHBG concentrations. No changes in serum estrones were seen in women supplemented with oat or corn bran (Rose *et al.* 1991).

Phytoestrogens, compounds with estrogenic activity, occur naturally in many edible plants and may exert an antiestrogenic effect by competing with estradiol for estrogen receptors in breast tissue and, thus, may beneficially affect breast cancer risk (Rose, 1992). A recent case-control study of diet and breast cancer in Singapore showed decreased risk to be associated with high intake of soy products, which are rich in precursors for biosynthesis of equol, a potent phytoestrogen (Lee *et al.* 1991). Fiber may also interfere with breast tumorigenesis through the formation of mammalian lignans, estrogen-like compounds that result from structural modifications of plant lignans by intestinal microflora (Adlercreutz, 1990). Urinary excretion of the two lignans enterolactone and enterodiol has been found to be positively associated with fiber intake and is significantly reduced in breast cancer patients (Adlercreutz *et al.* 1982). Overall, the limited data concerning the relationship between dietary fiber and breast cancer indicate that the degree of protection due to fiber intake from whole grains, fruits, and vegetables is unclear, and that the exact mechanism by which fiber may act is unknown.

A limited number of studies have demonstrated protection from consumption of fiber-rich foods against cancer of the esophagus, mouth, pharynx, stomach, rectum, endometrium, and ovary (Shankar *et al.* 1991).

Publicizing the Message

NCI Interim Guidelines as a First Step. Although a causal relationship between high fiber intake and reduced risk of cancer has not been unequivocally established, NCI believes it is prudent to provide dietary guidelines to increase fiber intake as the research continues. The NCI first published general dietary guidelines for cancer risk reduction in

1979. The guidelines advocated reducing total fat, increasing consumption of dietary fiber and vegetables and fruits, avoiding obesity, and using alcohol only in moderation. In 1980, NCI commissioned the National Research Council (NRC) of the National Academy of Sciences (NAS) to conduct a comprehensive review of the scientific information about diet, nutrition, and cancer and, if justified, to develop interim dietary guidelines for the public consistent with good nutritional practices and cancer risk reduction. This study resulted in the report by the committee on diet, nutrition, and cancer published by NAS in 1982. The report concluded that although it may never be possible to specify a diet that would protect everyone against all forms of cancer, interim dietary guidelines for the public would be prudent on the strength of existing evidence (National Academy of Sciences *et al.* 1982). The current NCI Dietary Guidelines for cancer prevention were derived in part from the NAS report and were augmented by NCI workshops and a comprehensive review of the data on dietary fiber. The current NCI guideline for dietary fiber, issued in 1987, recommends intake of 20 to 30 grams per day, not to exceed 35 grams (Butrum *et al.* 1988).

Cooperation With Industry. Governments, industry, and the research community need to work together to provide the soundest nutritional information available. At present, our practical knowledge related to reducing diet-related cancer may rest largely in the area of dietary change. In 1984, the Kellogg Company, using fiber statements endorsed by the NCI, began an advertising campaign about the possible benefits of a high-fiber, low-fat diet for preventing some types of cancer. Both Kellogg and non-Kellogg high-fiber cereals increased market share as a result of this campaign (Levy *et al.* 1987). During the period of the campaign, the Kellogg Company and NCI's Cancer Prevention Awareness Campaign favorably modified American dietary patterns by these efforts. Positive findings were documented in Wave II of the Cancer Prevention Awareness Survey and in the FDA/NHLBI survey. Purchasing behavior change was observed in the food sales data from Giant food stores.

Tracking of phone calls to the Cancer Information Service (CIS) further confirmed that the Kellogg campaign was reaching the public. Both cereal box messages and television commercials resulted in dramatically increased use of the CIS toll-free phone number. The Kellogg/NCI collaboration also increased advertising of high-fiber products by other cereal companies. Furthermore, eight new bran cereal products were introduced, and fiber became a selling point for other food products, notably fruits, beans, and bread (Freimuth *et al.* 1988).

Food Labeling. The Kellogg campaign reopened the FDA issue regarding health claims on food labels. In 1938 by congressional mandate, the Food, Drug, and Cosmetic Act determined that health claims for foods or food constituents classified them as drugs, thus subjecting the substance or food containing the substance to the safety and efficacy testing requirements of the drug law (U.S. Food and Drug Administration, 1991). Since FDA permitted Kellogg to continue their successful high-fiber campaign, other food companies began using food/health claims to promote their products. Numerous groups then began pressuring the FDA to issue guidelines for these health claims (Freimuth *et al.* 1988).

In 1987, the FDA formalized its approval of the use of health claims by issuing criteria for their use on food labels. The FDA has determined that the criteria were not specific enough to prevent misleading claims and thus proposed to re-evaluate the evidence for health claims. This re-evaluation, the controversy surrounding the misleading food labels, and the potential for nutrition education on food labels led to the introduction and passage of the 1990 Nutrition Food Labeling and Education Act. Ten diet-disease relationships have been identified for health claim examination, including fiber and cancer. Responses to the published proposed regulations are being evaluated. Final regulations are due in November, 1992 (U.S. Food and Drug Administration, 1991).

NCI strongly endorses health claims on foods and food labeling for fiber-containing foods such as fruits, vegetables, and whole grains, but does not endorse health claims on the labeling of dietary fiber supplements primarily because the supporting research is based largely on foods that contain naturally occurring fiber. Further, NCI has expressed support of third party endorsements in the form of government/private sector partnerships for health messages (with appropriate caveats—scientific standards, internal clearance procedures, and legal counsel) for their demonstrated impact on favorably changing attitudes and behavior regarding diet and health.

Directions in Research

From 1974 to 1990 the funding for diet and cancer research in the Division of Cancer Prevention and Control increased from 3 million to 67 million dollars. About 5 million of this current amount is allocated to dietary fiber and cancer research. A survey of the publication dates cited in three comprehensive reviews (Shankar *et al.* 1991; Greenwald *et al.* 1987; Trock *et al.* 1990) indicates that the number of studies examining the relationship between dietary fiber and cancer risk has more than doubled over the past two decades. A shift in the type of study conducted has also occurred. Fewer international correlation studies are published in comparison to case-control and metabolic epidemiologic studies, representing a natural progression of citing possible relationships on a population level to testing those relationships at the level of the individual, and then investigating potential biological mechanisms of the relationships.

Investigator-initiated research is the core of NIH-sponsored research. One of the mechanisms through which NCI supports this research is through Clinical Nutrition Research Units (CNRUs), which bring together laboratory and clinical investigators to enrich the effectiveness of research in nutritional science and related metabolic disorders through multidisciplinary approaches. The CNRUs are established at institutions that have in place ongoing, independently supported, peer-reviewed research programs in nutritional science. Other ongoing clinical research includes the multicenter Polyp Prevention Trial, described earlier; the analysis of dietary fiber and fiber components in food; a comparison in humans of the physical properties, chemical compositions, and biological effects of three different sources of dietary fiber; a clinical chemoprevention trial of adenomatous polyp recurrence with wheat bran fiber supplementation in subjects at high risk for colorectal cancer; and a diet, estrogen, and breast cancer study assessing the effects of three experimental diets—low-fat/high-fiber, high-fat/low-fiber, and high-fat/high-fiber—on plasma estrogens, androgens, SHBG, prolactin, progesterone, and 2-hydroxyestrone. Furthermore, health promotion projects to promote cancer prevention dietary changes are being conducted at worksites and in certain minority populations.

The numerous epidemiologic studies supporting the hypothesis that a diet high in fiber decreases the risk of colon cancer needs to be corroborated by controlled clinical trials. Basic research studies to achieve a better understanding of the determinants of protection from fiber sources are needed. Although it appears that consumption of fiber-rich foods may be protective against certain cancers, more research is needed on whether these effects are due to the dietary fiber component in general, or to specific fiber types, or to other constituents, such as micronutrients, within these foods. Standardization of the methods for the collection and analysis of dietary data may allow better distinction of the effects of the various components in high-fiber foods on cancer prevention.

References

Adlercreutz, H., 1990, Diet, breast cancer, and sex hormone metabolism, *Ann. NY Acad. Sci.* 595:281-290.

Adlercreutz, H., 1990, Western diet and Western diseases: Some hormonal and biochemical mechanisms and associations, *Scand. J. Clin. Lab. Invest.* 50:3-23.

Adlercreutz, H., Fostis, T., Heikkinen, R., and et al, 1982, Excretion of the lignans enterolactone and enterodiol and of equol in omnivorous and vegetarian post-menopausal women and in women with breast cancer, *Lancet* 2:1295-1299.

Adlercreutz, H., Fotsis, T., Hockerstedt, K., Hamalainen, E., Bannwart, C., Bloigu, S., Valtonen, A., and Ollus, A., 1989, Diet and urinary estrogen profile in pre-menopausal omnivorous and vegetarian women and in premenopausal women with breast cancer, *J. Steroid. Biochem.* 34(1-6):527-530.

Adlercreutz, H., Hamalainen, E., Gorbach, S. L., Goldin, B. R., Woods, M. N., and Dwyer, J. T., 1989, Diet and plasma androgens in postmenopausal vegetarian and omnivorous women and postmenopausal women with breast cancer, *Am. J. Clin. Nutr.* 49:433-442.

Alberts, D. S., Einspahr, J., Rees-McGee, S., Ramanujam, P., Buller, M. K., Clark, L., and et al, 1990, Effects of dietary wheat bran fiber on rectal epithelial cell proliferation in patients with resection for colorectal cancer, *J. Natl. Cancer Inst.* 82:1280-1285.

Bingham, S., 1987, Definitions and intakes of dietary fiber, *Am. J. Clin. Nutr.* 45:1226-1231.

Burkitt, D. P., 1971, Epidemiology of cancer of the colon and rectum, *Cancer* 28:3-13.

Butrum, R. R., Clifford, C. K., and Lanza, E., 1988, Dietary guidelines: Rationale, *Am. J. Clin. Nutr.* 48:888-895.

Carroll, K. K., and Khor, T. T., 1971, Effects of level and type of dietary fat on inci-dence of mammary tumors induced in female Sprague-Dawley rats by 7,12-dimethylbenz(a)anthracene, *Lipids* 6:415-520.

Cohen, L. A., Kendall, M. E., Zang, E., and et al, 1991, Modulation of n-nitroso-methylurea-induced mammary tumor promotion by dietary fiber and fat, *J. Natl. Cancer Inst.* 83:496-500.

Council on Scientific Affairs, 1989, Dietary fiber and health, *JAMA.* 262(4):542-546.

Decosse, J. J., Miller, H. H., and Lesser, M. L., 1989, Effect of wheat fiber and vi-tamins C and E on rectal polyps in patients with familial adenomatous poly-posis, *J. Natl. Cancer Inst.* 81:1290-1297.

Freimuth, V. S., Hammond, S. L., and Stein, J. A., 1988, Health advertising: Pre-vention for profit, *Am. J. Public. Health.* 78(5):557-561.

Freudenheim, J. L., Graham, S., Horvath, P. J., and et al, 1990, Risks associated with source of fiber and fiber components in cancer of the colon and rectum, *Cancer Res.* 50:3295-3300.

Giovannucci, E., Stamfer, M. J., Colditz, G., Rimm, E. B., and Willett, W. C., 1992, Relationship of diet to risk of colorectal adenoma in men, *J. Natl. Cancer Inst.* 84(2):91-98.

Greenwald, P., Lanza, E., and Eddy, G. A., 1987, Dietary fiber in the reduction of colon cancer risk, *J. Am. Diet. Assoc.* 87:1178-1188.

Howe, G. R., Hirohata, T., Hislop, T. G., and et al, 1990, Dietary factors and risk of breast cancer: Combined analysis of 12 case-control studies, *J. Natl. Cancer Inst.* 82:561-569.

Hursting, S. D., Thornquist, M., and Henderson, M. M., 1990, Types of dietary fat and the incidence of cancer at five sites, *Prev. Med.* 19:242-253.

Jain, M., Cook, G. M., Davis, F. G., Grace, M. G., Howe, G. R., and Miller, A. B., 1980, A case control study of diet and colorectal cancer, *Int. J. Cancer* 26:757-768.

Jensen, O. M., MacLennan, R., and Wahrendorf, J., 1982, Diet, bowel function, fecal characteristics, and large bowel cancer in Denmark and Finland, *Nutr. Cancer* 4:5-19.

Lanza, E., Jones, D. Y., Block, G., and et al, 1987, Dietary fiber intake in the U.S. population, *Am. J. Clin. Nutr.* 46:790-797.

Lee, H. P., Gourley, L., Duffy, S. W., Esteve, J., Lee, J. S., and Day, N. E., 1991, Dietary effects on breast-cancer risk in Singapore, *Lancet.* 337:1197-1200.

Levy, A. S., and Stokes, R. C., 1987, Effects of a health promotion advertising campaign on sales of ready-to-eat cereals, *Public. Health. Rep.* 104(4):398-403.

MacLennan, R., Jensen, O. M., Mosbech, J., and Vuori, H., 1978, Diet, transit time, stool weight, and colon cancer in two Scandinavian populations, *Am. J. Clin. Nutr.* 31:S239-S242.

McKeown-Eyssen, G. E. and Bright-See, E., 1984, Dietary factors in colon cancer: International relationships, *Nutr. Cancer* 6:160-170.

National Academy of Sciences, National Research Council, and Committee on Diet, Nutrition and Cancer, 1982, Diet, Nutrition and Cancer National Academy Press, Washington, DC.

National Academy of Sciences, National Research Council, Commission on Life Sciences, and Food and Nutrition Board, 1989, Diet and Health. Implications for Reducing Chronic Disease Risk. National Academy Press, Washington, DC.

National Cancer Institute, and NCI Division of Cancer Prevention and Control, 1991, Cancer Statistics Review: 1973-1988. U.S. Department of Health and Human Services, Public Health Service, National In, Bethesda, MD.

Nigro, N. D., and Bull, A. W., 1987, The impact of dietary fat and fiber on intestinal carcinogenesis, *Prev. Med.* 16:554-558.

Pilch, S., 1987, Physiological Effects and Health Consequences of Dietary Fiber. Federation of American Societies for Experimental Biology, Life Sciences Research, Bethesda, MD.

Potter, J. D., and McMichael, A. J., 1986, Diet and cancer of the colon and rectum: A case-control study, *J. Natl. Cancer Inst.* 76:557-569.

Reddy, B. S., 1986, *Diet and colon cancer: Evidence from human and animal model studies.* In: Diet, Nutrition and Cancer: A Critical Evaluation. Volume 1. Reddy, B. S. and Cohen, L. A., eds. CRC Press, Boca Raton, FL, pp. 47-65.

Reddy, B. S., 1987, Dietary fiber and colon cancer: Animal model studies, *Prev. Med.* 16:559-565.

Reddy, B. S., Engle, A., Katsifis, S., and et al, 1989, Biochemical epidemiology of colon cancer: Effects of types of dietary fiber on fecal mutagens, acid, and neutral sterols in healthy subjects, *Cancer Res.* 49:4629-4635.

Reddy, B. S., Hedges, A. R., Laakso, K., and Wynder, E. L., 1978, Metabolic epidemiology of large bowel cancer: Fecal bulk and constituents in high-risk North American and low-risk Finnish populations, *Cancer* 42:2832-2838.

Rose, D. P., 1990, Dietary fiber and breast cancer, *Nutr. Cancer* 13:1-8.

Rose, D. P., 1992, Dietary fiber, phytoestrogens, and breast cancer, *Nutrition* 8:47-51.

Rose, D. P., and Connolly, J. M., 1990, Dietary prevention of breast cancer, *Med. Oncol. Tumor. Pharmacother.* 7:121-130.

Rose, D. P., Goldman, M., Connolly, J. M., and et al, 1991, High-fiber diet reduces serum estrogen concentrations in premenopausal women, *Am. J. Clin. Nutr.* 54:520-525.

Shankar, S. and Lanza, E., 1991, Dietary fiber and cancer prevention, *Hematol. Oncol. Clin. North. Am.* 5:25-41.

Slattery, M. L., Sorenson, A. W., Mahoney, A. W., and et al, 1988, Diet and colon cancer: Assessment of risk of fiber type and food source, *J. Natl. Cancer Inst.* 80:1474-1480.

Steinmetz, K. A. and Potter, J. D., 1991, Vegetables, fruit, and Cancer I. epidemiology, *Cancer Causes and Control* 2:325-357.

Trock, B., Lanza, E., and Greenwald, P., 1990, Dietary fiber, vegetables, and colon cancer: Critical review and meta-analyses of the epidemiologic evidence, *J. Natl. Cancer Inst.* 82:650-661.

U.S. Department of Health and Human Services, 1988, The Surgeon General's Report on Nutrition and Health. Public Health Service, Washington, D.C., pp. 1-78.

U.S. Department of Health and Human Services, Office of Cancer Communications, NCI, National Institutes of Health, 1986, Management Summary. Cancer Prevention Awareness Survey, Wave II. Public Health Service.

U.S. Department of Health and Human Services, Public Health Service, National Institutes of Health, NCI, 1986, Cancer objectives for the nation: 1985-2000, *NCI. Monographs.*

U.S. Food and Drug Administration, 1991, Food labeling: Health claims; dietary fiber and cancer(21 CFR Part 101 [Docket No.91N-0098], *Fed. Register* 56(229):60566-60578.

Van't-Veer, P., Kilb, C. M., Verhoef, P., and et al, 1990, Dietary fiber, beta-carotene and breast cancer: Results from a case-control study, *Int. J. Cancer* 45:825-828.

Welsh, S. O. and Marston, R. M., 1982, Review of trends in food use in the United States, 1909 to 1980, *J. Am. Diet. Assoc.* 81:120-125.

Willett, W. C., Stampfer, M. J., Colditz, G. A., Rosner, B. A., and Speizer, F. E., 1990, Relation of meat, fat, and their fiber intake to the risk of colon cancer in a prospective study among women, *N. Engl. J. Med.* 323:1664-1672.

Fiber and Cancer: Historical Perspectives

John Higginson, M.D.

Clinical Professor
Department of Community and Family Medicine
Georgetown University Medical Center
Washington, DC 20007

Introduction

Early studies associating fiber with human cancer have been fully documented by Kritchevsky and Klurfeld (1990), Cummings and Bingham (1987), the National Research Council (National Academy of Sciences, 1982), and Leeds (1985, 1990). Accordingly, this paper will be limited to my own perceptions as an oncologist, interested in the causes of human cancer and the developments in dietary carcinogenesis, especially during the fifties and sixties.

Historical views on the association of diet and human cancer are of interest since they significantly influenced concepts on the role of multistage mechanisms and lifestyle factors in carcinogenesis and consequently the orientation of present research on diet and cancer preventative policies.

Customarily, physicians have repeatedly recommended simple, natural diets rich in vegetables to the affluent. The first epidemiological study, carried out over 2,500 years ago, was to test the health benefits of fibrous pulses and vegetables. Samuel Johnson described oats in his dictionary as, "... a grain in England that generally is given to horses, but in Scotland supports the people," to which Boswell replied, "Did you ever see such horses, and such men?" Prevention of constipation has always been linked to the fiber or roughage story. Throughout Victorian times numerous ills were ascribed to this complaint, and appropriate medicines were prescribed by dispensary doctors, at least in Ireland. Oatmeal porridge was considered "good," especially for children, and bowel regularity had a high priority in the Irish and Scottish nursery.

Such anecdotal views on the benefits of fiber continued into the 20th century. In the forties, William Pearson, professor of surgery at Trinity College in Dublin, taught medical students that roughage in the diet was responsible for the low frequency of appendicitis, colitis, and bowel cancer in West Africa. Thus, to my generation, the concept, although nebulous, that roughage, i.e., fiber, was beneficial to health was not completely foreign. Nonetheless, in the mind-set of the mid-20th century, associated with the exciting developments in chemical and viral carcinogenesis, the possibility that dietary components, which were perceived as relatively inert, could indirectly modify neoplastic disease was largely ignored.

Diet and Cancer

Direct Carcinogens

In the thirties, early studies on diet and cancer largely were directed to ingested carcinogens, following work in Japan on certain azo-dyes. Later, research was undertaken on the effects of feeding polycyclic aromatic hydrocarbons (PAH's) in rodents as possible causes of gastrointestinal cancer. These chemicals, which were among the most studied of early carcinogens, were widespread in the environment, for example, in cooked foods. Although intestinal tumors were produced, these studies were relatively unsuccessful, in general, a fact attributed to the relative insolubility of these compounds. It was not until the advent of the N-nitroso compounds in the late 1950's, however, that convenient experimental morphological models of gastro-intestinal cancer became available. Although the role of these compounds in humans still remains obscure, except possibly for stomach, such carcinogens have permitted the experimental investigation of modifying factors, such as bile salts, fiber, and macronutrients.

Nutritional Deficiency and Cancer

This early period of chemical carcinogenesis development coincided with the growth of modern nutritional science. Early nutritional studies, however, were largely directed toward defining an adequate diet, preventing nutritional deficiencies, and establishing the requirements of various micro- and macro-nutrients. The role of diet in chronic disease including cancer received little attention with certain exceptions. Early work in the thirties, however, had demonstrated that riboflavin deficiency was essential to "butter yellow" (DAB) hepatocarcinogenesis in rodents and, later, choline deficiency was reported to cause liver cancer. Accordingly, interest in nutritional deficiency in carcinogenesis began to emerge. The discovery of kwashiorkor, a protein calorie deficiency disease in infants, associated with a fatty liver, in Asia and Africa, led to the attractive hypothesis that this disease was the major factor in explaining the high incidence of liver cancer in such countries. It is ironic to note that the cancers reported in the early choline studies are now considered to have been caused by aflatoxin contamination of the experimental diet used.

The forties had also seen the outstanding studies by Tannenbaum (1945a, 1945b) and Tannenbaum and Silverstone (1957) indicating that excesses of macronutrients and calories enhanced cancer but, in contrast, deficiency inhibited tumors. Nonetheless, the predominant research effort on diet and cancer in the fifties and sixties was driven by the concept of ingested chemical or viral carcinogens. Fear of cancer and the perceived importance, especially in gastro-intestinal cancer, of ingested synthetic chemicals increased and gave rise to the passing, by the U.S. Congress, of the famous Delaney Clause. The general role of diet, including fiber, however, did not arouse great interest, although, in the fifties, researchers began to add fiber to pure experimental diets as it was found to improve the health of rodents.

South African Epidemiological Studies

In 1951, George Oettlé and I established a cancer registry in South Africa covering urban Johannesburg and the rural Transvaal (Higginson and Oettlé, 1960). Our aim was to determine the impact on cancer patterns, especially in the black community in that country, of a rapidly changing environment. These changes included industrialization, ambient pollution, but also a more Western style diet, as compared to a more pastoral lifestyle. In this context, it was decided to document and analyze general cultural, occupational, and lifestyle habits, including dietary and food habits of the community. We were fortunate at this time to have a window of opportunity, as the population was relatively well-served with free medical services and modern hospitals with first-class medical staffs. Alex Walker was also developing the nutritional unit at the SAIMR into an internationally recognized resource and the Gillman brothers were actively emphasizing nutrition in human disease. There appeared to be deficiencies of tumors of the gastrointestinal tract and breast.

The registry was successful and later incidence studies have been confirmatory. In black Africans, cancer of the esophagus, liver, and cervix were very common as compared to Europe and white North Americans. Prostate cancer was about the same as in Denmark but much lower than in American black men.

It was established, after standardization for age and sex, that the colo-rectal cancer frequency in the Bantu was about one-tenth, and stomach cancer was about half that anticipated in the United States and Denmark. We were aware that high rates of colo-rectal cancer were present in most European countries, although somewhat lower in Scandinavia, and the fall in gastric cancer in the United States had already been noted. On the other hand, reports based on relative frequency studies appeared of low frequencies of colo-rectal cancer from other parts of Africa and Asia. In Japan, colo-rectal rates were reported low in contrast to high gastric cancer rates.

It was clear that the causes of esophageal, stomach, and colo-rectal cancers were different. Further, certain differences between rectal and colon cancer were beginning to emerge. It was suggested that some hypothetical carcinogenic stimulus was operating at lower intensity in the Bantu than in Western populations in relation to colo-rectal cancer, the reverse being true for liver and esophagus. There was some evidence that hepatitic viruses were involved in the former and alcoholic beverages in the latter.

Earlier, Walker (1947) had discussed the role of diet on bowel habits in the Bantu. Accordingly, it required no great intellectual effort to make the comment that the Bantu consumed a large amount of roughage with few reports of constipation, and that colo-rectal cancer appeared to be rare in countries with natural diets and large amounts of roughage (Higginson and Oettlé, 1960). In Johannesburg, it was also observed that appendicitis, diverticulosis, and adenoma of the large bowel were also very rare in pathological material (Higginson and Simson, 1958). We only saw one case of diverticulosis in over 789 autopsies over 45 years of age (as compared to about 6% in comparable series in the United States). Only one solitary adenoma of the large bowel was found in our records, which contrasted with European and North American experience.

In a later follow-up, it was pointed out that Bantu stools were more bulky and frequent and the complaint of constipation indicated no more than the frequency of bowel movements had fallen to two or less per day (Oettlé, 1964). It also was suggested that the roughage content of the Bantu diet with the greater use of cereal and physical exercise might explain the lower incidence of rectal cancer. In Uganda, Trowell (1960) pointed out that the African was rarely constipated in the Western sense and consumed a bulky diet that might explain the rarity of bowel diseases and certain chronic diseases that he attributed to Western diets. In India, Malhotra (1967) described variations in bowel cancer and had suggested differences between the north and south parts of the country might be due to the level of cellulose and fiber in the diet. Cleave (1956) was probably the first to formulate such views.

It was clear that a low level of chronic bowel diseases existed over the whole of the African continent south of the Sahara. Whites and other races, for example, the Cape Colored population who lived in these areas, however, showed much higher frequencies, comparable to Europe. These early cancer studies were reported in the United States in 1954 at the same time as the findings on the rareness of atherosclerotic heart disease, which was attributed to the low fat content of the diet.

By this time, we became convinced that these differences were largely environmental and not ethnic. From our registry material we calculated that 70 to 80% of all cancers had an environmental component (Higginson and Oettlé, 1960).

Although we were familiar with the concept of multi-stage carcinogenesis and the growing work on nutrition, our initial impulse had been to attribute cancer variations between countries to the presence of environmental carcinogens, especially man-made. However, we became convinced that diet and lifestyle (including smoking) were the predominant factors involved. However, it was easier to establish incidence rates than etiology, and we pointed out the problems of carrying out appropriate analytical epidemiological studies on lifestyle, especially diet, in view of the lack of a specific hypothesis for testing. It was believed that the number of ill-defined confounding variables was so great as to make studies through traditional methods unsatisfactory until exposures could be measured more accurately. Since liver and esophagus appeared easier to study, especially following the discovery of aflatoxin in 1960, we transferred our interest to that field.

Later Studies

In the early sixties in Kansas, I organized a case history study to cover 340 patients with colo-rectal cancer and 93 patients with cancer of the stomach (Higginson, 1966). Results showed no significant differences from controls in dietary habits for colo-rectal cancer, whereas gastric cancer showed the suspected lower intake of dairy products and fresh fruit and vegetables. No significant differences in bowel habits and laxative use could be demonstrated, although Boyd and Doll (1954) had reported a slight increased association of colon cancer with the use of mineral oil. Laxatives, however, were quite widely used in Kansas.

It was concluded that a carcinogenic risk factor prevalent in the overall environment was involved which could not readily be identified by traditional epidemiological approaches. It was also considered possible that cancer differences might represent variations in susceptibility, rather than in exposures. It was hypothesized that bowel habits including constipation might modify the action of the hypothetical carcinogenic factor either "through mobility, concentration, or dilution." The role of differing dietary oils in modifying experimental PAH carcinogenesis was considered relevant. It was believed unlikely, however, that insoluble hydrocarbons in food were important in colo-rectal cancers in humans, but that, theoretically, water soluble carcinogens might be of greater significance. Despite the negative association of colo-rectal cancer with roughage, we could not, at that time, propose any satisfactory methods for investigating the problem further.

The Kansas survey illustrated the many technological problems in carrying out an epidemiological study on diet and cancer, and others have had similar problems. These include measurement of past dietary intakes and establishing a convincing association with a chronic disease with a long latent period. The difficulty of using any single component to define dietary complexities is well known. Thus, diets high in fiber tend to be low in fat and high in fruits and vegetables which contain high levels of anticarcinogens, carotenes, anti-oxidants, etc. Confounding cannot be avoided.

The Modern Period

In 1971, Burkitt defined several hypotheses susceptible to epidemiological testing. He described in detail the epidemiology of colon cancer, its close relationship with other noninfectious diseases of the bowel and the association of the latter with refined diets characteristic of economic development. His views aroused great interest and resulted in increased studies on fiber and its biological effects.

It is not my intention to discuss these extensive studies, to which many members of this symposium have contributed. Thus the concept of dietary inhibition of cancer became fully established and many hypotheses were advanced relevant to potential mechanisms through which dietary fiber could operate (Hill, 1985; Cummings and Bingham, 1987; Klurfeld, 1992). These include: 1) physical dilution of gut contents, 2) more rapid transit time, 3) protective effects of butyrate on colon epithelium, 4) lower pH, 5) reduced availability of N-compounds through stimulation of bacterial growth, and 6) altered bile acid and metabolism.

Moreover, the modern classifications of fiber or non-starch polysaccharides have been vastly improved so that study of the biological effects of fibers of varying origin is now possible.

Further epidemiological studies have confirmed the low frequency of colo-rectal cancer in Africa and Asia. In North America and part of Europe, slight temporal increases in colon without an increase in rectal cancer have been observed. In contrast, there have been significant increases in both colon and especially rectal cancer in Japan, but also in Japanese migrants to the United States. These changes contrast with the fall in rates in gastric cancer. Further, coronary disease, which is suspected to have some commonality in etiology, has also decreased.

Animal studies to date have been of relatively little assistance in identifying the nature of the relationship between fiber and colon cancer (Angres and Beth, 1990). The chemical compounds of greatest importance in reproducing morphological large bowel cancer in animals still have not been convincingly demonstrated to be significant in humans. Such models tend to use very high doses (almost toxicological) of suspected factors that may not be relevant to human dietary conditions. Thus, such models may be more valuable in providing better tools for studying the molecular biology of colo-rectal disease exploring mechanisms possibly relevant to humans.

It is difficult to see how further epidemiological or ecological studies using traditional techniques will add significant new data, unless individual population groups can be more adequately defined in terms of genetic susceptibility and their lifetime intake of dietary components measured more accurately. While the development of long-term follow-up studies are theoretically attractive, they pose significant logistic problems as dietary patterns change over time. Modification of one nutrient automatically may modify a second with confounding. Certain foods tend to be associated, making the identification of the effects of individual dietary components difficult. It is necessary to distinguish cereal fibers from those in fruits or vegetables. The latter are also associated with increased inhibitory factors (Wattenberg, 1992). Long term prospective studies also will require that susceptible populations be identified at the beginning.

It may be possible to study geographic or ethnic communities differing markedly in incidence and to determine whether or not the differences show any correlation with biomarkers for susceptibility. The use of some of the newer biomarkers, such as mutant *ras* gene, while attractive, may prove expensive and not offer immediate solutions (Sidransky, et al., 1992). Other approaches include attempts to modify diet in individuals with familial polyposis or the follow-up of individuals with adenomas. Again, problems may arise as indicated by the recent report that sigmoidoscopy alone and the removal of an adenoma may impact on mortality rates. Nonetheless, it must be remembered that colo-rectal cancer is unique in that the risk can change during the lifetime of an individual as evidenced by migrant studies (Haenszel, 1982).

Conclusion

My talk has largely referred to colo-rectal cancer since data are even less certain regarding the role of fiber in cancers of the breast and prostate. Such studies are also confounded by fats and other macro-nutrients in the diet. Thus, while I am convinced of the role of diet in cancer of the large intestine and believe fiber almost certainly plays a part, I am disappointed that so far the data remain inconclusive.

The early period of fiber research and enthusiastic acceptance as a preventative is finished and we are entering a period when more cautious interpretations are prevalent and the need for systematic mechanistic studies are appreciated. It must be realized that although much epidemiological investigation supports a causal association in terms of geographical differences, religious variations, temporal changes, etc. there are still inconsistencies which require explanation (Higginson, et al., 1992). Thus, modern studies must attempt to apply a rigorous scientific disciplinary approach to provide hard data to justify public health recommendations and significant modification of an enjoyable habit to which people have become accustomed.

Studies as to the role of fiber continue to be confusing despite increasing technological sophistication and little can be added to the conclusions of the National Academy of Sciences (1982) that the role of fiber in carcinoma of the large intestine "remains far from compelling." In conclusion, the role of dietary components, including fiber, in large intestinal cancer in humans remains uncertain (Higginson et al., 1992).

References

Angres, G. and Beth, M., 1990, Effects of dietary constituents on carcinogenesis in different tumor models, *in:* "Nutrition and Cancer," D. Kritchevsky and R. B. Alfin-Slater, eds., Plenum Press, New York.

Boyd, J. T. and Doll, R., 1954, Gastro-intestinal cancer and the use of liquid paraffin, *Brit J Cancer* 8:231.

Burkitt, D. P., 1971, Epidemiology of cancer of the colon and rectum, *Cancer* 28:3.

Cleave, T. L., 1956, The neglect of natural principles in current medical practice, *J R Nav Med Serv.* 42:55.

Cummings, J. H. and Bingham, S. A., 1987, Dietary fibre, fermentation and large bowel disease, *Cancer Surv.* 6:601.

Haenszel, W., 1982, Contribution of migrant population to study of cancer risk, *in:* "Cancer Prevention in Developing Countries," Proceedings of the first UICC

Conference on Cancer Prevention in Developing Countries, K. Aoki, S. Tominaga, T. Hirayama, and Y. Hirota, eds., University of Nagoya Press, Nagoya.

Higginson, J., 1966, Etiological factors in gastrointestinal cancer in man, *J Natl Cancer Inst.* 37:527.

Higginson, J. and Oettlé, A.G., 1960, Cancer incidence in the Bantu and "Cape Colored" races of South Africa: report of a cancer survey in the Transvaal (1953-55), *J Natl Cancer Inst.* 23:589.

Higginson, J. and Simson, I., 1958, Lesions of the gastro-intestinal tract in the non-white population of South Africa, *Schweiz Zeit Path Bakt.* 21:577.

Higginson, J., Muir, C. and Muñoz, N., 1992, "Human Cancer: Epidemiology and Environmental Causes," Cambridge University Press, Cambridge.

Hill, M. J., 1985, Mechanisms of colorectal carcinogenesis, *in*: "Diet and Human Carcinogenesis," J. V. Joossens, M. J. Hill, and J. Geboers, eds., Excerpta Medica, Amsterdam.

Klurfeld, D. M., 1992, Dietary fiber-mediated mechanisms in carcinogenesis, *Cancer Res.*52(Suppl.):2055s.

Kritchevsky, D. and Klurfeld, D.M., 1990, Dietary fiber and cancer, *in*: "Nutrition and Cancer," D. Kritchevsky, and R. B. Alfin-Slater, eds., Plenum Press, New York.

Leeds, A. R. (ed.), 1985, "Dietary Fibre Perspectives: I," John Libbey & Co., London.

Leeds, A. R. (ed.), 1990, "Dietary Fibre Perspectives: II," John Libbey & Co., London.

Malhotra, S. L., 1967, Geographical distribution of gastro-intestinal cancers in India with special reference to causation, *Gut* 8:361.

National Academy of Sciences, Committee on Diet, Nutrition, and Cancer, Commission on Life Sciences, National Research Council, 1983, "Diet, Nutrition, and Cancer: Directions for Research," National Academy Press, Washington, DC.

National Academy of Sciences, Committee on Diet, Nutrition, and Cancer, Assembly of Life Sciences, National Research Council, 1982, "Diet, Nutrition, and Cancer," National Academy Press, Washington, DC.

Oettlé, A.G., 1964, Cancer in Africa, especially in regions south of the Sahara, *J Natl Cancer Inst.* 33:383.

Sidransky, D., Tokino, T., Hamilton, S. R., Kinzler, K. W., Levin, B., Frost, P. and Vogelsten, B., 1992, Identification of *ras* oncogene mutations in the stool of patients with curable colorectal tumors, *Science* 256:102.

Tannenbaum, A., 1945a, The dependence of tumor formation on the degree of caloric restriction, *Cancer Res.* 5:609.

Tannenbaum, A., 1945b, The dependence of tumor formation on the composition of the calorie-restricted diet as well as on the degree of restriction, *Cancer Res.* 5:616.

Tannenbaum, A. and Silverstone, H., 1957, Nutrition and the genesis of tumours, *in*: "Cancer," Volume 1, R.W. Raven, ed., Butterworth, London.

Trowell, H.C., 1960, "Non-Infective Disease in Africa," Edward Arnold Ltd., London.

Walker, A. R. P., 1947, The effects of recent changes of food habits on bowel motility, *S Afr Med J.* 55:495.

Wattenberg, L. W., 1992, Inhibition of carcinogenesis by minor dietary constituents, *Cancer Res.* 52(Suppl.):2085s.

Dietary Fiber and Colon Cancer Risk: The Epidemiologic Evidence

Tim Byers, M.D., M.P.H.

Centers for Disease Control
Division of Nutrition
1600 Clifton Road, NE
Mailstop K-26
Atlanta, GA 30333

Introduction

Ecological evidence suggests that dietary fiber may protect against cancers, especially cancer of the colon (1–5). Animal experimental evidence for a role of dietary fiber in the prevention of colon cancer is mixed, however (5–7).

Many dietary factors have been hypothesized to be associated with colorectal cancer risk. These include caloric balance, total dietary fat, saturated fat, polyunsaturated fat, anti-oxidant micronutrients including vitamins E, C, and beta-carotene, selenium, calcium, and dietary fiber. This review will examine dietary fiber and fiber-containing foods as factors in colon cancer in case-control and cohort epidemiologic studies.

Methods

All epidemiologic case-control and cohort studies published in the English language were reviewed. Only those case-control studies including 100 or more cases and those cohort studies yielding 50 or more incident cases are included in this review. Likewise, only studies that presented findings for dietary fiber, vegetables, fruits, and/or cereal grain products were included. Because investigators have used many different methods for defining nutrient exposures, presentations in this review were standardized to facilitate comparisons. The measure of association

COLON CANCER AND CEREAL GRAINS

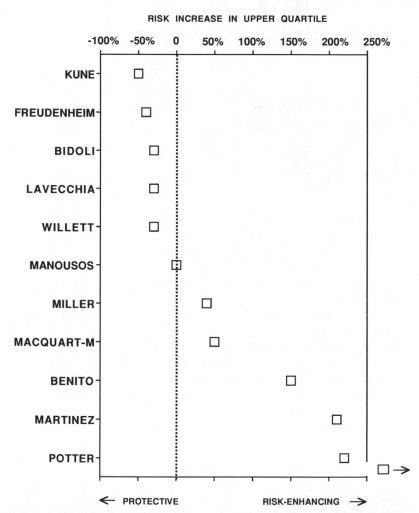

Figure 1. Findings from case-control and cohort studies of colon cancer as related to intakes of fiber and cereal grains. Each point represents the increase in risk for the highest quartile compared to the lowest quartile.

lon cancer risk for the highest category of intake within each study divided by that in the lowest category. For most studies, the highest intake category compared the approximate upper quartile of the distribution of dietary intake, and the lowest category was the approximate lowest quartile. Average values were computed when sex-specific analyses were presented. These estimates of relative risk were then converted to "percent of excess risk" for the highest quartile as compared to the lowest quartile by the formula: "percent excess risk" = (RR-1)100. Because this review is intended to present an overview of the findings of fibers and foods in various studies, this review does not focus on the question of statistical significance of the findings from individual studies, and because of the diversity in study methods, a meta-analytical approach is not used to compute combined quantitative effect estimates.

Results

More studies have shown a protective effect of fibers against colon cancer than have shown a risk-enhancing effect (Figure 1). Many of the effect estimates are very small, however, including the large case-control studies by Miller (20) and Graham (19) and the large cohort study by Willett (17). The two Australian studies are both large and

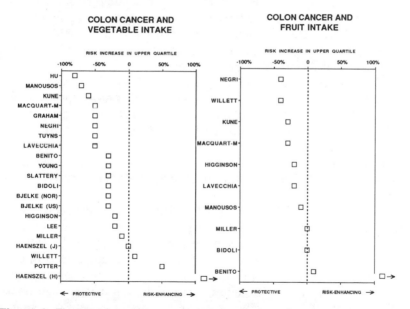

Figure 2. Findings from case-control and cohort studies of colon cancer as related to intakes of vegetables and fruits. Each point represents the increase in risk for the highest quartile compared to the lowest quartile.

seem to have been well-conducted, yet their findings are discrepant (8,23). In studies that have examined the relationship between colon cancer and cereal grain intake, a similar number of studies found increased risk with higher cereal grain intake as have found decreased risk (Figure 1).

As compared to findings for fiber, findings for vegetable intake as related to colon cancer are more consistently in the "protective" direction (Figure 2). The only exceptions are an Australian study (23) and a study of Hawaiian Japanese (33). Another way to contrast the findings for fiber with those for vegetables is to compare their effects in studies that have presented data on both fiber and vegetable intake. Though the pattern of effect for fiber and vegetables is similar, vegetables are slightly more protective than are indices of dietary fiber within those studies (8–11,17,18,20,23). Fruit is also associated with colon cancer in the "protective" direction in most studies (Figure 2). However, contrasting the effects of fruits and vegetables within those studies that have examined both shows that vegetables seem to be more protective against colon cancer than are fruits (8,11,17,20,25–28,30,32).

Discussion

There are many important limitations in epidemiologic studies of fiber intake. The definition of fiber is inconsistent across the set of studies, in part because the quantitative assays differ. Considerable attention has been focused on the problem created by the difference between crude fiber and dietary fiber measurements in foods (36,37). However, this difference is not likely to be a serious limitation in comparing epidemiologic studies because indices of crude fiber and dietary fiber are very highly correlated. Hence, the rank-order of study subjects according to crude fiber is very similar to that for dietary fiber, so effect estimates according to categorized ranking (as in this review) would be similar for crude and dietary fiber. Older studies using crude fiber as the nutrient index are therefore still quite informative for dietary fiber effects.

The more serious limitations of all epidemiologic studies derive from measurement errors of food intake and from the narrow range of fiber intake within populations. Measurement error of dietary intake will tend to bias effect estimates towards a null value. Hence, true effects of even a halving (or doubling) of risk might appear to be very weak effects as estimated in epidemiologic studies. The variation of dietary fiber intake within a population is usually not as great as that seen between populations in ecological studies. Hence, if an effect threshold exists of 15 to 20 grams of dietary fiber, then this effect could not easily be seen when the extreme quantiles compared in a study conducted in a single population might differ by as little as 5 to 10 grams of intake.

An additional problem in epidemiologic studies is the difficulty in interpretation created by multi-variable analysis. Dietary fiber covaries with both micronutrients and macronutrients in the diet. Because all nutrients are found in combinations within foods, observational epidemiologic research is limited by the problem of multi-collinearity between nutrients (38). Estimating food intake, then computing indices of nutrient intake using information on the nutrient content of foods, is a commonly used method to attempt to assess the effects of individual nutrients on cancer risk. However, analyses in which the effects of dietary fiber are estimated in mathematical models containing other nutrient indices derived from the same set of foods can be very hard to interpret. For instance, relative risk estimates for dietary fiber intake are often quite different with and without statistical adjustment for caloric intake or dietary fat (19,34). It is hard to be certain whether the appearance of fiber effects only after statistical adjustment for fat or calories represents a true effect of fiber or whether statistical multi-collinearity accounts for the difference. Multi-variable modeling has created many interpretation problems in nutritional epidemiology which are yet to be resolved. This is a particular problem when we are uncertain of the biologic model we are testing in epidemiologic research, as is often the case in nutritional epidemiology.

It may well be that understanding independent effects of single nutrients is irrelevant to cancer prevention, however, because proper nutrient combinations in the diet are almost certainly needed to resolve cancer risks. The teleological argument seems compelling: that we have evolved with plants as a major source of food, and we therefore evolved to be dependent on a complex mixture of nutrients to maintain our normal state of health. The reductionistic tendencies of the scientific approach to attempt to understand the relationships between nutrition and human biology in a univariate way may therefore fail us in our attempt to understand the relationships between disease risk and the consumption of whole foods in the population.

If the slight reduction in colon cancer incidence in U. S. men seen in recent years continues, there will surely be many who will argue for this as an effect of changes in their favorite factor: decreasing saturated fat intake, increasing fiber intake, and/or increased endoscopic screening. Recent studies suggest that low-dose aspirin intake may have a surprisingly strong protective effect for colorectal cancer (39). Low-dose aspirin has been advocated for coronary heart disease prevention in recent years, and many older Americans, especially men, are taking aspirin in the hope of preventing heart disease. Salicylates naturally present in fruits and vegetables can now be added to the list of possible colon cancer-protective dietary factors.

The goals for the United States for the year 2000 include three important goals to reduce chronic disease risk through improved diet: to reduce obesity prevalence from 26% to 20% of adults, to reduce dietary fat intake from 36% of kilocalories to 30%, and to increase fruit and vegetable intake from 2.5 servings per day to 5 servings per day (40). Achieving this goal of doubling fruit and vegetable intake over the next eight years will require a concerted effort by many sectors of the U. S. society. With endoscopic screening every 5 years, with prophylactic aspirin intake for cardiovascular disease prevention for adults over 50, with a doubling of fruit and vegetable intake in the U. S. diet, and with continued improvements in colorectal cancer treatment, there is every reason to believe that as we begin the 21th century, colorectal cancer will be a condition very much on the decline as a cause of mortality in the United States.

References

1. D. Burkitt. Epidemiology of cancer of the colon and rectum. Cancer 28:3-13 (1971).
2. P. Greenwald, E. Lanza, and G. Eddy. Dietary fiber in the reduction of colon cancer risk. JADA 87:1178-1188 (1987).
3. B. Trock, E. Lanza, and P. Greenwald. Dietary fiber, vegetables, and colon cancer: critical review and meta-analyses of the epidemiologic evidence. JNCI 82:650-661 (1989).
4. R. G. Ziegler. Vegetables, fruits, and carotenoid and the risk of cancer. AJCN 53:251S-259S (1991).
5. M. C. Boutron, M. Wilpart, and J. Faivre. Diet and Colorectal Cancer. European Journal Cancer Prev. 1 (suppl 2), 13-20 (1991).
6. L. R. Jacobs. Fiber and colon cancer. Gastroenterology clinics of North America 17:747-760 (1988).
7. D. Klurfeld. Dietary fiber-mediated mechanisms in carcinogenesis. Cancer Res. 52:2055s-2059s (1992).
8. S. Kune, G. Kune, and L. Watson. Case-control study of dietary etiologic factors: The Melbourne Colorectal Cancer Study. Nutrition and Cancer 9:21-42 (1987).
9. A. Tuyns, M. Haelterman, and R. Kaaks. Colorectal cancer and the intakes of nutrients: Oligosaccharides are a risk factor, fats are not. A case-control study in Belgium. Nutrition and Cancer 10:181-196 (1987).
10. M. L. Slattery, A. W. Sorenson, A. W. Mahoney. Diet and colon cancer: Assessment of risk by fiber type and food source. JNCI 80:1474-1480 (1988).
11. C. La Vecchia, E. Negri, A. Decarli, et al. A case-control study of diet and colo-rectal cancer in Northern Italy. Int J. Cancer 41:492-498 (1988).
12. B. Modan, V. Barell, F. Lubin, et al. Low-fiber intake as an etiologic factor in

cancer of the colon. JNCI 55:15-18 (1975).

13. D. W. West, M. L. Slattery, L. M. Robinson, et al. Dietary intake and colon cancer: sex and anatomic site-specific associations. Am J Epidemiol. 130:883-894 (1989).

14. L. K. Heilbrun, A. Nomura, J. H. Hankin, and G. N. Stemmerman. Diet and colorectal cancer with special reference to fiber intake. Int J Cancer 44:1-6 (1989).

15. A. S. Whittemore, A. H. Wu-Williams, M. Lee, et al. Diet, physical activity, and colorectal cancer among Chinese in North America and China. JNCI 82:915-926 (1990).

16. M. G. De Verdier, U. Hagman, G. Steineck, et al. Diet, body mass and colorectal cancer: A case-referent study in Stockholm. Int J Cancer 46:832-838 (1990).

17. W. C. Willett, M. J. Stampfer, G. A. Colditz, et al. Relation of meat, fat, and fiber intake to the risk of colon cancer in a prospective study among women. NEJM 323:1164-1172 (1990).

18. H. Lee, L. Gourley, S. Duffy, et al. Colorectal cancer and diet in an American population in a case-control study among Singapore Chinese. Int J Cancer 43:1007-1016 (1989).

19. S. Graham, J. Marshall, B. Haughey, et al. Dietary epidemiology of cancer of the colon in Western New York. Am J Epidemiol 128:490-503 (1988).

20. A. B. Miller, G. R. Howe, M. Jain, et al. Food items and food groups as risk factors in a case-control study of diet and colo-rectal cancer. Int J Cancer 32:155-161 (1983).

21. J. L. Lyon, A. W. Mahoney, D. W. West, et al. Energy intake: Its relationship to colon cancer risk. JNCI 78:853-861 (1987).

22. I. Martinez, R. Torres, Z. Frias, et al. Factors associated with adenocarcinomas of the large bowel in Puerto Rico. Adv. Med. Onc. Rea. Edve. 3:45-52 (1975).

23. J. D. Potter and A. J. McMichael. Diet and cancer of the colon and rectum: A case-control study. JNCI 76:557-569 (1986).

24. J. Hu, Y. Lin, Y. Yu, et al. Diet and cancer of the colon and rectum: A case-control study in China. Int J. Epidemiology 20:362-367 (1991).

25. O. Manousos, N. E. Day, D. Trichopoulos, et al. Diet and colorectal cancer: A case-control study in Greece. Int J Cancer 32:1-5 (1983).

26. G. Macquart-Moulin, E. Riboli, J. Cornee, et al. Case-control study on colorectal cancer and diet in Marseilles. Int J. Cancer 38:183-191 (1986).

27. E. Negri, C. La Vecchia, S. Franceschi, et al. Vegetable and fruit consumption and cancer risk. Int J. Cancer 48:350-354 (1991).

28. E. Benito, A. Obrador, A. Stiggelbout, et al. A population-based case-control study of colorectal cancer in Marjorca. I. dietary factors. Int J Cancer 45:69-76 (1990).

29. T. B. Young and D. A. Wolf. Case-control study of proximal and distal colon cancer and diet in Wisconsin. Int J. Cancer 42:167-175 (1988).

30. E. Bidoli, S. Franceschi, R. Talamini, et al. Food consumption and cancer of the colon and rectum in Northern-Eastern Italy. Int J. Cancer 50:223-29 (1992).

31. E. Bjelke. Dietary factors and the epidemiology of cancer of the stomach and large bowel. Aktuelle Ernaehrungsmedizin 2:10-17 (1978).

32. J. Higginson. Etiological factors in gastrointestinal cancer in man. JNCI 37:527-545 (1966).

33 W. Haenszel, J. W. Berg, M. Segi, et al. Large-bowel cancer in Hawaiian Japanese. JNCI 51:1765-1779 (1973).

34. J. L. Freudenheim, S. Graham, P. J. Horvath, et al. Risks associated with source of fiber and fiber components in cancer of the colon and rectum. Cancer Research 50:3295-3300 (1990).

35. S. Graham, H. Dayal, M. Swanson, et al. Diet in the epidemiology of cancer of the colon and rectum. JNCI 61:709-714 (1978).

36. M. A. Eastwood. What does the measurement of dietary fibre mean? Lancet 1487-1488 (1986).

37. G. A. Spiller. Beyond dietary fiber. AJCN 54:615-617 (1991).

38. K. R. Smith, M. L. Slattery, and French. Collinear nutrients and the risk of colon cancer. J Clin Epid 44:715-723 (1991).

39. M. J. Thun, M. M. Namboodiri, and C. W. Heath, Jr. Aspirin use and reduced risk of fatal colon cancer. NEJM 325:1593-1596 (1991).

40. U. S. Department of Health and Human Services. Healthy People 2000: National Health Promotion and Disease Prevention Objectives. DHHS Publication No. (PHS) 91-50213. (1991) Washington, D.C.

Your Mother was Right—Eat Your Vegetables: The Role of Plant Foods in Cancer

John D. Potter, MD PhD
Kristi Steinmetz, RD PHD

Division of Epidemiology
School of Public Health
University of Minnesota

Introduction

Humanity has always believed in the relevance of plants to health and disease. In fact, the roots of medicine in our culture, and the practice of medicine in many parts of the world today, involve the prescription of specific foods (plant-foods in particular) for a large number of illnesses. Historically, foods ascribed healing properties in and around the Mediterranean and Middle East included cruciferous vegetables, which were cultivated primarily for medicinal purposes (Fenwick 1983), and members of the allium (onion) family; Pliny declared that consumption of cabbage would cure as many as 87 diseases and that consumption of onions would cure as many as 28 (Kohman 1947). Other therapeutic plants included celery, cucumber, endive, parsley, radish, and legumes. The ancient Romans believed that lentils were a cure for diarrhea and conducive to an even temper. A variety of fruits including citrus fruits, raisins, and grapes were incorporated into oral preparations, enemas, inhalations, and topical applications (see Darby 1977).

It has been estimated that from 10 to 70% of all cancer is attributable to diet (Doll 1981). Relevant dietary hypotheses include possible roles for dietary fat and fiber in the etiology of colon cancer, for alcohol in upper digestive tract cancers, and for inadequate intake of various vitamins and minerals, including vitamins A, C, and E and selenium spe-cifically, in several cancers. High intakes of vegetables and fruit appear to be protective against cancers at many sites. This hypothesis may be better supported by the scientific literature than most of the other, better known, dietary hypotheses.

An answer to the question of the role of vegetables and fruit in cancer is important for making dietary recommendations. The Basic Four Food Groups, with which most Americans are familiar as a guideline for eat-ing, includes the Fruit and Vegetable Group. Until recently, four serv-ings per day from this group have been recommended. It has been es-timated from the Second National Health and Examination Survey (NHANES II) that the average American consumes only about 0.7 serv-ings of vegetables (1.5 servings when potatoes and salads are included), 0.7 servings of fruit, and 0.3 servings of legumes and nuts per day (Lanza 1987), although U.S. Department of Agriculture statistics show that annual per capita consumption of fruits and vegetables increased by 23% between 1970 and 1985 (Pearl 1990). If, in fact, consumption of vegetables and fruit reduces cancer risk, public health and economic interventions to increase the current U. S. consumption level would be well justified and, given the low current intake, relatively effective.

The Epidemiologic Evidence

We have recently reviewed the epidemiologic evidence regarding the association of cancer risk and vegetables and fruit (Steinmetz and Potter 1991a). A summary follows.

Cohort Studies

Of the 6 cohort studies in the scientific literature, all but 1 (Phillips 1985) show an inverse association (higher consumption–lower risk) between consumption of vegetables or fruits and cancer. The bulk of the evidence for such an association covers green and yellow vegetables (Hirayama 1982a, 1982b, 1986, and Colditz 1985) and soy products and legumes (Hirayama 1982a, 1982b, 1986, and Mills 1988). Lung cancer is the cancer for which there is the most cohort study evidence for a lower risk with vegetable and fruit consumption, but it is also the most-studied cancer (Hirayama 1982a, 1982b, 1986, Kväle 1983, Long-de 1985).

Case-Control Studies

Summary by cancer site

Separate consideration of case-control studies by each cancer site is necessary when attempting to sort out possible causal relationships for cancer at different sites. Different cancers have very different non-dietary risk factors and appear to have different dietary risk (and risk-reduction) factors also. Major differences exist between tissues of the body in the amount of cancer-causing and protective substances they are likely be exposed to (and how it gets there—eaten, via blood, breathed in etc.) and major differences, too, in the chemicals (enzymes) that protect it against (or, sometimes, activate) those carcinogens.

Lung Cancer   Consumption of carrots and green leafy vegetables appear to be particularly associated with a lower risk of lung cancer.

Colon Cancer   Cruciferous vegetables (the cabbage family) and carrots appear to be particularly beneficial in relation to colon cancer. Both are especially high in a number of specific anti-carcinogenic substances (see below) and appear to be more effective in colon cancer than vegetables that are not particularly high in these substances, but that, nonetheless, contain similar amounts of fiber. Thus, the case-control evidence for colon cancer seems to suggest a lower risk associated with vegetables over and above that associated with fiber alone.

Rectal Cancer   For rectal cancer, although an association with consumption of 1 or more vegetables and/or fruits has been consistently reported, no patterns emerge.

Upper Aerodigestive Tract Cancer   Consumption of fruit appears to be strongly associated with lower risk of esophageal, laryngeal, and oral and pharyngeal cancers. This may relate to a common etiology of these cancers of the upper aerodigestive tract (the strongest and most consistent risk factors are tobacco and alcohol). Consumption of vegetables appears to be especially associated with lower risk of laryngeal cancer.

Stomach Cancer   Several vegetables and fruits have been found quite consistently associated with lower risk of stomach cancer. These include fruit in general, lettuce, onions, tomatoes, celery, and squash. Fruit and lettuce have been particularly commonly reported. Consumption of vegetables and fruit raw, rather than cooked or preserved, also appears to be a consistent pattern. Canned fruit and potatoes have been positively related to stomach cancer risk in some studies.

Pancreas Cancer   For pancreatic cancer, almost every case-control study has reported that consumption of 1 or more vegetables and/or fruits is associated with lower risk, but no specific patterns are apparent.

Bladder Cancer   Consumption of vegetables and fruit in general, and of carrots in particular appear associated with lower risk of bladder cancer.

Hormone-dependent Cancers   In contrast to cancers at each of the above epithelial sites, the so-called hormone-dependent cancers appear less associated with vegetable and fruit consumption. There is some evidence for an inverse relationship with cancers of the breast and uterus, but the evidence is not as consistent as that for the above cancers. For ovarian and prostate cancers, virtually no evidence exists for an association.

Summary by types of vegetables and fruits

Although a site-specific review of the vegetable and fruit data is useful, particularly for understanding mechanisms, an overall assessment of which vegetables and fruits are associated in the most consistent way with cancer at all sites is of the greatest importance for developing dietary recommendations. To this end, the Table shows a summary of the 108 case-control studies of all cancer sites, which we have reviewed, and presents the number of studies finding increased or decreased risk, or no association between cancers and specific types of vegetables and fruits. Overall, the case-control evidence strongly suggests that consumption of the following vegetables and fruits is lower in those with cancer: raw and fresh vegetables, leafy green vegetables, cruciferae, carrots, broccoli, cabbage, lettuce, raw and fresh fruit, and citrus fruit. Raw and fresh vegetables is the outstanding food category with 93% of studies showing a negative association and only 8% (just 1 study) showing a positive association. The proportion of all case-control studies reporting a lower risk is greater than 70% for the following: raw or fresh vegetables, leafy green vegetables, cruciferae, carrots, lettuce, and citrus fruit. In addition, greater than 80% of the associations for these foods were either in the reduced-risk direction or had no association, thus showing that there is very little likelihood of harm arising from consumption of these foods. For broccoli, 100% of the associations showed a lower risk or no association. Even the "no-associations" should not necessarily be interpreted as evidence against a lower risk, as a variety of factors tend to ensure that the associations seen in epidemiologic studies—whether with increased or decreased risk—are conservative.

The evidence for consumption of potatoes is more equivocal, with only 53% of the studies finding an inverse or null relationship. The summation of the findings for legume consumption are contrary to what might be expected in that 73% of the studies actually found a positive or null association with cancer.

A comment must be made regarding the positive associations presented in this table. Approximately half of the 35 positive associations listed (excluding those for legumes) come from studies by Tajima (1985), who consistently found positive associations for consumption of almost all vegetables and fruits studied in a series of methodologically similar case-control studies of cancers of the colon, rectum, and stom

Table 1. Summary of the studies in the epidemiologic literature that have reported on the relationship between vegetables and fruit and risk of cancer at any site

Type of vegetable or fruit	Total number of studies	Number of studies showing a negative association[a,b]	Number of studies showing no association	Number of studies showing a positive association[a,c]
Raw or Fresh Vegetables[d]	14	13 (93%)	0 (0%)	1 (7%)
Leafy Green Vegetables[e]	39	30 (77%)	3 (8%)	6 (15%)
Cruciferous Vegetables	22	16 (72%)	3 (14%)	3 (14%)
Allium Vegetables[f]	12	8 (67%)	1 (8%)	3 (25%)
Carrots[g]	32	25 (78%)	4 (13%)	3 (9%)
Broccoli[h]	10	7 (70%)	3 (30%)	0 (0%)
Cabbage[i]	19	12 (63%)	3 (16%)	4 (21%)
Lettuce[j]	18	15 (83%)	0 (0%)	3 (17%)
Potatoes	15	8 (53%)	0 (0%)	7 (47%)
Legumes[k]	11	3 (27%)	1 (9%)	7 (64%)
Raw or Fresh Fruit	16	9 (56%)	4 (25%)	3 (19%)
Citrus Fruit[l]	16	12 (75%)	2 (13%)	2 (13%)

[a] Number in parentheses is the percentage of total studies.
[b] Number of studies in which the inverse association was statistically significant (expressed as significant studies/total studies); raw or fresh vegetables — 11/13, leafy green vegetables — 18/30, cruciferous vegetables — 10/16, allium vegetables — 7/8, carrots — 12/24, broccoli — 3/6, cabbage — 4/12, lettuce — 8/14, potatoes — 3/8, legumes — 1/3, raw or fresh fruit — 6/9, and citrus fruit — 8/12.
[c] Number of studies in which the positive association was statistically significant (expressed as significant studies/total studies): raw or fresh vegetables — 1/1, leafy green vegetables — 2/6, cruciferous vegetables — 1/3, allium vegetables — 3/3, carrots — 0/3, broccoli — 0/0, cabbage — 1/4, lettuce — 0/3, potatoes — 2/7, legumes — 4/7, raw or fresh fruit — 1/3, & citrus fruit — 0/2.
[d] Includes categories titled raw vegetables, fresh vegetables, uncooked vegetables, salad vegetables, and raw yellow-green vegetables.
[e] Includes categories titled leafy green vegetables, green leafy vegetables, dark green vegetables, green vegetables, raw green vegetables, kale, chicory, and spinach.
[f] Includes categories titled allium vegetables, onions, raw onions, and cooked onions.
[g] Includes categories titled carrots, raw carrots, and cooked carrots.
[h] Includes categories titled broccoli and raw broccoli.
[i] Includes categories titled cabbage and raw cabbage.
[j] Includes categories titled lettuce, lettuce and endive, lettuce salad, and romaine lettuce.
[k] Includes categories titled legumes, dried beans, beans, kidney beans, peas and beans, seeds and legumes, and soybeans.
[l] Includes categories titled citrus fruit and fresh citrus fruit.

ach in Japan. Such positive associations were not limited to vegetable and fruit consumption, but were seen for almost all foods studied. In these studies, the control group included patients with gastritis, ulcers, polyps, and other diseases; only 48% of the control group did not have abnormal clinical findings. Thus, the case-control differences are likely to have been affected by decreased intake of food and energy intake in general, or of vegetables and fruit specifically, by the diseased persons in the control group. Tajima and colleagues found their own results "unexpected" in light of "the results of most previous epidemiological and experimental studies."

If the studies by Tajima are removed from the Table, the proportion of studies finding inverse associations for consumption of vegetables is increased. In particular, the proportion of studies finding an inverse association for consumption of cabbage is 100%. The proportions of studies finding consumption of leafy green vegetables, allium vegetables, carrots, cabbage, and potatoes to be associated with lower risk is increased from 77, 67, 78, 63, and 53%, respectively, to 84, 89, 86, 74, and 67%. Further, the number of associations with increased risk for allium vegetables, carrots, and lettuce is reduced to zero.

Strength of the Associations

The majority of the studies show no more than a halving of risk with high consumption of vegetables and fruit. As noted above, a variety of factors tend to ensure that the strength of the associations seen in nutritional epidemiologic studies—whether risk is increased or decreased— are conservative. Therefore, odds ratios consistently suggesting a halving of risk may, in fact, be signalling stronger relationships. Even if the risk of cancer were only doubled by low vegetable and fruit consumption, this would still be a major influence on the overall burden of cancer in the community because exposure to low vegetable and fruit consumption is so widespread. Diet is modifiable, and thus, a potential target for intervention.

Caveat

While every attempt has been made to include every study that has investigated the relationship, there are undoubtedly data that are not included (see Steinmetz and Potter 1991a). Such information would be useful in order to present the complete picture of the relationship between vegetable and fruit consumption and cancer. Nonetheless, if the associations were only chance, there would be a similar number of data points suggesting an increased risk as those suggesting a decreased risk.

Mechanisms

Phytochemicals

There are many biologically plausible reasons why consumption of vegetables and fruit might slow or prevent the appearance of cancer. These include the presence of potentially anticarcinogenic substances such as carotenoids, vitamin C, vitamin E, selenium, dietary fiber, dithiolthiones, isothiocyanates, indoles, phenols, protease inhibitors, allium compounds, plant sterols, limonene, and others—these are increasingly being called, collectively, phytochemicals—chemicals of plant origin that play a crucial role in metabolism. In a companion paper to the review of the epidemiology, we have considered what is known, at present, about some of these phytochemicals (Steinmetz and Potter 1991b).

Steps from pro-carcinogen exposure to a cancer-prone cell

Many carcinogens are not in their fully active form when first encountered; the steps from exposure to this pro-carcinogen form to the ultimate conversion of a normal cell into a cancer-prone cell (transformation) can be considered to go through the following steps: the pro-carcinogen is activated to the ultimate carcinogen form by enzyme systems normal to the body, particularly the systems collectively known as P450 enzymes (It is worth keeping in mind that the body is not trying to make carcinogens—it is trying to make insoluble foreign compounds soluble and therefore to enable their easy excretion in the urine. It is also complicated by the fact that the same enzyme can often make one compound less carcinogenic and another more carcinogenic); either of these forms of the carcinogen (pro-carcinogen or ultimate carcinogen) may be converted by other enzyme systems into a form that is relatively inert and even more easily excreted. These enzymes usually are called Phase II enzymes and are typified by glutathione S-transferase; if not excreted, the carcinogen can pass through the cell membrane and the membrane of the nucleus; the carcinogen can then interact with the DNA—perhaps forming adducts and/or producing mutations; DNA synthesis and replication (or DNA repair) subsequently occur; repair may have varying degrees of fidelity; if the DNA is not repaired accurately and it is a crucial piece of DNA that has been mutated, cell replication—producing daughter cells with copies of the mutated DNA—occurs; these cells then synthesize an abnormal protein or fail, altogether, to synthesize a protein crucial to normal function of the cell or even crucial to controlling cell replication itself (this is almost certainly what happens when a tumor suppressor gene [e.g., p53] mutates or is lost).

This sequence of stages brings a cell a step closer to becoming a cancer cell (alternatively, even with abnormal DNA, the cell may cease to replicate and then undergoes differentiation—a step away from becoming a cancer cell). DNA damage probably has to occur several times before a cell becomes completely free of growth restraint and a fully cancerous cell. Finally, by mechanisms that are poorly understood, the abnormal cells obtain a growth advantage over the normal cells and steadily increase in numbers (promotion)—often becoming more malignant and able to spread (progression).

Specific anti-carcinogenic phytochemicals

At almost every one of the above stages, known phytochemicals can alter the likelihood of carcinogenesis, occasionally in a way that enhances risk, but usually in a favorable direction. For example, such substances as glucosinolates and indoles, isothiocyanates and thiocyanates, phenols, and coumarins can induce a multiplicity of solubilizing and (usually) inactivating enzymes; ascorbate and phenols block the formation of carcinogens such as nitrosamines; flavonoids and carotenoids can act as antioxidants, essentially disabling carcinogenic potential; lipid-soluble compounds such as sterols may alter membrane structure or integrity; some sulphur-containing compounds can suppress DNA- and protein-synthesis; carotenoids suppress DNA-synthesis and enhance differentiation. More detail follows.

The variety of substances in vegetables and fruits for which protective mechanisms have been postulated and, in many cases, shown experimentally, lends plausibility to the view that a diet high in plant foods is protective against cancer. Evidence for the anticarcinogenic effects of carotenoids, vitamins C and E, folate, selenium, dietary fiber, dithiolthiones, glucosinolates and indoles, isothiocyanates, flavonoids, phenols, isoflavones, protease inhibitors, plant sterols, allium compounds, saponins, inositol hexaphosphate, and limonene is reviewed. Because some of these substances are the subject of entire fields of research themselves and a complete reference list would be intolerably long, review articles are the major sources of data for the more intensively investigated substances.

Carotenoids Investigation of the relationship between carotenoids and retinol and cancer has produced an extensive literature. Reviews have been prepared by Fontham (1990), Willett (1990), Ziegler (1989), Olson (1986), Graham (1984), Hennekens (1986), Krinsky (1991), the National Research Council (1989). More than 500 carotenoids occur in nature. They are present in dark green leafy vegetables and in yellow and orange vegetables and fruits. β-Carotene is found in most of these, but it is not the predominant carotenoid in most vegetables; however, carrots, sweet potatoes, and red palm oil are especially high. The predominant carotenoids in green leafy vegetables are the oxygenated carotenoids (xanthophylls), of which the major representative is lutein. β-Carotene, α-carotene, and lycopene are hydrocarbon carotenoids. Lycopene is found in large amounts in tomatoes and red palm oil, but is otherwise relatively scarce. Carotenoids are heat-labile, particularly the xanthophylls. Micozzi (1990) has compiled vegetable carotenoid values.

One of the mechanisms by which carotenoids may reduce risk of cancer is via conversion to vitamin A. In the U. S., one-third or less of dietary intake of vitamin A comes from carotenoids (Subcommittee on the Tenth Edition of the RDAs, Food and Nutrition Board 1989); the majority comes from retinol, which is found in animal products. Functions of retinol include a role in epithelial cell differentiation. Because dedifferentiation is a feature of cancer cells, low serum vitamin A may plausibly be invoked as a relevant agent. A different anti-cancer role for carotenoids (unrelated to pro-vitamin A activity, which is, in fact, a property of only a subset of carotenoids) may be related to their capacity to quench singlet oxygen. Carotenoids can deactivate mono-oxygen molecules generated as by-products of normal metabolic processes and can trap free radicals. β-Carotene may also enhance immunologic function (Krinsky 1991, Bendich 1988).

In vitro, retinoids can reverse or prevent malignant changes in cells exposed to a number of carcinogens (see Hennekens 1986). Retinoic acid has antiproliferative capacity, can induce differentiation, and may influence oncogene expression (see Prasad 1990). Most animal research on cancer and vitamin A has also involved retinoids, not carotenoids. Retinol deficiency predisposes animals to pre-malignant changes and to enhance the development of chemically induced tumors; a few investigators have reported that retinoids may enhance tumor production. (see Hennekens 1986, Bertram 1987, Graham 1984).

Protective effects of carotenoids without vitamin A activity (Mathews-Roth 1985) and a mechanism of inhibition for carrots unrelated to β-carotene (Rieder 1983) have been reported. The epidemiologic evidence showing an inverse association between green vegetable consumption and cancer risk suggests xanthophylls (approximately 90% of carotenoids in green vegetables) as the potential anticarcinogens. The finding that consumption of raw vegetables appears to be associated more often, with lower risk, than consumption of cooked vegetables is consistent with a role for these oxygenated carotenoids.

Population studies of dietary carotenoids include prospective studies by Shekelle (1981) and Paganini-Hill (1987) and a large sequence of case-control studies; see Le Marchand (1989), Ziegler (1989), and

Fontham (1990) for references to nine studies of lung cancer. Each of these has shown an inverse association between carotenoid intake and risk. Two studies (Hirayama 1982b, 1986) of lung cancer have attempted to distinguish which vegetables associated with which carotenoids are most related to risk; they found consumption of dark green vegetables (high in lutein), tomatoes (high lycopene), and total vegetables to be as strong as, or stronger than, carrots or β-carotene as risk predictors. Howe's 1990 meta-analysis of breast cancer case-control studies showed an odds ratio of 0.8 (P < 0.003) for high β-carotene intake for post-menopausal breast cancer (eight studies). All five prospective studies (Stähelin 1991, Nomura 1985, Menkes 1986, Wald 1988, Connett 1989) examining blood β-carotene levels and lung cancer risk reported an inverse association (4 statistically significant). Three studies (Stähelin 1991, Nomura 1985, Wald 1988) of stomach cancer showed similar results (only one statistically significant). Associations of cancer risk with blood retinol have not been as consistent as those with β-carotene. Burney (1989), Helzlsouer (1989) and Comstock (1990) reported studies of pancreas, bladder, and rectum cancer showing lycopene associated with lower risk. Hsing (1990) and Stryker (1988) found no associations for a variety of carotenoids with melanoma and prostate cancer.

Clinical trials, using carotenoids and retinoids both as treatment and chemoprevention (see Bertram 1987, Hennekens 1983, Stich 1984a, 1984b), should begin to clarify the place of these compounds in the overall inverse association between vegetables and fruit and the risk of epithelial cancers.

Vitamin C There are a large number of recent reviews of the literature on vitamin C and cancer (National Research Council [1989], Bertram [1987], Willett [1984a], Chen [1988], Colditz [1987], Block [1991]). Vitamin C is found in highest quantities in fruits and vegetables, (particularly citrus fruits and juices, broccoli, peppers, tomatoes, strawberries, melons, cabbage, and green, leafy vegetables). Vitamin C is heat-labile, easily oxidized and water-soluble and therefore readily lost in cooking. Substantial amounts of this vitamin can be provided by supplements and fortified foods.

Wattenberg (1985) has categorized vitamin C as preventing the formation of carcinogens from precursors. An important mechanism by which ascorbate may reduce cancer occurrence, particularly stomach cancer, is through the capacity to reduce nitrite; nitrite reacts readily with secondary amines to form nitrosamines (National Research Council 1989). Ascorbate is also an antioxidant and can enhance immune response. Vitamin C is also involved in the hydroxylation of lysine and proline in collagen synthesis; a deficiency may therefore disrupt connective tissue integrity and thus produce a permissive environment for tumor growth or prevent effective tumor encapsulation (Cameron 1979).

In vitro, ascorbate lowers the mutagenicity of gastric juice (O'Connor 1985). It has also been shown to induce regression of malignant changes in hamster lung cells and to increase survival of radiation-exposed ovarian tumor cells (see Willett 1984a). Feeding vitamin C to animals pre-treated with carcinogens largely results in a reduction of tumors or no evidence of effect. Some ascorbate salts have been shown to promote bladder cancer in rodents. (See National Research Council [1989] for references to animal studies). Guinea pigs, who, like humans, require exogenous ascorbate, showed either no effect or an enhancing effect of ascorbate following induction of sarcomas (see Bertram 1987).

Case-control studies of cancer in some directly exposed epithelial tissues shows risk to be inversely related to ascorbate intake (see Bertram 1987, Willett 1984a, Fontham 1990). Howe (1990) reported a similar finding for breast cancer. Chemoprevention trials are under way (see Bertram 1987).

Vitamin E Although less-studied than vitamins A and C, there are several reviews of the area available: National Research Council (1989), Chen (1988), Bertram (1987), Colditz (1987), Willett (1986), Fiala (1985), and Diplock (1991). Major dietary sources of Vitamin E are vegetable oils and margarine. Other sources include whole grains, wheat germ, seeds, nuts, and green vegetables, such as lettuce and asparagus. Its most active form in foods is α-tocopherol; other tocopherols and tocotrienols have some vitamin E activity.

Vitamin E is a significant intracellular antioxidant. It protects cell-membrane polyunsaturated fatty acids from oxidative damage. Further, it maintains selenium in the reduced state and has been shown to inhibit nitrosamine formation, especially at low pH (see Bertram 1987 and Fiala 1985). More speculative mechanisms have been proposed (see National Research Council 1989). Wattenberg (1985) characterizes vitamin E as a cancer inhibitor, its major effect being prevention of carcinogen formation from precursors.

In vitro, tocopherols have been shown to modify the expression of the oncogenes, *myc* and H-*ras*; (see Prasad 1990). Overall, animal experimental results have been inconclusive (see National Research Council 1989). Epidemiologic studies of dietary vitamin E are inconsistent, perhaps because of methodologic limitations (see National Research Council [1989], Bertram [1987]). Of 13 studies where blood was collected prospectively, seven showed a statistically significant difference between cases of all or site-specific cancer and controls (see Knekt 1988). Chemoprevention studies are under way (Bertram 1987).

Folic Acid Folate is an essential vitamin found in high concentrations in green leafy vegetables, asparagus, broccoli, beets, and a variety of beans. Oranges and orange juice contain moderate amounts, and are major contributors of folate to the U. S. diet because of high consumption. Mild to moderate folate deficiency is surprisingly prevalent. MacGregor (1990) has recently discussed a possible anticarcinogenic role.

In vitro and animal studies show that folate deficiency causes increased formation of micronuclei and chromosomal damage; cancer-related breakpoints, including certain fragile sites associated with oncogenes have also been shown to be increased. Dysplasia in cervical and lung cells can be reversed by administration of folate. Finally, caffeine consumption may act synergistically with folate deficiency to produce these effects (MacGregor 1990). For references to animal and in vitro studies, see MacGregor (1990).

Selenium Reviews of the association between dietary selenium and cancer include those by Bertram (1987), Willett (1986), the National Research Council (1989), and Diplock (1991). Selenium is found in foods in amounts proportional to soil-content and is often present as an amino-acid compound. Selenium is a cofactor for glutathione peroxidase, an enzyme that protects against oxidative damage. At high levels, it suppresses cell proliferation. It may also enhance immune response (see National Research Council [1989] and Colditz [1987]). Wattenberg (1985) has classified selenium as an agent that prevents the expression of neoplasia.

In vitro, selenium decreases the mutagenicity of many compounds (see Willett 1986). Conversely, several selenium compounds, specifically selenites, are known to damage DNA (National Research Council 1989). Animal experiments on both deficiency and high dietary intake of selenium are inconsistent. Where very high doses of selenium (many times the nutritional requirement and, in some cases, near toxic doses) have been fed, an inhibition of induced carcinogenesis results. Ip (1985), in a review, noted that 31 of 35 studies have resulted in such a finding (see also Bertram 1987, Fiala 1985, Milner 1985, Willett 1984).

Geographically, there is an inverse relationship between crop selenium level and cancer mortality (see National Research Council 1989 for references). In 9 of 13 cohort studies with prospectively collected blood, low selenium was a risk factor for cancer (see Helzlsouer [1989], Knekt [1988]). This relationship is relatively more consistent for men than women, and seen most consistently for stomach cancer.

Dietary Fiber Jacobs (1988), the National Research Council (1989), Potter (1990), Trock (1990), and Greenwald (1986, 1987) recently have reviewed the evidence for an association between cancer and dietary fiber, particularly in relation to colorectal cancer. This volume contains some further thoughts on the evidence from Byers (1994).

This area of research is troubled particularly by the lack of a universally accepted definition of "dietary fiber" (see Potter 1990 and Pilch 1987) and by a lack of consistent, well-accepted food-fiber analysis methods. Dietary fiber is found in vegetables, fruits, legumes, nuts, seeds, and unrefined grains. (For fiber values for foods, see Lanza 1986.)

Several mechanisms have been proposed for dietary fiber in colon carcinogenesis (see Jacobs 1988). The data appear to support a protective effect of high fecal bulk, but not rapid transit time. In general, insoluble fibers tend to decrease transit time and increase fecal bulk; soluble fibers are less effective (see National Research Council 1989 for references). Fermentation by colonic bacteria leads to more acid pH in the colon as the production of short-chain fatty acids increases; this inhibits the conversion of primary to secondary bile acids. Further, at low pH, free bile acids are less soluble and thus less available as co-carcinogens. Fermentation may also release bound calcium, which is then free to bind bile acids and fatty acids. Finally, fermentation in the proximal colon leads to production of butyrate, a short-chain fatty acid with antineoplastic properties.

The results of case-control studies on fiber and colon cancer are inconsistent. Of 13 case-control studies, 5 provide strong support and 4, moderate support, for a reduced risk. Two studies give support for no association and 2 equivocally suggest increased risk (for references to case-control studies see Potter [1990] and Trock [1990]). Howe (1990) has recently completed a formal meta-analysis of 13 case-control studies where dietary fiber was measured, and concludes that there is a lower risk with higher consumption; the data show a dose-response (p for trend < 0.0001) and an approximate halving of risk for the uppermost quintile versus the lowermost.

The prospective study of Willett (1990b) examined the associations with fiber intake and with other dietary variables, on incidence of colon cancer over a 6-year period among female nurses. A dose-related decrease in risk was associated with fruit fiber (expressed as crude fiber); an odds ratio of 0.6 (0.4–1.1) was reported for the uppermost vs. lowermost intake quintile. None of the other fiber variables—total dietary fiber, total crude fiber, vegetable fiber, and cereal fiber—were associated with risk of colon cancer.

Dithiolthiones   Bueding (1986) has reviewed the data on the effect of dithiolthiones on carcinogenesis. Cruciferous vegetables contain these compounds. Studies in animals given the synthetic dithiolthione, oltipraz, show reduced numbers of carcinogen-induced tumors of lung and forestomach. Oltipraz reduces DNA-aflatoxin adducts in liver and kidney (Kensler 1985, 1987) in rats, and chromosome breaks and lipid peroxidation in elderly mice (Stohs 1986). Other experiments show that oltipraz and other dithiolthiones increase levels of glutathione and activities of a variety of Phase II enzymes (see Bueding 1986). Wattenberg 1985 has classified dithiolthiones as agents that protect against cancer by blocking the reaction of electrophilic carcinogens with cellular macromolecules. No clinical trials have been undertaken.

Glucosinolates and Indoles   The effects of indoles on carcinogenesis were reviewed by Hocman (1989). Glucosinolates are found in cruciferae; brussels sprouts, rutabaga, mustard greens, and dried horseradish are particularly high. More than 20 different glucosinolates have been isolated. Glucobrassicin and sinigrin each make up approximately 30% of the glucosinolates in cruciferous vegetables. Glucobrassicin is found in plant cells in a separate compartment from the enzyme myrosinase, which, when plant cells are damaged, catalyzes its hydrolysis to indoles, including indole-3-carbinol and indole-3-acetonitrile. The average daily intake of glucosinolates in Japan is estimated to be over 100 mg (Bailey 1987); in Britain, daily intakes of glucobrassicin and indoles are about 30 mg and 10 mg, respectively (Wattenberg 1986).

Indole-3-carbinol, but not indole-3-acetonitrile, increases microsomal mixed function oxidase activity (especially that of aryl hydrocarbon hydroxylase) in dose-response fashion (see Loub 1975, Salbe 1986 and reviews by Bailey 1987 and Hocman 1989). The aggregate effect is probably anticarcinogenic (Carr 1985). A further mechanism against the development of hormone-related cancers involves estrogen metabolism directly. In rodents and humans (at approximately 50 times the U. S. average daily intake), indoles increase hepatic estradiol 2-hydroxylation (Michnovicz 1990). To the degree that indoles are able to produce a shift from 16-hydroxylation to 2-hydroxylation, they may reduce risk of estrogen-related cancers (Michnovicz 1986, 1988, Schneider 1983, Bradlow 1985, 1986, Fishman 1984). Animal studies suggest that indoles are protective against a variety of tumors (Wattenberg 1978, 1986, Morse 1988, Bailey 1987, Dashwood 1989), but not all (Salbe 1986, Morse 1988).

Isothiocyanates and Thiocyanates   Isothiocyanates are found in large amounts in cruciferous vegetables. Others have been made synthetically. Animal experiments show that the naturally occurring and synthetic compounds inhibit both DNA-methylation and the early and late stages of carcinogenesis; see Wattenberg (1978b, 1977, 1981, 1987), Morse (1989). Wattenberg (1985) has defined benzyl isothiocyanate as an agent that prevents the reaction of carcinogens with critical sites and as an inhibitor of expression of neoplasia. One relevant mechanism involves the capacity of isothiocyanates to induce Phase II xenobiotic-metabolizing enzymes, including glutathione S-transferase (Sparnins 1982).

Coumarins are found in vegetables and citrus fruits. Their mechanism of action also may involve induction of glutathione S-transferase activity (Sparnins 1982). Wattenberg (1985) classified coumarins as blocking agents. Animal experiments show tumor inhibition (see Wattenberg 1978b).

Flavonoids, including quercetin, kaempferol, myricetin, and chrysin are found in most fruits and vegetables. Tangeretin, nobiletin, and rutin are found in citrus fruits. Berries, tomatoes, potatoes, broad beans, peapods, and colored onions are relatively high in quercetin; radishes and horseradish are relatively high in kaempferol. Food values for specific flavonoids have been published by Hermann (1976). The average daily intake of flavonoids for Americans is approximately 1 gram (Brown 1980).

Flavonoids are, to varying degrees, antioxidants. Some flavonoids induce mixed function oxidase activity—with potentially mixed results for carcinogenesis. In vitro and animal experiments have also produced mixed results; see Brown (1980), Jansen (1982), Friedman (1984), and Fiala (1985).

Phenols Stich (1984c) has published a review of the anticarcinogenic properties of phenols. Certain of these compounds, α-tocopherol and quercetin, were discussed above. Caffeic, ferulic, and ellagic acids are phenols that are widely distributed in plants. Chlorogenic acid is the quinic acid conjugate form of caffeic acid and is the most common form of caffeic acid. It is the most prevalent phenolic compound and is found in almost all fruits and vegetables. Phenol levels are highest in freshly harvested fruits and vegetables because phenolic compounds are readily oxidized during processing and storage. Values for the amounts of phenolic compounds in some fruits have been published by Hermann (1973) and Stich (1984c). It has been estimated that humans consume approximately 1 gram of plant phenols daily (Hocman 1989). Their probable mechanism of action involves the induction of Phase II conjugation enzymes. They also inhibit N-nitrosamine production (Stich 1984c). Wattenberg (1985) classified caffeic and ferulic acids as agents that prevent carcinogen formation and that block the reaction of carcinogens with macromolecules. *In vitro*, phenolic compounds inhibit mutagenicity and, in animals, decrease lung and skin tumors (see Fiala 1985).

Isoflavones Messina (1991a,1991b) and Adlercreutz (1990) have proposed that isoflavones are important cancer-preventive agents. They are found in soybeans and at least 300 other plants (Messina 1991a). Genistein and daidzein are soy isoflavones that are found at high levels in human urine (Messina 1991a). Equol is found in mammalian urine and is derived from plant precursors (Messina 1991a). One proposed anticarcinogenic action of isoflavones is a consequence of their weak estrogenic activity; they bind to estrogen receptors, blocking binding by more potent estrogens, and eliciting only a minor estrogenic response— generally about 0.1% of that of conjugated endogenous estrogens (Messina 1991b, 1991a). Isoflavones also stimulate production of sex hormone-binding globulin, resulting in a decrease in free estrogen (Adlercreutz 1990). Thus, isoflavones may thwart the progression of the hormone-dependent cancers—breast, endometrium, ovary, even prostate. These phytoestrogens could be considered as a class of "naturally occurring Tamoxifens," to which some isoflavones are structurally similar. Other mechanisms have been proposed: genistein inhibits tyrosine kinases that are associated with signal-transduction from cellular growth factor receptors and that are highly expressed in transformed cells (Messina 1991b, Adlercreutz 1990). Some cytochrome P450 enzymes may also be inhibited (Messina 1991a).

Studies in rodents have shown a decreased incidence of carcinogen-induced breast tumors with diets high in soybeans. One study reported that the effect was seen for both cooked and raw soybeans, probably ruling out protease inhibitors as the relevant agents. (See Messina 1991a, Adlercreutz 1990.) Human observational data are also consistent with a cancer preventive role for isoflavones. Vegetarians excrete higher levels of isoflavones (probably from soy) and have lower risk of many cancers. Asian women generally consume more soy than Americans and have lower rates of breast cancer—both in their countries of origin and, for one or two generations, as immigrants. Seventh-day Adventist and Hawaiian Japanese men, both of whom consume relatively large amounts of tofu and legumes, have lower rates of prostate cancer. Of course, differences in other factors may also contribute to the explanation of these ecologic observations. (See Messina 1991a, Adlercreutz 1990.) Premenopausal women fed large amounts of soy showed greater length of menstrual cycle, suggesting alterations in hormone metabolism in a manner likely to decrease the risk of hormone-related cancers (see Messina 1991b).

Saponins   Messina (1991a) and Oakenfull (1989) have discussed saponins as potential anticarcinogenic agents. These compounds are common to a number of plants and are found in soy in particularly significant amounts; approximately five percent of the dry weight of soybeans is accounted for by saponins. A suggested mechanism of action is the ability of saponins to bind bile acids and cholesterol (Messina 1991a). Animal and in vitro studies show that saponins reduce cell proliferation in the gut and decrease growth-rate and rate of DNA synthesis in some tumor cells (see Messina 1991a).

Inositol Hexaphosphate, which is found particularly in soybeans and cereals, is proposed by Messina (1991a) as an anticarcinogen. It accounts for more than 1% of the dry weight of soybeans. The suggested mechanism involves the ability of inositol hexaphosphate to bind dietary minerals, a property with potentially adverse, as well as, beneficial effects. The binding of iron may reduce the production of hydroxyl radicals. The compound decreases both lipid peroxidation and induced colon cancer in animals. (Messina 1991a).

Protease Inhibitors   Seeds and legumes are especially rich sources of protease inhibitors. Soybeans contain at least 5 types of these compounds. Although soy protease inhibitors are destroyed by heat, some survive the processing into tofu. Some, in kidney beans and chickpeas, remain unchanged after canning. Grains, including barley, wheat, oats, and rye, also contain protease inhibitors—these enzymes total 5 to10% of the water soluble protein and are concentrated in the embryo and endosperm. Trypsin inhibitors are the most studied and are found in the highest levels in potatoes and sweet corn; they are found also in spinach, broccoli, cucumbers, brussels sprouts, and radishes (see Richardson 1977 and Fiala 1985). Endogenous synthesis also occurs; this is increased in cancer and other conditions (Schelp 1988).

Most protease inhibitors are proteins of 70–90 amino acids; their action involves competitive inhibition of proteases via the formation of complexes (see Richardson 1977). A possible mechanism involves an effect on proteases produced by cancer cells; the actions of cancer-associated proteases include the destruction of the extracellular matrix, cellular detachment, and subsequent local invasion (Schelp 1988). Wattenberg (1985) describes protease inhibitors as agents with the capacities for suppression of the expression of neoplasia and inhibition of tumor promotion. *In vitro,* they inhibit growth of transformed cells (see Schelp 1988). Animal studies show that protease inhibitors reduce the occurrence of tumors (see Schelp 1988, Wattenberg 1985, 1987). No human research has yet been undertaken on protease inhibitors.

Plant Sterols   Vegetables are rich sources of plant sterols, including β-sitosterol, campesterol, and stigmasterol; together, these make up about 20% of dietary sterols. Intake of plant sterols has been estimated to be approximately 250 mg per day in the U. S. diet. They are similar in structure to cholesterol but pass through the gastrointestinal tract almost completely unabsorbed. (see Raicht 1980 and Fiala 1985).

Raicht (1980) found that inclusion of 0.2% β-sitosterol in the diet resulted in decreased occurrence of N-methyl-N-nitrosourea (NMNU)-induced colonic tumors in rats. Because NMNU is direct-acting, the authors suggest that the anticarcinogenic mechanism probably does not involve alteration of carcinogen metabolism. Fecal concentrations of cholesterol and bile acids in this study were not affected by β-sitosterol. Because of their structural similarity to cholesterol, plant sterols may affect cellular membranes. No human research has been done on the effects of plant sterols but it has been reported that vegetarians have higher levels of fecal β-sitosterol (see Raicht 1980).

Allium Compounds Onions, garlic and chives, are some of the allium vegetables. Diallyl sulfide and allyl methyl trisulfide are components of garlic oil. The anticarcinogenic mechanism may involve the induction of detoxification systems. Activation of microsomal monooxygenase enzymes and glutathione S-transferase has been observed in response to allium compounds (see further below). Antibacterial properties of onions and garlic may suggest a mechanism for protection against stomach cancer, specifically by inhibiting the bacterial conversion of nitrate to nitrite.

In vitro work has shown that onion extracts decrease tumor proliferation (see You 1989). Several animal studies have shown reduced occurrence of tumors at several alimentary tract sites and increased activity of enzymes such as glutathione S-transferase as a result of dosing with allium compounds (Wargovich 1988, Wattenberg 1986) and onion extracts (You 1989). No experimental human research has been undertaken on allium compounds in humans, but ecologic studies have shown that an area of northern China, where garlic production is high, has the lowest national rate of mortality from stomach cancer in a country where gastric cancer, in general, is high; and that an area of Georgia, where vidalia onions are grown, has a stomach cancer mortality rate about one half the U. S. national level (among the lowest rates in the world). Case-control studies in Greece, China, and Hawaii, have shown that high consumption of allium vegetables is associated with reduced risk of stomach cancer (see You 1989).

Limonene The major component of citrus fruit oils is D-limonene. Wattenberg (1983) has shown that, in mice, citrus oils added to a semipurified diet induce glutathione S-transferase activity and inhibit tumors of forestomach, lung, and mammary (see Wattenberg 1986 and Hocman 1989).

Adaptation and Maladaptation

The relation of cancer risk to consumption of plant foods is probably most usefully considered in an evolutionary/adaptational context. For the purposes of understanding the vegetable, fruit, and cancer data in the broader context, this paper takes, as a starting point, the existence of a seasonally variable diet to which humans are well adapted, especially focusing on intakes of substances for which we are dependent on the environment and intakes of substances to which we have little or infrequent exposure. The following argument is explicated in more detail elsewhere (Potter and Graves 1991, Potter 1992).

Human dietary adaptation?

We cannot be certain to what kind of diets humans are best adapted (although the length and structure of the digestive tract, dental structure, and enzyme patterns provide some clues). Nonetheless, it is reasonable to attempt some tentative description of our early dietary patterns. Significant variability in details must have existed in the same way that extensive geographic and temporal variability are seen today.

Some common features of our early diet include: a high intake of a wide variety of plant foods—roots, leaves, nuts, seeds, fruit (grains could have only become a staple in the last 10 to 15 thousand years but were probably gathered regularly in season); sporadic intake of lean meat low in saturated fat (a more secure and regular supply of fish and seafood for coastal dwellers); an intake of insects, grubs, bone marrow, and organ meats; very low intake of alcohol; little refining or fractionation of food; low and irregular intake of eggs, and very little non-human milk; variability, by season, both of total amount of food available and of kinds of foods resulting in variability in intake of particular nutrients. Other variations in this overall intake pattern would have been defined by climate as it varied over time and from place to place including the consumption of high-fat (but not high saturated-fat) diets in extreme northern populations. In general, until very recently, saturated fat and alcohol intake would have been low, plant food (but not grain) intake high, and food sources highly varied and seasonally variable.

The adaptation argument that helps us make sense of the diet and cancer story, in the light of the idea of an "original" diet, is this: the essential nutrients—both energy-bearing and micronutrients—are available to varying degrees in nature; they have important functions in growth, development, and reproduction; the organism is dependent on their ready availability; deficiencies or excesses impair growth, development, and reproduction. This is the way we already understand the role of essential vitamins, fatty acids, amino acids, etc. There is a plausible analogy for this argument in relation to the presence of substances necessary for the *maintenance* of the organism including, especially, dietary patterns that reduce the risk of cancer. It goes like this: the normal long-term functioning of cells is dependent on the presence of a variety of widespread dietary constituents including, but not confined to, those necessary for growth and development. In their long-term absence, cells malfunction. This malfunctioning state may make the cells more susceptible to exposure to carcinogens or may impair some specific protective mechanisms, such as the responsiveness of enzyme systems that eliminate carcinogens and toxins from the body. It may also be characterized by higher cell replication rates as somatic cells seek to adapt to the new (unprotected) conditions. Some of the substances described above, while not yet usually thought of as "essential nutrients", are probably best described in this way: these substances are the naturally occurring chemicals that, in concert with our own detoxifying enzymes, we rely on to keep us cancer-free.

A converse argument applies to those dietary constituents which are rare in nature: if substances are normally met with only occasionally (or not at all), high intake may have detrimental consequences. This applies both to very rare exposures that produce acute poisoning and to unaccustomed high intakes that overwhelm the metabolic processes which normally handle them. Bacterial, plant, and fungal toxins are members of the first class. Several examples exist of the second: a high fat/high calorie intake has consequences for cholesterol and insulin metabolism, adipose storage, and sex steroid hormone production; a high grain diet (found, particularly, in agricultural communities) is often associated with a reduced intake of other plant foods (and of animal foods) and contains large amounts of abrasive material that may increase cell replication rates particularly in the upper digestive tract; a high intake of alcohol, which together with a generally reduced range of foods, is associated with a wide variety of metabolic abnormalities. There may be differing degrees of adaptation in long-exposed vs unexposed populations in each of these cases.

Objection to the Relevance of an Adaption Argument for Diet and Cancer

An objection to an adaptation argument, in relation to chronic disease, is that natural selection influences reproductive success and that, as chronic diseases are largely diseases of post-reproductive years, a dietary adaptation to ensure long-term maintenance of the organism is an unnecessary postulate. There are four responses to this: the first is to argue that humans have a long period of infant and juvenile dependence and that survival of parents in a healthy state is likely to be selected for. The second response requires consideration of the unit of evolutionary selection. If the issue is the survival of tribes or bands, then those bands would have survived better that had sufficient elders who knew how to respond to infrequently met hazards—food or water shortage, epidemic disease, and natural hazards such as fire or extreme weather. The tribal wisdom maintained by the old would have meant survival of the tribe. Tribes without elders and without knowledge would be more likely to perish. Therefore the tribes in which longevity had appeared would, in turn, have survived other threats to pass on their wisdom, their adaptive eating habits, their adapted metabolisms, their genes, and their tendency to longevity.

Third, to argue that chronic diseases are a phenomenon of older age and therefore that resistance to them cannot have been selected for, is to ignore that these diseases are not a phenomenon of younger ages and that, therefore, some resistance (at least to the point of postponing them to older ages) has been selected for. Fourth, a diet that reduces risk of cancer may also improve reproductive success. There are a wide variety of substances that increase—and some compounds that reduce—both teratogenicity and carcinogenicity. So selection for a diet that improved reproductive success could directly select for reduced risk of cancer.

Summing Up

There are a variety of ways in which diet may influence the development of human cancers. We propose here a theoretical framework for understanding why a high plant food intake lowers cancer risk and indeed for understanding diet and cancer more generally; it is expressed in the form of an argument that, although not yet fully developed, has the following features:

a) There is a dietary pattern to which humans are well-adapted—an "original diet";

b) This original dietary pattern had specific features that included regular exposure to a variety of substances found in plants on which human metabolism, in the long run, is dependent but which are not usually explicitly labelled as "essential nutrients." We would argue that this is now worthy of serious consideration—that is, some of these compounds are essential to the maintenance of a cancer-free organism in a manner exactly analogous to the essential nature of a variety substances to the growth and development of that same organism;

c) Conversely, the original dietary pattern was low in highly abrasive cereal products with less resultant damage and less need for frequent cell repair particularly to the upper gastrointestinal tract;

d) The diet involved variability in intake which was accompanied by variability in cell replication rates particularly in the lower gastrointestinal tract, and little risk of obesity;

e) There was little intake of alcohol and therefore little capacity for its solvent and chronic cell damage capacities;

f) Abandonment of each of these aspects of diet to which we are adapted has consequences for carcinogenesis. Most notable is the reduction of intake of vegetables and fruit (with subsequent loss of increased enzyme "tuning", carcinogen inactivation, suppression of DNA and protein synthesis etc.) and a generally increased rate of cancer at a number of sites. A high intake of fat, of grains, and of alcohol, and increased obesity are each associated with an identifiable pattern of cancers. Further, the plant-derived substances may be most beneficial when the metabolism is exposed to high levels of carcinogenic products and endogenous co-carcinogenic compounds—most associated with eating a diet high in cooked animal foods, living in an industrial society, and using tobacco and alcohol;

g) Testable consequences follow. For instance, increasing vegetables and fruit should reduce the risk of colon cancer and perhaps of colonic adenomatous polyps even in the presence of a high fat intake, and of esophageal cancer even with exposure to specific carcinogenic compounds including those from cigarette smoke. Testing *in vitro* and *in vivo* will provide more definitive answers regarding the specific compounds and their sites and modes of action.

Reduction of consumption of vegetables and fruit means reduced intake of a wide variety of substances that keep enzyme systems "tuned" to handle occasional high intakes of carcinogens; that block the activation of other carcinogens; that act as substrates for endogenous production of anticarcinogens; that reduce the capacity of transformed cells to proliferate, etc. Vegetables and fruit contain the anticarcinogenic cocktail to which we are adapted. We abandon it at our peril.

References

Adlercreutz, H. Western diet and western diseases: some hormonal and biochemical mechanisms and associations. *Scand J Clin Lab Invest* 1990; 50 Suppl 201:3-23.

Bailey G S, Hendricks J D, Shelton D W, Nixon J E, Pawlowski N E. Enhancement of carcinogenesis by the natural anticarcinogen indole-3-carbinol. *J Natl Cancer Inst* 1987; 78:931-4.

Bendich A, Shapiro S S. Effect of beta-carotene and canthaxanthin on the immune responses of the rat. *J Clin Nutr* 1988; 116:2254-62.

Bertram J S, Kolonel L N, Meyskens F L. Rationale and strategies for chemoprevention of cancer in humans. *Cancer Res* 1987; 47:3012-31.

Block G. Vitamin C and cancer prevention: the epidemiologic evidence. *Am J Clin Nutr* 1991; 53:270S-82S.

Bradlow H L, Hershcopf R, Martucci C, Fishman J. 16 alpha-hydroxylation of estradiol: a possible risk marker for breast cancer. *Ann N Y Acad Sci* 1986; 464:138-51.

Bradlow H L, Hershcopf R J, Martucci C P, Fishman J. Estradiol 16 alpha-hydroxylation in the mouse correlates with mammary tumor incidence and presence of murine mammary tumor virus: a possible model for the hormonal etiology of breast cancer in humans. *Proc Natl Acad Sci USA* 1985; 82:6295-9.

Brown J P. A review of the genetic effects of naturally occurring flavonoids, anthraquinones and related compounds. *Mutation Res* 1980; 75:243-77.

Bueding E, Ansher S, Dolan P. Anticarcinogenic and other protective effects of dithiolthiones. In: *Basic Life Sciences* vol. 39. 1986:483-9.

Burney, P G J, Comstock, G W, and Morris, J S: Serologic precursors of cancer: serum micronutrients and the subsequent risk of pancreatic cancer. *Am J Clin Nutr* 1989 49:895-900.

Cameron E, Pauling L. Cancer and vitamin C. Palo Alto, California: Linus Pauling Institute of Science and Medicine, 1979.

Carr B I. Chemical carcinogens and inhibitors of carcinogenesis in the human diet. *Cancer* 1985; 55(Suppl. 1):218-24.

Chen L H, Boissonneault G A, Glauert H P. Vitamin C, vitamin E, and cancer (review). *Anticancer Res* 1988; 8:739-48.

Colditz, G A, Branch, L G, Lipnick, R J, Willett, W C, Rosner, B, Posner, B M, and Hennekens, C H. Increased green and yellow vegetable intake and lowered cancer deaths in an elderly population. *Am J Clin Nutr* 1985 41:32-36.

Colditz G A, Stampfer M J, Willett W C. Diet and lung cancer. A review of the epidemiologic evidence in humans. *Arch Intern Med* 1987; 147:157-60.

Comstock, G W, Menkes, M S, Schober, S E, Vuilleumier, J-P, and Helsing, K J. Serum levels of retinol, beta-carotene, and alpha-tocopherol in older adults. *Am J Epidemiol* 1990 127:114-123.

Connett J E, Kuller L H, Kjelsberg M O, et al. Relationship between carotenoids and cancer: The Multiple Risk Factor Intervention Trial (MRFIT) Study. *Cancer* 1989;64:126-34.

Darby, W J, Ghalioungui, P, and Grivetti, L: Food: The Gift of Osiris, vol. 2. Academic Press Inc., New York, 1977.

Dashwood R H, Arbogast D N, Fong A T, Pereira C, Hendricks J D, Bailey G S. Quantitative interelationships between aflatoxin B1 carcinogen dose, indole-3-carbinol anti-carcinogen dose, target organ DNA adduction and final tumor response. *Carcinogenesis* 1989; 10:175-81.

Diplock A T. Antioxidant nutrients and disease prevention: an overview. *Am J Clin Nutr* 1991; 53:189S-93S.

Doll, R, and Peto R. The Causes of Cancer. Oxford University Press, New York, 1981, p. 1256.

Fenwick, G R, Heaney, R K, and Mullen, W J. Glucosinolates and their breakdown products in foods and food plants. *CRC Crit Rev Food Sci Nutr* 1983 18:123-201.

Fiala E S, Reddy B S, Weisburger J H. Naturally occurring anticarcinogenic substances in foodstuffs. *Annual Rev Nutr* 1985; 5:295-321.176.

Fishman J, Schneider J, Hershcope R J, Bradlow H L. Increased estrogen-16 alpha-hydroxylase activity in women with breast and endometrial cancer. *J Steroid Biochem* 1984; 20:1077-81.

Fontham E T H. Protective dietary factors and lung cancer. *Int J Epidemiol* 1990; 19(Suppl. 1):S32-S42.

Friedman M, Smith G A. Factors which facilitate inactivation of quercetin mutagenicity. *Adv Exp Med* 1984; 177:527-44.

Graham S. Epidemiology of retinoids and cancer. J Natl Cancer Inst 1984; 73:1423-8.

Greenwald P, Lanza E, Eddy G A. Dietary fiber in the reduction of colon cancer risk. J Am Dietetic Assoc 1987; 87:1178-88.

Greenwald P, Lanza E. Dietary fiber and colon cancer. Contemporary Nutrition, published by the General Mills Nutrition Department, vol. 11, no. 1, 1986.

Helzlsouer, K J, Comstock, G W, and Morris, J S. Selenium, lycopene, α-tocopherol, β-carotene, retinol, and subsequent bladder cancer. *Cancer Res* 1989 49:6144-6148.

Hennekens C H, Mayrent S L, Willett W. Vitamin A, carotenoids, and retinoids. *Cancer* 1986; 58(Suppl. 8):1837-41.

Hennekens C H, Physicians Health Study Research Group. Strategies for a primary prevention trial of cancer and cardiovascular disease among U.S. physicians. *Am J Epidemiol* 1983; 118:453-4.

Herrmann K. Flavonols and flavones in food plants: a review. *J Food Tech* 1976; 11:433-8.

Herrmann K. The phenolics of fruits. I. Our knowledge of occurrence and concentrations of fruit phenolics and of their variations in the growing fruit. *Zeitschrift fur Lebensmittel-Untersuchung und -Forschung* 1973; 151:41-51.

Hirayama T. Relationship of soybean paste soup intake to gastric cancer risk. *Nutr Cancer* 1982a 3:223-233.

Hirayama T. Does daily intake of green-yellow vegetables reduce the risk of cancer in man? An example of the application of epidemiologic methods to the identification of individuals at low risk. *IARC Sci Publ* 1982b; 39:531-40.

Hirayama T. Nutrition and cancer—a large scale cohort study. *Prog Clin Biol Res* 1986; 206:299-311.

Hocman G. Prevention of cancer: vegetables and plants. *Comp Biochem Physiol* 1989; 93:201-12.

Howe G R, Hirohata T, Hislop, et al. Dietary factors and risk of breast cancer: combined analysis of 12 case-control studies. *J Natl Cancer Inst* 1990; 82:561-9.

Hsing, A W, Comstock, G W, Abbey, H, and Polk B F. Serologic precursors of cancer. Retinol, carotenoids, and tocopherol and risk of prostate cancer. *J Natl Cancer Inst* 1990 82:941-946.

Ip C. The chemopreventive role of selenium in carcinogenesis. Presented at the NCI workshop on "Strategies Needed to Develop Selenium Compounds for Cancer Preventive Agents," Bethesda, Maryland, 1985.

Jacobs L R. Fiber and colon cancer. *Gastroenterol Clin North Am* 1988; 17:747-60.

Jansen J D. Nutrition and cancer. *World Rev Nutr Diet* 1982; 39:1-22.

Kensler T W, Egner P A, Dolan P M, Groopman J D, Roebuk B D. Mechanisms of protection against aflatoxin tumorigenicity in rats fed 5-(2-pyrazinyl)-4-methyl-1,2-dithiol-3-thione (oltipraz) and related 1,2-dithiol-3-thiones and 1,2-dithiol-3-ones. *Cancer Res* 1987 47:4271-7.

Kensler T W, Egner P A, Trush M A, Bueding E, Groopman J D. Modification of aflatoxin B1 binding to DNA in vivo in rats fed phenolic antioxidants, ethoxyquin, and a diothiolthione. *Carcinogenesis* 1985; 6:759-63.

Knekt, P, Seppanen R, and Aaran, R K. Determinants of alpha-tocopherol in Finnish adults. *Prev Med* 1988 17:725-735.

Kohman, E F. The chemical components of onion vapors responsible for wound-healing qualities. *Science* 1947 106:625-627.

Krinsky N. Effects of carotenoids in cellular and animal systems. *Am J Clin Nutr* 1991:53:238S-46S.

Kväle G, Bjelke E, Gart J J. Dietary habits and lung cancer risk. *Int J Cancer* 1983; 31:397-405.

Lanza E, Butrum R R. A critical review of food fiber analysis and data. *J Am Dietetic Assoc* 1986; 86:732-40.

Lanza E, Jones D Y, Block G, Kessler L. Dietary fiber intake in the U.S. population. *Am J Clin Nutr* 1987; 46:790-7.

Le Marchand L, Yoshizawa C N, Kolonel L N, Hankin J H, Goodman M T. Vegetable consumption and lung cancer risk: a population-based case-control study in Hawaii. *J Natl Cancer Inst* 1989; 81:1158-64.

Long-de W, Hammond E C. Lung cancer, fruit, green salad and vitamin pills. *Chin Med J* 1985; 98:206-10.

Loub W D, Wattenberg L W, Davis D W. Aryl hydrocarbon hydroxylase induction in rat tissues by naturally occurring indoles of cruciferous plants. *J Natl Cancer Inst* 1975; 54:985-8.

MacGregor J T, Schlegel R, Wehr C M, Alperin P, Ames B N. Cytogenetic damage induced by folate deficiency in mice is enhanced by caffeine. *Proc Natl Acad Sci USA* 1990; 87:9962-5.

Mathews-Roth M M. Carotenoids and cancer prevention—experimental and epidemiological studies. *Pure Appl Chem* 1985; 57:717-22.

Menkes M S, Comstock GW, Vuillemier J P, Helsing K J, Rider A A, Brookmeyer R. Serum beta-carotene, vitamins A and E, selenium, and the risk of lung cancer. *N Engl J Med* 1986;315:1250-4.

Messina M, Barnes S. The role of soy products in reducing risk of cancer. *J Natl Cancer Inst* 1991a; 83:541-6.

Messina M, Messina V. Increasing use of soyfoods and their potential role in cancer prevention. *J Am Dietetic Assoc* 1991b; 91:836-40.

Michnovicz J J, Bradlow H L. Induction of estradiol metabolism by dietary indole-3-carbinol in humans. *J Natl Cancer Inst* 1990; 82:947-9.

Michnovicz J J, Hershcopf R J, Naganuma H, Bradlow H L, Fishman J. Increased 2-hydroxylation of estradiol as a possible mechanism for the anti-estrogenic effect of cigarette smoking. *N Engl J Med* 1986; 315:1305-9.

Michnovicz J J, Naganuma H, Hershcopf R J, Bradlow H L, Fishman J. Increased urinary catechol estrogen excretion in female smokers. *Steroids* 1988; 52:69-83.

Micozzi M S, Beecher G R, Taylor P R, Khachlik F. Carotenoid analyses of selected raw and cooked foods associated with a lower risk for cancer. *J Natl Cancer Inst* 1990; 82:282-5.

Mills, P K, Beeson, W L, Abbey, D E, Fraser, G E, Phillips, R L. Dietary habits and past medical history as related to fatal pancreas cancer risk among Adventists. *Cancer* 1988 61:2578-2585.

Milner J A. Dietary antioxidants and cancer. Contemporary Nutrition, published by General Mills Nutrition Department, vol. 10, no. 10, 1985.

Morse M A, Wang C, Stoner G D, et al. Inhibition of 4-(methlynitrosamino)-1-(3-pyridyl)-1-butanone-induced DNA adduct formation and tumorigenicity in the lung of F344 rats by dietary phenethyl isothiocyanate. *Cancer Res* 1989; 49:549-53.

Morse M A, Wang C X, Amin S G, Hecht S S, Chung F L. Effects of dietary sinigrin or indole-3-carbinol on 06-methylguanine-DNA-transmethylase activity and 4-(methylnitrosamino)-1-(3-pyridyl)-1-butanone-induced DNA methylation and tumorigenicity in F344 rats. *Carcinogenesis* 1988; 9:1891-5.

National Research Council (U.S.), Committee on Diet and Health: Diet and Health: Implications for Reducing Chronic Disease Risk. National Academy Press, U.S., 1989.

Nomura A M Y, Stemmerman G N, Heilbrun L K, Salkeld R M, Vuilleumier J P. Serum vitamin levels and the risk of cancer of specific sites in men of Japanese ancestry in Hawaii. *Cancer Res* 1985;45:2369-72.

O'Connor H J, Habibzedah N, Schorah C J, Axon A T, Riley S E, Garner R C. Effect of increased intake of vitamin C on the mutagenic activity of gastric juice and intragastric concentrations of ascorbic acid. *Carcinogenesis* 1985; 6:1175-6.

Oakenfull D, Sidhu G S. Saponins. In: Toxicants of Plant Origin, Cheeke P R, ed., Boca Raton, Florida: CRC Press, Inc., 1989.

Olson J A. Carotenoids, vitamin A and cancer. *J Nutr* 1986;116:1127-30.

Paganini-Hill A, Chao A, Ross R K, Henderson B E. Vitamin A, beta-carotene, and the risk of cancer: a prospective study. *J Natl Cancer Inst* 1987; 79:443-8.

Pearl, R C: Trends in consumption and and processing of fruits and vegetables in the United States. *Food Tech* 1990 44:102-104.

Phillips R L, Snowdon D A. Dietary relationships with fatal colorectal cancer among Seventh-Day Adventists. *J Natl Cancer Inst* 1985; 74:307-17.

Pilch S M, ed. Physiological effects and health consequences of dietary fiber. Bethesda, Maryland: Life Sciences Research Office, Federation of American Societies for Experimental Biology, 1987.

Potter J D. The epidemiology of diet and cancer. Evidence of human maladaption. In Moon TE, Micozzi MS (eds): Nutrition and Cancer Prevention. Investigating the Role of Macronutrients. Dekker: New York, 1992. pp. 55-84.

Potter J D. The epidemiology of fiber and colorectal cancer: why don't the epidemiologic data make better sense? In: Kritchevsky, D, Bonfield, C, Anderson, J W, eds. Dietary Fiber. Plenum Press: New York, 1990:431-446.

Potter J D, Graves K L. Diet and cancer: Evidence and mechanisms—an adaption argument. In Rowland I R (ed): Nutrition, Toxicity, and Cancer. CRC Press: Boca Raton, 1991:379-412.

Prasad K N, Edwards-Prasad J. Expressions of some molecular cancer risk factors and their modification by vitamins. *J Am Coll Nutr* 1990; 9:28-34.

Raicht R F, Cohen B I, Fazzini E P, Sarwal A N, Takahashi M. Protective effect of plant sterols against chemically induced colon tumors in rats. *Cancer Res* 1980; 40:403-5.

Richardson M. The proteinase inhibitors of plants and micro-organisms. *Phytochemistry* 1977; 159-69.

Rieder A, Adamek M, Wrba H. Delay of diethylnitrosamine-induced hepatoma in rats by carrot feeding. *Oncology* 1983; 40:120-3.

Salbe A D, Bjeldanes L F. Effects of brussels sprouts, indole-3-carbinol and in vivo DNA binding of aflatoxin B1 in the rat. *Fed Proc* 1986; 45:970.

Schelp F P, Pongpaew P. Protection against cancer through nutritionally-induced increase of endogenous protease inhibitors—a hypothesis. *Int J Epidemiol*

1988; 17:287-92.

Schneider J, Bradlow H L, Strain G, Levin J. Effects of obestity on estradiol metabolism: decreased formation of nonuterotrophic metabolites. *J Clin Endocrinol Metab* 1983; 56:973-8.

Shekelle R B, Lepper M, Liu S, et al. Dietary vitamin A and risk of cancer in the Western Electric Study. *Lancet* 1981; 2:1185-90.

Sparnins V L, Venegas P L, Wattenberg L W. Glutathione S-transferase activity: enhancement by compounds inhibiting chemical carcinogenesis and by dietary constituents. *J Natl Cancer Inst* 1982; 68:493-6.

Stähelin H B, Gey K F, Eichholzer M, Lüdin E. β-Carotene and cancer prevention: the Basel study. *Am J Clin Nutr* 1991; 53:263S-9S.

Steinmetz K A, Potter J D. Vegetables, fruit, and cancer. I. Epidemiology. *Cancer Causes and Control* 1991a; 2:325-357.

Steinmetz K A, Potter J D. Vegetables, fruit, and cancer. II. Mechanisms. *Cancer Causes and Control* 1991b; 2:427-442.

Stich H F, Rosin M P, Vallejera M O. Reduction with vitamin A and beta-carotene administration of the proportion of micrinucleated buccal mucosal cells in Asian betel nut and tobacco chewers. *Lancet* 1984a; 2:1204-6.

Stich H F, Stich W, Rosin M P, Vallejera M O. Use of the micronucleus test to monitor the effect of vitamin A, beta-carotene and canthaxanthin on the buccal mucosa of betel nut/tobacco chewers. *Int J Cancer* 1984b; 34:745-50.

Stich H F, Rosin M P. Naturally occurring phenolics as antimutagenic and anticarcinogenic agents. *Adv Exp Med* 1984c; 177:1-29.

Stocks P, Karn M N. A co-operative study of the habits, home life, dietary and family histories of 450 cancer patients and of an equal number of control patients. *Ann Eugenics* 1933; 5:30-280.

Stohs S J, Lawson T A, Anderson L, Bueding E. Effects of oltipraz, BHA, ADT, and cabbage on glutathione metabolism, DNA damage and lipid peroxidation in old mice. *Mech Ageing Development* 1986; 37:137-45.

Stryker, W S, Kaplan, L A, Stein, E A, Stampfer, M J, Sober, A, Willett, W C. The relation of diet, cigarette smoking and alcohol consumption to plasma betacarotene and alpha-tocopherol levels. *Am J Epidemiol* 1988 127:283-296.

Subcommittee on the Tenth Edition of the RDAs, Food and Nutrition Board, National Research Council. Recommeded Dietary Allowances, 10th Ed. Washington, D.C. National Academy of Sciences, 1989.

Tajima, K, and Tominaga, S: Dietary habits and gastro-intestinal cancers: a comparative case-control study of stomach and large intestinal cancers in Nagoya, Japan. *Jpn J Cancer Res* 1985 76:705-716.

Trock B, Lanza E, Grennwald P. Dietary fiber, vegetables, and colon cancer: critical review and meta-analyses of the epidemiologic evidence. *J Natl Cancer Inst* 1990; 82:650-61.

Wald N J, Thompson S G, Densem J W, Boreham J, Bailey A. Serum β-carotene and subsequent risk of cancer: results from the BUPA study. *Br J Cancer* 1988; 57:428-33.

Wargovich M J, Woods C, Eng V W S, Stephens L C, Gray K. Chemoprevention of N-nitrosomethylbenzylamine-induced esophageal cancer in rats by the naturally occurring thioether, diallyl sulfide. *Cancer Res* 1988; 48:6872-5.

Wattenberg L W. Chemoprevention of cancer. *Cancer Res* 1985; 45:1-8.

Wattenberg L W. Inhibition of neoplasia by minor dietary constituents. *Cancer Res* 1983 43(Suppl.):2448s-53s.

Wattenberg L W. Inhibition of chemical carcinogenesis. *J Natl Cancer Inst* 1978b; 60:11-18.

Wattenberg L W. Inhibition of carcinogen-induced neoplasias by sodium cyanate, tert-butyl isocyanate, and benzyl isothiocyanate administered subsequent to carcinogen exposure. *Cancer Res* 1981; 41:2991-4.

Wattenberg L W. Inhibitory effects of benzyl isothiocyanate administered shortly before diethylnitrosamine or benzo[a]pyrene on pulmonary and forestomach neoplasia in A/J mice. *Carcinogenesis* 1987; 8:1971-3.

Wattenberg L W, Hanley A B, Barany G, Sparnins V L, Lam L K T, Fenwick G R. Inhibition of carcinogenesis by some minor dietary constituents. In: Hayashi, Y, ed. Diet, Nutrition, and Cancer. Tokyo: Japan Sci. Soc. Press, 1986:193-203.

Wattenberg L W, Loub W D. Inhibition of polycyclic aromatic hydrocarbon-induced neoplasia by naturally occurring indoles. *Cancer Res* 1978a; 38:1410-3.

Willett W C, Mac Mahon B. Diet and cancer—an overview I. *N Engl J Med* 1984a; 310:633-638.

Willett WC, Mac Mahon B. Diet and cancer—an overview II. *N Engl J Med* 1984b; 310:697-703.

Willett W C, Stampfer M J, Colditz G A, Rosner B A, Speizer F E. Relation of meat, fat, and fiber intake to the risk of colon cancer in a prospective study among women. *N Engl J Med* 1990b; 323:1664-72.

Willett W C. Selenium, vitamin E, fiber, and the incidence of human cancer: an epidemiologic perspective. *Adv Exp Med Biol* 1986; 206:27-34.

Willett W C. Vitamin A and lung cancer. *Nutr Rev* 1990a; 48:201-11.

You W C, Blot W J, Chang Y S, et al. Allium vegetables and the reduced risk of stomach cancer. *J Natl Cancer Inst* 1989; 81:162-4.

Ziegler R G. A review of epidemiologic evidence that carotenoids reduce the risk of cancer. *J Nutr* 1989; 119:116-22.

The Polyp Prevention Trial: Rationale and Design

Arthur Schatzkin, M.D., Dr.P.H.
Elaine Lanza, Ph.D.
Laura Kruse, R.D., M.P.H.

Cancer Prevention Studies Branch
Division of Cancer Prevention and Control
National Cancer Institute
Bethesda, Maryland 20892

A great deal of evidence suggests that diet plays an important role in the etiology of large bowel cancer. However, causality is not yet proven, and may questions remains unanswered.

The study being discussed here, the Polyp Prevention Trial (PPT) is designed to answer some of these questions. The PPT is a multi institutional randomized controlled dietary intervention study of large bowel adenomatous polyp recurrence. It is an intramural trial originating in the Cancer Prevention Studies Branch in the Division of Cancer Prevention and Control at NCI. The study chairpersons are Dr. Elaine Lanza and myself.

We should remember that large bowel cancer is a particularly nasty disease. In this country alone over 150,000 cases will be diagnosed this year and the disease will kill of over 60,000 men and women (1).

The Likely Role of Environmental Factors

Three lines of evidence indicate that environmental factors are important in the genesis of large bowel cancer:

First, the frequency of the disease varies widely throughout the world, there being over a 10-fold difference in colon cancer mortality between countries with the highest and those with the lowest rates (2).

Second, time trend studies show substantial changes in large bowel cancer rates in relatively short periods of time, as in Japan (3).

Third, a number of studies have shown among migrants a convergence in cancer rates from those in the country of origin to those in the country of destination (4). Moreover, and this is particularly relevant to our study, this convergence can occur within the lifespan of the migrants themselves (5).

Diet and Large Bowel Cancer

Among the many environmental exposures to consider, diet is a strong candidate. In accord with the ecologic data just cited, diet varies widely across countries, dietary intake has changed over time in several countries, and diet changes with migration and acculturation (6,7). Furthermore, dietary etiology makes sense biologically: food or its various metabolites reaches the bowel mucosa directly and various nutrients affect several physiologic processes implicated in large bowel carcinogenesis, such as bile acid metabolism (8,9).

Although in our study we emphasize an overall dietary pattern, it is necessary to specify individual nutrients or foods in order to characterize the dietary pattern and make an intervention concrete and practical. There are three aspects of diets from low risk populations that have received a great deal of attention: dietary fat, dietary fiber and fruits and vegetables.

Only a few remarks will be made here about dietary fat and fruits and vegetables. Although the data are not entirely consistent, animal studies, human metabolic studies, and epidemiological evidence generally point to a role for dietary fat in large bowel carcinogenesis (10). Rather compelling data have been produced by the Nurse's Health Study, a prospective cohort study of over 90,000 nurses yielding about 150 colon cancers (11). There was about a doubling of colon cancer risk among those nurses in the highest, compared to those in the lowest, category of animal fat intake, as well as a significant dose-response relation. Most epidemiologic studies show that intake of vegetables and (to a lesser extent) fruits is protective against large bowel cancer (12).

Although there is something about fiber that lends itself to cartoons, there is a good deal of hard science to back up the hypothesis that dietary fiber intake protects against large bowel malignancy. For example, there is a strong international correlation between colon cancer mortality and per capita fiber consumption (13) (though not as strong as that for fat [9]). In a recent meta-analysis of case-control studies of dietary fiber and large bowel cancer, Trock and colleagues found approximately a 35% reduction in risk for persons in the highest compared to those in the lowest quantile of fiber intake (14).

In the PPT the intervention involves changes in an overall eating plan, rather than a modification of a single nutrient. There are several rationales for this comprehensive dietary pattern approach:

1. Nutrients are intercorrelated. In epidemiologic studies it is difficult to disentangle, for example, associations with fiber and vegetables.

2. As yet unidentified nutrients (in vegetables and other plant foods, for example) may play a role in large bowel carcinogenesis, and a single-nutrient intervention might not capture these.

3. There may be important interactions among several food constituents.

4. Finally, given the evidence for each of the three dietary components—fat, fiber and fruits and vegetables, we want to intervene with an eating plan comprising all three, to maximize the possibility of showing an effect.

Certainly one can conceive of a broad range of dietary patterns that correspond to those from, for example, low and high risk areas around the world.

Adenomatous Polyps as Study Endpoint

There are at least three reasons why adenomatous polyps make a food endpoint:

First, they are very common in the U. S. population, with a prevalence of more than 30% in men and women over the age of 50 (15).

Second, they recur often (recurrence referring to the development of a polyp anywhere in the large bowel after an earlier polypectomy), with annual rates of 10% and up being reported from various studies (16).

Third, considerable evidence has accumulated in support of what is known as the adenoma-carcinoma sequence. It is generally held today that adenomas are necessary precursors for most large bowel malignancies (15, 17).

It follows, therefore, that factors diminishing polyp recurrence are likely to reduce the incidence of large bowel cancer. This is an underlying premise of the PPT.

Trial Design

The primary objective of the PPT is to determine whether the recurrence rate of large bowel adenomatous polyps will be lower in persons adopting a low fat, high fiber, high fruit and vegetable eating plan than in those with the customary high fat, low fiber, low fruit and vegetable U.S. dietary pattern.

One of the things that makes this trial possible is the standard of care for colonoscopic post-polypectomy surveillance. Many gastroenterologists have adhered to a scheme whereby patients undergo colonoscopy one and four years after the initial polypectomy. This scheme is incorporated into the PPT, as reflected in the trial flow chart (Figure 1).

Men and women at least 35 years of age who have had at least one adenoma removed will fill out a 4DFR and FFQ as part of a quasi-"run-in" phase. Only those persons successfully completing this run-in and meeting other eligibility criteria will be randomized. (Examples of these other eligibility criteria are not having a prior history of large bowel cancer, inflammatory bowel disease, or colorectal resection; age 35 and above; not consuming a dietary pattern similar to the intervention eating plan; not having any dietary practice, behavior or attitude that would substantially limit adherence to the intervention program.)

Participants will be randomized, to T_0, to either the intervention or control group, with 1000 participants in each group. One year and 4 years after T_0 participants will be endoscoped, and follow-up is complete at the T_4 procedure. Randomization of the 2000 participants at the Clinical Centers is expected to take 2 years and should be completed before the end of 1994. The trial is currently taking place at eight clinical centers around the country: Bowman Gray School of Medicine, Winston-Salem, North Carolina; University of Pittsburgh School of Medicine, Pennsylvania; Kaiser Foundation Research Institute, Oakland, California; Memorial Sloan-Kettering Cancer Center, New York; University of Buffalo School of Medicine and Biomedical Sciences, New York; Walter Reed Army Medical Center, Washington Center, Hines, Illinois. The data and Nutrition Coordinating Center is Westat, Inc., located in Rockville, Maryland.

Although recurrence of one or more adenomas is our primary endpoint, we can also look at number, size and histology of adenomas. The sample size of 2000 in the PPT permits detection of approximately a

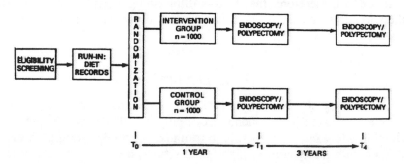

Figure. 1. Flow chart for Polyp Prevention Trial.

24% reduction in the annual polyp recurrence rate. This corresponds to an expected recurrence proportion over three years of 21% in the intervention group, compared to 27% in the control group.

Nutrition Program

The nutrition program is a critical component of the PPT. The dietary targets for the intervention group are 20% calories from fat, 18g dietary fiber per 1000 kcal.; and 508 servings per day of fruits and vegetables. You will note that the targets for each of the three dietary elements—fat, fiber, fruits and vegetables—has been adjusted for total energy intake (Table 1).

You can see in the last two rows that it is anticipated that about half of the fiber will come from fruits and vegetables and half from grains.

The Polyp Prevention nutrition program is modeled after that for the Women's Health Trial (18). It involves individual counseling in the first year with group counseling being introduced in the second year and, in fact, even earlier at some Centers. There will be 6 weekly counseling sessions, 3 biweekly and 9 monthly sessions in the first year. Beginning in the second year sessions will take place every other month and we may maintain that for the duration of the trial. The program involves the integration of both nutritional and behavioral principles, including self-management in the development of a specific eating plan; an emphasis on the positive, e.g., those foods that may be added to one's dietary repertoire; gradual change in adopting the new eating plan; and finally, the involvement of social supports in adopting and maintaining the eating plan.

With regard to the organization and focus of the intensive counseling program, fat is introduced first, then fruits and vegetables, eating plan; an emphasis on the positive, e.g., those foods that may be added to one's

Table 1. Dietary goals for intervention participants at different levels of total energy intake

Calories	1,300	1,700	2,100	2,400
Fat (g/day)	29	38	47	53
Fruit/Veg servings	5	6	7	8
Total Fiber (g/day)	23	31	38	43
Fiber (g/day: fruit/veg)*	13	15	18	20
Fiber (g/day: grains)*	10	16	20	23

*The distribution of fiber from each of the two major sources, fruits/vegetables and grains, will be monitored but is not an explicit dietary goal. The figures here are estimates of the likely amounts of total dietary fiber coming from these two sources.

dietary repertoire; gradual change in adopting and maintaining the eating plan.

With regard to the organization and focus of the intensive counseling program, fat is introduced first, then fruits and vegetables, and then fiber. Each participant receives a nutrition manual with chapters tailored to each counseling visit.

Dietary assessment is an important aspect of the PPT nutrition program. Given the strengths and limitations of various assessment instruments, we will use each of three different instruments: the four-day food record (4DFR), food frequency questionnaire (FFQ) (specially modified given the low fat, high fiber eating plan), and the unannounced 24-hour recall. The FFQ will be analyzed for 100% of participants, the 4DFR for 20% and the 24-hour recall for 10% of the participants.

Biologic Specimens and Intermediate Endpoints

We are collecting and storing bloods for subsequent analysis of lipids, carotenoids, hormones. White cells are being collected for possible DNA analysis. We are also obtaining rectal biopsy specimens for cell proliferation studies, particularly labeling index determinations with the bromodeoxuyuridine (19) and proliferating cell nuclear antigen (PCNA) (20) assays.

There are 3 secondary objectives in integrating these putative intermediate endpoints into the Polyp Prevention Trial. These are to investigate

1) the relation between diet and the proliferation markers,

2) the relation between the markers and polyps—does epithelial cell proliferation predict polyp recurrence, and

3) whether the intermediate endpoints, these markers of proliferation, mediate any observed relation between diet and neoplasia.

Conclusion

The PPT has a good chance of demonstrating definitively that dietary modification affects large bowel neoplasia, in particular, the key precursor lesion for malignancy. This would go a long way toward establishing the scientific basis of a rational prevention strategy for large bowel cancer.

References

1. Ries L A G, Hankley B F, Miller B A, Hartman A M, Edwards B K. Cancer Statistics Review 1973-88. National Cancer Institute. NIH Pub. No. 91-2789, 1991.
2. Kurihara M, Aoki K, Tominaga S. Cancer mortality statistics in the world,

Nagoya, Japan: University of Nagoya Press, 1984.

3. Kazuo T, Hirose K, Nakagawa N, et al. Jpn J Cancer Res. (Gann) 1985; 76: 717-28.

4. Ziegler R G, Devesda. S S, Fraumeni J F. Epidemiologic patterns of colorectal cancer. In DeVita V T, Jr., Hellman S., Rosenberg S A, eds. Important advances in oncology. Philadelphia: J.P. Lippincott, 1986, pp. 209-32.

5. McMichael A J, Giles G G. Cancer in migrants to Australia: extending the descriptive epidemiological data. Can Res 1988; 48: 751-6.

6. Drasar B S, Irving D. Environmental factors and cancer of the colon and breast. Br J Cancer 1973; 27: 167-72.

7. Weisburger J H, Wynder E L. Etiology of colorectal cancer with emphasis on mechanism of action and prevention. In DeVita V T, Jr., Hellman S., Rosenberg S A, eds. Important advances in oncology. Philadelphia: J. P. Lippincott, 1987, pp.197-220.

8. Bruce W R. Recent hypotheses for the origin of colon cancer. Can Res 1987; 47:4237-42.

9. Hill M J. Mechanisms of colorectal carcinogenesis. In Joosens J V et al., eds. Diet and human carcinogenesis. Elsevier Science Publishers, 1985, pp. 149-163.

10. Kolonel L. Fat and colon cancer; how firm is the epidemiologic evidence. Am. J. Clin Nutr. 1987; 45: 336-41.

11. Willett W C, Stampfer M J, Colditz G A, Posner B A, Speizer F E. Relation of meat, fat and fiber intake to the risk of colon cancer in a prospective study among women. New Engl J Med 1990; 323: 1164-72.

12. Steinmetz K A, Potter J D, Vegetables, fruit and cancer. I. epidemiology. Steinmetz K A, Potter J D. Cancer Causes and Control 1991; 2: 325-57.

13. McKeown G E, Bright-SEE E. Dietary factors in colon cancer: international relationships. Nutr Cancer; 1984; 6: 160-170.

14. Trock B, Lanza E, Greenwald P. Dietary fiber, vegetables and colon cancer: critical review and meta- analyses of the epidemiologic evidence. J Natl Cancer Inst 1990; 82: 650-61.

15. Berg J W. Epidemiology, pathology, and the importance of adenomas. In Steel G, Jr., Burt R W, Winawer, S J, Karr J P, eds. Basic and clinical perspectives of colorectal polyps and cancer. New York: Alan R. Liss, Inc. 1988, pp. 13-21.

16. Neugut A I, Johnsen C M, Forde K A, Treat Mr. Recurrence rates for colorectal polyps. Cancer 1985; 55:1586-9.

17. Muto T., Bussey J H R, Morson B C. The evolution of cancer of the colon and rectum. Cancer 1975; 36:2251-70.

18. Henderson M M, Kushi K H, Thompson D J, Gorbach S L, Clifford C K, Insull W, Moskowitz M, Thompson R S. Feasibility of a randomized trial of a low-fat diet for the prevention of breast cancer: dietary compliance in the Women's Health Trial Vanguard Study. Preventive Medicine 1990; 19:115-33.

19. Potten C S, Kellett M, Roberts S A, Rew D A, Wilson G D. Measurement of in vivo proliferation in human colorectal mucosa using bromodeoxyuridine. Gut 1992; 33:71-8.

20. Galand P, Degraef C. Cyclin/PCNA immunostaining as an alternative to tritiated thymidine pulse labelling for marking S. phase cells in paraffin sections from animal and human tissues. Cell Tissue Kinetics 1989; 22:383-92.

ECP Trial of Fibre in Precancerous Lesion of the Large Bowel

Michael J. Hill

European Cancer Prevention Organization
PO Box 1199, Andover, Hants SP1 1YN, UK

Background

Within the European Community cancer causes more than 700,000 deaths per year, and a high proportion of these must be preventable. There is also a wide range in cultures and in cancer patterns between the various component countries; this range is illustrated in Tables 1 and 2. Table 1 shows the varying cancer patterns between the European countries; colorectal cancer tends to be more common in the north and west than in the south and east of Europe, whilst the reverse tends to be true of cancer of the oesophagus, stomach and liver. Lung cancer mortality is relatively low (but falling) in the Benelux countries and the UK. Table 2 illustrates the variation in incidence of colorectal cancer between and within European countries; there is a 3-fold range in incidence between Saarland and Zaragoza, but within the major European countries the incidence in the highest registry is more than 50% in excess of that in the lowest registry. These ranges are accompanied by equally wide ranges in dietary patterns, smoking habits, exposure to sunlight, etc., and these ranges in exposures to putative carcinogens and in cancer incidences make Europe an ideal "laboratory" for the study of cancer causation and prevention.

For this reason in 1981 the European Cancer Prevention organization was set up, its aim being to organize multinational concerted action studies of causation and prevention of cancer.

The work programme is divided under 7 headings, one of which is the colon cancer group, headed by Professor Jean Faivre (Dijon, France). The structure of ECP is discussed in more detail elsewhere (Hill, 1991).

The ECP Colon Cancer Group

The group took as its starting point the mechanism of the adenoma carcinoma sequence as set out by Hill et al (1978) and as further elaborated by Faivre et al (1985). There is a large mass of information on the role of diet in the overall process of colorectal carcinogenesis, but there are many inconsistencies and few studies have yielded strong correlations. Table 3 lists some areas of consistency and some of inconsistency. An intriguing observation is that, whilst data from the United States and Australia tend to support a major role for fat, a series of recent case-control studies have failed to obtain similar findings, all showed strong protective effects of vegetables and of fresh fruit (Table 4). Perhaps the reasons for this are that, not only are the separate stages of the adenoma-carcinoma sequence caused by different factors, but that also the factors causing an individual stage are not the same in all locations. This is plausible, but there is at present little evidence for or against any of it.

Table 1. Mortality (per 100,000 males, age adjusted) from cancer at various sites in a sample of European countries (data from Levi *et al*, 1989)

	Mouth	Oesophagus	Stomach	Colo-rectum	Liver	Lung
Sweden	2.7	2.9	12.8	16.5	3.7	24.6[+]
Denmark	3.1	3.5	12.2[+]	24.3**	2.4	53.4
Norway	2.5	2.6[+]	14.6	18.1	1.6	26.4
Germany FRG	3.9	4.0	21.2	18.0	1.6	49.0
Germany DDR	3.2	3.1	21.7	23.7*	1.9	50.9
France	15.6**	13.3**	12.5	22.9	2.8	42.1
England & Wales	2.8	5.9	16.8	21.1	1.1[+]	69.9
Scotland	3.2	8.1*	17.4	23.1	1.5	83.5**
Belgium	3.5	4.3	16.4	22.6	3.1	77.8*
Netherlands	2.0[+]	3.4	17.5	20.0	1.2	77.6
Portugal	5.0	5.8	29.7*	16.9	0.9[+]	20.1[+]
Spain	4.0	5.3	19.8	11.8	9.1**	33.9
Greece	1.7[+]	1.9[+]	12.1[+]	7.7[+]	1.7	45.1
Italy	6.2*	4.8	22.7	18.2	4.7	52.9
Yugoslavia	4.5	3.6	21.1	11.8	6.4	39.3
Poland	4.8	4.2	30.4**	11.7[+]	7.7*	54.6

** and * are the two highest mortality rates for a cancer site whilst the two lowest are marked [+].

ECP therefore decided to carry out a multi-centre concerted action study of the relation between diet and adenoma causation, adenoma growth, and adenoma progression to carcinoma. At the same time, since there is evidence that carcinoma of the right colon, the left colon and the rectum have differences in epidemiological behaviour, the results of the

Table 2. Variation within European countries in age-standardized incidence of colorectal cancer

Country	Registry	Cancer incidence (per 100,000)	
		Males	Females
FRG	Saarland	43.1	30.7
	Hamburg	30.6	25.2
France	Bas-Rhin	41.6	23.4
	Isere	31.9	21.4
	Calvados	27.8	17.8
UK	NE Scotland	39.9	32.1
	NW England	33.5	24.0
	SW England	30.0	23.5
	S Thames	27.6	22.7
Italy	Varese	38.9	25.9
	Porma	32.6	21.5
	Ragusa	22.0	15.8
Spain	Navarre	22.9	15.8
	Zaragoza	13.8	10.7

Table 3. Epidemiology and aetiology of colorectal adenomas

Geographical distribution	Prevalence is high in North America, Australia and Western Europe; low in Asia and the Andean countries; very low in Africa.
Prevalence in comparison with colorectal cancer incidence	There are groups of countries with similar prevalence of adenomas but very different cancer incidence and *vice versa*
Subsite distribution	Adenomas evenly distributed along the large bowel (carcinomas are concentrated in the left colon and rectum)
Sex ratio	Prevalence in males:females = 1.5
Relation to diet	Very little information
Relation to lifestyle	Prevalence higher in smokers

study are being stratified by subsite as well as by stage in the adenoma-carcinoma sequence. The results are currently being analysed, but examples of some of the early results (Boutron et al, 1991) are that both alcohol and tobacco have been associated with individual stages. Tobacco was strongly associated with adenoma formation but not with adenoma growth or progression to carcinoma (hence the difficulty is detecting an association with the overall process). Alcohol was associated with adenoma growth but not with adenoma formation or progression; it was much more strongly associated with distal colonic adenomas than with those in the proximal colon. The results of the main dietary analysis should be available later this summer.

Strategy for the Design
of the ECP Intervention Study

On the basis of the adenoma-carcinoma sequence, it can be seen that colon carcinogenesis can be prevented either by inhibiting adenoma formation or by inhibiting adenoma progression through increasing serenity of epithelial dysplasia to carcinoma. Since large adenomas are very much more sensitive to dysplasia-causing agents, inhibiting adenoma growth should also inhibit carcinogenesis in the colon.

Table 3 summarizes our knowledge of the causation of adenomas. It is not impressive and certainly does not, at this stage, justify a reasoned intervention study. However, studies of the effect of dietary changes on the rate of formation of new adenomas are easy to design and to conduct and so, despite the lack of scientific background information, most primary prevention studies are of this type. In 1987 ECP organized a work-

Table 4. Epidemiology and aetiology of large colorectal adenomas

Geographical distribution	Large adenomas are a higher proportion of the total in the UK, US and Sweden than in Japan or Colombia
Prevalence in relation to colorectal cancer incidence	Epidemiology very similar to colorectal cancer
Subsite distribution	Similar to that of colorectal cancers rather than adenomas
Sex ratio	Prevalence in males:females $= 1.5$
Relation to diet	Associated with high fat/low fibre and with alcohol
Relation to lifestyle	Excess risk in smokers less than for all adenomas but more than for carcinomas

shop on colorectal carcinogenesis (Faivre and Hill, 1987) in which the evidence on the normal rate of growth of adenomas was presented (Hoff et al, 1986, 1987, 1991), together with evidence that small adenomas could safely be left in situ for 3 years without developing dysplasia or growing to more than 10 mm diameter. This made it feasible to study the effect of dietary intervention on adenoma growth—about which we know a considerable amount from indirect evidence (Table 4). In fact, almost all that we know about dietary colorectal carcinogenesis concerns the adenoma-growth stage because this is the rate-limiting step.

Choice of Intervention

On the basis of what we know abut colorectal carcinogenesis, there are a number of possible intervention strategies including (a) dilution of colonic contents, (b) decrease of colonic pH, (c) change to a low fat/high fibre diet, (d) high calcium diet.

The evidence that adenoma growth is caused by factors in the gut lumen has been discussed in detail elsewhere. Some of the most persuasive evidence comes from the demonstration that diversion of the faecal stream (as a result of colostomy, for example) causes the regression of rectal polyps. The distribution of large adenomas in the colon is consistent with them being caused by a luminal factor concentrated during colonic transit by the gradual dehydration of colonic contents. If this is so then any stool bulking agent which causes dilution of the colonic contents should decrease the rate of adenoma growth and progression to carcinoma.

There is a body of evidence that suggests that an acid environment in the colon protects against colorectal carcinogenesis (Thornton, 1981); this comes from epidemiological studies (Hill, 1971; McDonald et al, 1977; Petrouista et al, 1985) and from animal model experiments (Rafter et al, 1986). There is also a body of evidence implicating gut bacterial metabolites (Hill, 1971, 1987; Gorbach, 1984; Reddy et al, 1979). A possible mechanism for the effect of colonic pH could be through its effect on the activity of bacterial enzymes and the rate of production of adenoma growth factors. Regardless of the mechanism, interventions which cause acidification of the colonic contents should decrease the rate of adenoma growth and progression to carcinoma. There is a body of evidence from studies of populations that a high prevalence of large adenomas is associated with a diet rich in animal fat and relatively low in dietary fibre. This has yet to be supported (or refuted) by case-control studies, although in this respect the results of the ECP case-control study discussed earlier will be of interest. If this association is causal, then a low fat/high fibre diet should decrease the rate of adenoma growth. The postulated role for calcium has been discussed at length elsewhere (Wargovich et al, 1983; Newmark et al, 1984; Rafter, et al, 1986; Van der Meer et al, 1991). This suggests that dietary supplements of calcium should protect against the toxic and adenoma growth promoting effects of bile acids. These toxic effects can also be ameliorated by precipitation of the bile acids at acid pH values (Rafter et al, 1987)—a further possible mechanism by which colonic acidification might work.

On the basis of these mechanisms the interventions that were considered were (a) high fibre/low fat diet; (b) supplements of stool bulking dietary fibre; (c) supplements of lactulose; (d) supplements of calcium.

The first of these options was rejected quickly as being the least suitable for a large intervention trial. Such trials are most readily set up and monitored when the nature of the intervention is simplest and clearest. For example, administration of a vitamin is readily explained to the subject in terms of numbers of tablets per day and readily monitored from blood levels. It is relatively easy for volunteers to modify their diets by taking supplements without interfering with their social lives and family dining arrangements. Change of the whole diet to one low in fat and high in fibre either leads to the subject having to prepare meals for one and eating alone or else to the whole family taking the modified diet. Furthermore, the dietary change is not easy to validate and so requires an elaborate and expensive monitoring system. Finally, it is not amenable to double blind study.

In contrast, the calcium supplements provide the ideal intervention, being easy to administer as tablets to be taken with meals, easy to validate (via urinary or faecal calcium) and easy to match to a placebo allowing double blind studies. There is a large body of experience (and literature) to confirm the safety of the supplements and there is good evidence from animal experiments (Rafter et al, 1986) and from cell proliferation studies (Lipkin and Newmark, 1985) that it might be an effective intervention.

Supplements to promote stool bulking share the simplicity of study design of the calcium supplements and are easy to administer, can be matched to a placebo and can be monitored if sufficient is given to yield measurable increase in stool bulk. Since many fibre supplements are readily fermented in the colon, it is possible to aim for both stool bulking and colonic acidification. This aim is most readily achieved with oligosaccharides or disaccharides (such as lactulose) or sugar alcohols (such as mannitol). However, such saccharides proved, in pilot studies, to be unacceptable to healthy persons as long-term supplements because of the level of colonic unease, which made people reluctant to go far from a toilet.

The acceptable supplements were therefore calcium and fibre, and these are being used in the ECP intervention study. The rationale for the calcium and the fibre interventions have been described by Faivre et al (1991).

The ECP Intervention Study

As has been discussed earlier, my personal view is that we have little information on adenoma formation and so no justification at this stage for a dietary intervention to inhibit new adenoma formation. However, the simplicity of such an end-point makes it very suitable for inclusion in a study of adenoma growth. The primary aim of the intervention is therefore to determine the effects of the dietary supplements on: (a) a small adenoma left *in situ*; (b) the rate of formation of new adenomas in the large bowel. In addition to these primary aims, a number of other questions will be answered, including the importance of adenoma subsite on the efficacy of the treatment and the effect of the number of previous polypectomies; the effect of the treatment on the rate of colonic cell proliferation and on the stool fatty acid composition.

A diet history will be taken on all subjects to permit the evaluation of the effect of normal diet on the rate of adenoma and recurrence in the placebo group and on the effect of the supplements in the treatment groups. In addition, in the placebo group it will permit the study of the relation between diet and colonic cell proliferation rate and of the relation between colonic cell proliferation rate on recruitment on the rate of formation of new adenomas or growth of existing adenomas during the next 3 years.

The study that is currently in progress is a parallel design with 3 arms (calcium, fibre, placebo). Calcium is administered as 2 g calcium per day (as 13.6 g calcium gluconolactate and 0.6 g calcium carbonate), in the form of 4 sachets of orange flavoured evanescent capsules taken in water with meals. This did not give compliance problems in the preliminary organoleptic studies. Fibre (3.5 g per day) is given in the form of fybogel (ispaghula husk) as an orange flavoured drink. The placebo is also in the form of an orange flavoured drink and contains sucrose.

The study population will consist of persons aged 40–75 at entry, recruited from the polypectomy clinic and who at entry have at least two colorectal polyps, at least one of which must be an adenoma more than 5 mm in diameter (in order to be sure that the colonic environment contains the factors causing adenoma growth). During complete colonoscopy all of the polyps are removed except for one less than 5 mm diameter, situated in a subsite that makes it easy to locate and identify. The person is then given a study number and assigned to one of the treatment arms according to a computer established randomization list. Patients are only recruited to the study if it is established that they are able and willing to follow the protocol and after having given informed consent in writing. There is a long list of exclusions (eg polyposis coli, inflammatory bowel disease, colonic resection, life threatening disease, history which contra-indicates administration of fibre or calcium etc). The diet supplementation will be for 3 years.

It has been estimated that a cohort of 400 patients in each arm will be needed to detect a 10% reduction in rate of adenoma growth or of adenoma formation (the former takes account of the fact that a proportion of the tumours left in will not be non-adenomatous polyps).

Contact will be maintained with the patients principally through the study nurse who will talk to them regularly (ie, six monthly) when they are given their next supply of tablets. Blood will be taken (for calcium assay) annually and also a faecal sample for assay of calcium and of volatile fatty acids. A dietary questionnaire will be completed on recruitment to the study and at the end of 3 years treatment, because it is possible that the cohort will be exposed to healthy diet messages involving either fibre or calcium intake (or both). Biopsy samples will be taken from the sigmoid colon at the initial and final colonoscopies for cell proliferation assay. Faecal samples will be collected at regular intervals for faecal bile acid assay in order to document the effect of the intervention, the relation between faecal bile and cell proliferation (as suggested by the results of Biasco et al, 1991) and the relation between faecal bile acids and adenoma growth and new adenoma formation.

Conclusion

The study will yield a rich harvest of information on the relation between clinical, dietary, and analytical factors and the rate of growth of adenomas or the rate of formation of new tumours. If either intervention is successful, it will then be necessary to determine the best public health measures to achieve the same effect in the general population. It is widely assumed that this will be by promoting a major switch in the national diet accompanied by fortification of foods. However, it is likely that a proportion of the population willing to listen to advice on healthy eating would nevertheless prefer to continue with their current diet, supplemented by tablets.

References

Biasco G, Paganelli G, Owen R et al (1991). Faecal bile acids and colorectal cell proliferation. *Eur J Cancer Prevention* 1 (Suppl 2):63-8.

Boutron M-C, Wilpart M, Faivre J (1991). Diet and colorectal cancer. *Eur J Cancer Prev* 1 (Suppl 2):13-20.

Faivre J, Boutron M-C, Hillon P, Bedenne L, Klepping C (1985). Epidemiology of colorectal cancer. In Diet and Human Carcinogenesis (eds, J Joossens, M Hill,

J Geboers); Excerpta Medica, Amsterdam, pp 123-36.

Faivre J, Hill M (1987). Causation and Prevention of Colorectal Cancer, Excerpta Medica, Amsterdam.

Faivre J, Doyon F, Boutron M-C (1991). The ECP calcium fibre polyp prevention study. *Eur J Cancer Prev* 1 (Suppl 2):83-90.

Gorbach S L (1984). Estrogens, breast cancer and intestinal flora. *Rev Infect Dis* 6:85-9.

Hill M J (1971). The effect of some factors on the faecal concentration of acid steroids, neutral steroids and urobilins. *J Path* 104: 239-45.

Hill M J (1987). The role of bacteria in human carcinogenesis. *Anticancer Res* 7:1079-1084.

Hill M J (1991). Introduction and overview of ECP. In Causation and Prevention of Human Cancer (eds M Hill, A Giacosa); Kluwer Academic Publishers, Lancaster, pp 1-8.

Hill M J, Morson B C, Bussey H J R (1978). Aetiology of adenoma-carcinoma sequence in the large bowel. *Lancet* 1:245-7.

Hoff G, Moen E, Trygg K et al (1986). Epidemiology of polyps in the rectum and sigmoid colon. Evaluation of nutritional factors. *Scand J Gastroenterol* 21:199-204.

Hoff G, Vatn M, Larsen G (1987). Relationship between tobacco smoking and colorectal polyps. *Scand J. of Gastroenterol* 22:13-16.

Hoff G, Vatn M (1991). Colonic adenoma: natural history. Digestive Dis 9:61-9.

Levi F, Maisonneuve P, Filiberti R, La Vecchia C, Boyle P (1989). Cancer incidence and mortality in Europe. *Soz Priventiv Med* Supplement 2.

Lipkin M, Newmark H (1985). Effect of added calcium on colonic epithelium cell proliferation in subjects at high risk of familial colonic cancer. *N Eng J Med* 313:1381-4.

MacDonald I A, Webb G R, Mahoney D E (1978). Fecal hydroxysteroid dehydrogenase activities in vegetarian Seventh Day Adventists, control subjects and bowel cancer cases. *Am J Clin Nutr* 31:233- 8.

Newmark H L, Wargovich M J, Bruce W R (1984). Colon cancer and dietary fat, phosphate and calcium: a hypothesis. *JNCI* 72: 1323-6.

Petrouisti A, Caprilli R, Giuliano M, Serrano S, Vita S (1985). Faecal pH in colorectal cancer. *Ital J Gastroenterol* 17:88-91.

Rafter J, Eng V, Furrer R, Medline A, Bruce W R (1986). Effect of dietary calcium and pH on the mucosal damage produced by deoxycholic acid in the rat colon. *Gut* 27:1320-9.

Rafter J, Child P, Anderson A M, Alder R, Eng V, Bruce W R (1987). Cellular toxicity of faecal water depends on diet. *Am J Clin Nutr* 45:559-63.

Reddy B S, Watanabe K (1979). Effect of cholesterol metabolites and promoting effect of lithocholic acid in germfree and conventional F344 rats. *Cancer Res* 39:1521-4.

Thornton J R (1981). High colonic pH promotes colorectal cancer. *Lancet* 1:1081-2.

Van der Meer R, Kleibeuker J H, Lapré J (1991). Calcium phosphate, bile acids and colorectal cancer. *Eur J Cancer Prev* 1 (Supplement 2):55-62.

Wargovich M, Eng V, Newmark H, Bruce W R (1983). Calcium ameliorates the toxic effects of deoxycholic acid on colonic epithelium. *Carcinogenesis* 4:1205-7.

IV. Fiber's Nutritional Effects

Dietary Fiber and Digestive Tract Disorders

Albert I. Mendeloff, M.D., M.P.H. (deceased)

Of the eight major non-malignant digestive disorders (Table 1) clear evidence that dietary fiber intake has any relevance to prevention, treatment, or exacerbation is not available. Dr. Cleave in his book, *The Saccharine Disease* (1), classified five disorders as due to removal of fiber in food processing or cooking, four other disorders as due to over consumption, and peptic ulcer disease as caused by the removal of protein from natural foodstuffs. None of these assumptions or predictions have ever been supported by convincing evidence, and the behavior of populations harboring these disorders has been much more carefully studied since his book appeared in 1974. Only gallstone disease and diverticular disease of the colon have been identified as having some relevance to dietary intake of any nutrients, and these will be discussed later. Only two human digestive disorders have been definitely linked to nutritional intake; lactose intolerance and gluten-induced enteropathy,

Table 1. Major non-malignant gastrointestinal disorders

1. Acid-peptic disorders
   a. esophagitis
   b. peptic ulcer
   c. chronic gastritis
2. Pancreatitis
3. Gallstone disease
4. Hepatitis and cirrhosis
5. Appendicitis
6. Inflammatory bowel disease
7. Diverticular disease of the colon
8. Irritable bowel disease

generally called celiac disease. Acute Crohn's disease of the small intestine usually responds well to an elemental diet for 4–6 weeks, but relapse occurs in over 50% of these patients during the next few months. Aside from the obvious need to replete those rendered malnourished or dehydrated, no other digestive disorder can be said to depend for its treatment or its prevention on a particular nutritive program. When gastric surgery was in its heyday a generation ago, the "dumping syndrome" of unpleasantly rapid emptying into the jejunum was shown in a small number of cases to be relieved by the ingestion of pectin throughout the day (2). In recent years there have appeared no articles on this subject, we don't see any "dumpers," and very little gastric surgery for ulcer is being performed.

Much of the disappointment in assessing the role of any nutritional therapy for these common digestive disorders has to do with the very large range of measurable parameters, and their inconsistency, for digestive function. Swallowing, gastric emptying, gastric acid secretion, duodenal bicarbonate secretion, the three types of intestinal electrical activity, and such items as mouth-cecal transit times, colonic transit times, and the functions of the anorectal segment are all measurable by newer techniques, but exhibit a wide spectrum of measurements. Although it can be shown that various maneuvers, including changes in diet, and in dietary fiber components, can influence these measurements, none of them have been consistently predictive in the laboratory and even less so in the patient considered clinically.

A vast literature has accumulated on the metabolism and fate of the various bile acids in liver and gallbladder bile as influenced by nutritive intake of fiber and other nutrients. Thus far, except for the gross features of the epidemiology of gallbladder disease noted for many years by Burkitt and Trowell, there have been no therapeutic or prophylactic programs instituted anywhere that would give us reason to believe that an established dietary program could lessen the unhealthy impact of this very common disorder. Small (3) has classified the pathophysiology of cholesterol gallstones into four classes: 1) excessive bile salt loss, 2) oversensitive bile acid feedback, 3) excessive cholesterol secretion, and 4) a mixed defect of types 2 and 3. In addition, there may be extrahepatic reasons for gallstones, depending on altered intestinal absorption, primary problems in the extrahepatic biliary tract, etc. In any case, all efforts centered on the nonsurgical management of gallbladder disease at the present time have largely ignored nutritional manipulations in favor of direct administration of various bile salts. In addition, I have not mentioned the large problem of pigment gallstones, black to brown, which have many separate factors in genesis, but none by therapy (4).

With respect to appendicitis, there has been a 45% decrease in its incidence in the United States since 1940. Similar, although less impressive decreases have occurred in northern and western Europe. This disease has not changed in its population distribution (80% in those under 40), not in its clinical and laboratory manifestations (5). Furthermore, despite the fact that almost two generations of people now own an appendix that would have been removed in earlier years, the incidence of the disease in the elderly is unchanged. You will recall that Burkitt and his mentor, Randall Short, have attributed the pathogenesis of appendicitis to a spasm of the appendix, and suggested that a high fiber diet would prevent this (6). There has never been any supportive evidence for this concept, and, in view of the decline in the disease in the face of little or no change in the intake of dietary fiber, we can let this hypothesis die quietly. Other theories, especially the inflammatory and lymphoid hypotheses so well summarized by Walker and Segal (7) remain to be investigated further.

Peptic disorders, esophagitis, gastritis, and ulcer disease have had a phenomenal number of investigations over the past century, with no proven conclusions about the role of nutritional factors in their pathogenesis or treatment. In the past ten years we have discovered *H. pylori,* a spiral organism that lives in the stomach in populations all over the world, including those that dwell in the high Andes and eat large amounts of fiber (8). Although a complete clarification of its role in peptic disorders is not yet at hand, its ability to cause chronic gastritis and duodenitis is clear. Thus far, no nutritional interactions with its presence, absence or eradication have been established, although its eradication by antibiotics and by bismuth salts has been accomplished, and a reduction in recurrence rates of ulceration has ensued.

For colonic disorders, the impact of dietary fiber and resistant starch is obviously very great. In fact, the most important result of the interest in these two classes of nutrients has been a much more complete elucidation of fermentation and the importance of its products on colonic function (9). At present, a great deal more must be learned about the relationship of these products to bowel function and to the disease processes encountered in the human colon. A good place to start is the process known as diverticular disease of the colon. There are at least five categories into which the process of outpouchings of colonic mucosa may be classified, and we do not understand any one of the five (10). Theories as to how they have come about are almost totally unsupported by evidence, and the various measurements which have been applied to pressure-diameter relationships in the normal and diverticulotic colon have very poor correlation with symptoms, stool size, transit time, and concentrations of bile acids, short-chain fatty acids, and stool pH. It is not clear that any or all of these measurements play any part in the development of symptoms or complications of an underlying bowel problem. Most of the speculations about the relationship between dietary intake of fiber or resistant starch and diverticular disease are based on epidemiological data of questionable validity. Diverticula must be demonstrated by barium studies or by colonoscopy; they cannot be inferred from symptoms or stool size. We identify the disorder in patients complaining of problems physicians believe merit such a work-up. Too often, the presence of diverticulosis is assigned as the cause for lower gastrointestinal bleeding. Diverticula do not disappear, once formed. No one has yet shown that a diet high in fiber will change their appearance, or increase the caliber of the affected segment of colon in which they reside.

We have little information on so-called diverticular symptoms; most gastroenterologists believe these are essentially the same as those of the irritable bowel syndrome in a person with diverticula. Follow-up studies on the irritable bowel patients without diverticula show no changes in symptoms as diverticulosis supervenes (11). About 85% of persons with diverticulosis are asymptomatic through life; 15% have some pre-diverticulitic inflammatory process, usually resulting in a mild bout of fever, left-sided abdominal pain, and some change in bowel habit, usually constipation. The disease in the U. S. is responsible for fewer than 3000 deaths a year, most often in the very old population harboring a number of other disorders. After a bout of documented diverticulitic disease, it is not the custom to prescribe an insoluble fiber supplement; results of such therapy are expressed in terms of reduced recurrence rates of the same symptoms, although such data are very limited.

Whether such data are related to the same factors that lead to development of diverticulosis in the first place is not at all clear. Diverticular disease is the most age-related category of digestive diseases; it has been estimated but not shown conclusively that about 10% of the U.S. population have developed it by age 70; in Europe the figures are higher, as high as 35% in Germany, for example. In other populations, diverticulosis bear no direct relationship to polyps of the colon or to colonic cancer (12).

We can conclude with remarks directed to the irritable bowel syndrome, a term applied to a young population of patients complaining of abdominal pain relieved by defecation, more frequent stools with the onset of the pain, looser stools at the onset of pain, abdominal distention, increased mucus in the stools, and a feeling of incomplete evacuation after defecation. The so-called Manning criteria (13) are often increased by symptoms referable to the stomach and small intestine. This complex of symptoms, thought to be provoked by neuroendocrine receptors in the gut, obviously involves a complex of probably related conditions, with a female sexual preponderance. Often controlled clinical trials of different fibers, bran, ispaghula, psyllium, and methylcellulose, less than half showed any favorable effects compared to those of the placebo (14). At the present time we cannot distinguish the kind of patient who will have some benefit from a dietary change from those who will not. We usually end up by trying a combination of dietary fiber plus some drug therapy aimed at underlying anxiety-depression and at some antispasmodic effect on the colon. Over a one-year period it is difficult to say that we have made anyone better, except for the benefit frequent discussion with a physician may confer.

In summary, over the past twenty years we have thoroughly examined the original postulates of the fiber-inadequacy theory and have failed to confirm its validity for the usual range of digestive disorders. We fall back to the general advantages of the "prudent diet" designed especially for protection against coronary heart disease and diabetes. Despite the enormous importance of colonic fermentation and its dependence on the presence of fermentable polysaccharides and resistant starch, we have not yet been able to link these effects with the kinds of digestive symptoms patients complain of. We will simply have to try harder.

References

1. T. L. Cleave. "The Saccharine Disease." Keats Publishing, New Canaan (1975).
2. A. R. Leeds, D. N. L. Ralphs, F. Ebied, G. Metz, and J. B. Dilawari. Pectin and the dumping syndrome. *Lancet* 1:1075-1078 (1981).
3. D. M. Small. Pathogenesis of cholesterol stones, in: "Gastroenterology, 4th Ed.," J. E. Berk, ed., Saunders, Philadelphia (1985).
4. R. D. Soloway, P. F. Malet. Pigment stones, in: "Gastroenterology, 4th Ed.," J. E. Berk, ed., Saunders, Philadelphia (1985).
5. J. Berry, Jr. and R. A. Malt. Appendicitis near its century. *Ann. Surgery* 200:567-575 (1984).
6. D. P. Burkitt. The aetiology of appendicitis. *Brit. J. Surgery* 58:695-699 (1971).
7. A. R. P. Walker and I. Segal. Editorial: what causes appendicitis? *J. Clin. Gastro* 12:127-129 (1990).
8. B. J. Marshall, J. A. Armstrong, McGechie et al. Attempt to fulfill Koch's postulates for pyloric Campylobacter. *Med. J. Austral.* 142:426 (1985).
9. G. T. Macfarlane and J. H. Cummings. The colonic flora, fermentation, and large bowel digestive function, in: "The Large Intestine," S. F. Phillips, J. H. Pemberton, and R. G. Shorter, eds., Raven Press, New York (1991).
10. A. I. Mendeloff. Thoughts on the epidemiology of diverticular disease. *Clinics in Gastroenterology* 15:855-877 (1986).
11. T. Havia and R. Manner. The irritable colon syndrome, with respect to devel-

opment of diverticulosis. *Acta Chir Scand* 137:569-572 (1971).

12. P. E. Coode, K. W. Chan, Y. T. Chan. Polyps and diverticulosis of the large intestine; a necropsy survey in Hong Kong. *Gut* 26:1045-1048 (1985).

13. A. F. Manning, W. G. Thompson, K. W. Heaton, A. F. Morris. Towards positive diagnosis of the irritable bowel. *Brit. Med. J.* 2:653-654 (1978).

14. K. W. Heaton. Role of dietary fibre in irritable bowel syndrome, in: "Irritable Bowel Syndrome," N. W. Read, ed., Grune and Stratton, Orlando (1984).

Dietary Fiber and the Pattern of Energy Intake

Victoria J. Burley and John E. Blundell

BioPsychology Group
Department of Psychology
University of Leeds
Leeds, UK

Introduction

Recent data from the Office of Population Censuses and Surveys suggests that in Britain more of us are overweight than ever before (Gregory et al., 1990). The proportion of the population classified as overweight or obese has increased by 15% for men and 12% for women since a similar study was conducted in 1980. It is known of course, that the only way in which body adiposity can be reduced is for energy intake to fail to meet energy requirements. Does the dietary fiber component of food have any influence on the ease with which reductions in energy intake can be made?

The original 'fiber-depletion hypothesis' formulated by Surgeon Captain Cleave in the 1950's related the development of obesity to the consumption of highly refined foods, particularly sugar and white wheat flour. The hypothesis was concerned with dietary fiber merely as a consequence of increased consumption of 'refined' food products. Since then, however, the idea that fiber may play a direct role in obesity has developed. Unfortunately, interpretation of studies on the action of dietary fiber on obesity has often been hampered by methodological difficulties including a paucity of information on the type and dosage of fiber used, unbalanced study designs and a lack of control or placebo products. Furthermore, it is difficult to bring together results of studies which have administered fiber in different ways. There have been three different approaches: (1) use of isolates (capsules, slurries, bran, etc.), where the fiber is separated from the other food constituents (2) use of fiber-supplemented foods (3) and, the use of 'whole' or unrefined foods. Each of these forms of dietary fiber has very different physical and sensory properties and is therefore likely to generate varying physiological and behavioral responses. Is there any evidence that dietary fiber, delivered in the various forms increase satiety?

Satiety, Satiation and the Satiety Cascade

Firstly, it is essential to define what we mean by the term satiety. Satiety has previously been defined as 'the state of inhibition over eating' (Burley and Blundell, 1990). From our knowledge of the mechanisms which underlie satiety, it is possible to obtain some idea about the consequences of food consumption by an examination of the duration each phase of satiety. Figure 1 illustrates the proposed contribution of different processes to the intensity and time course of satiety. Thus, in the early phase of satiety, sensory and cognitive aspects (e.g., beliefs about how 'healthy' or 'filling' a food might be) of the food consumed may be responsible for activating and maintaining this state of inhibition over eating. Post ingestive properties such as the capacity of food to distend the stomach, to evoke the release of gut hormones and the rate at which it is emptied from the stomach, are likely to be involved in prolonging

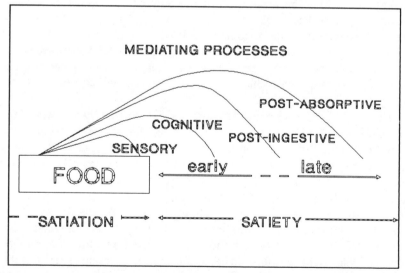

Figure 1. Conceptualization of the contribution of different processes to the intensity and time course of satiety.

satiety in its mid and late stages. Late stages of satiety may be extended by the properties of food which decrease the rate of digestion and/or absorption. Dietary fiber has the capacity to influence physiological processes at many sites in the gastrointestinal tract, including alterations in gastric emptying rate and total transit time, hormonal influences and effects on digestion rate. These properties of dietary fiber all have great potential for altering the time course or duration of satiety.

Fiber Isolates

In reviewing the literature on 'isolate' studies, we find that most evidence suggests that when sufficient quantities of dietary fiber are administered in this way, a reduction in hunger may be observed (Burley, 1992). Unfortunately, many studies have relied solely on changes in subjective motivation to eat, and have not generated any objective measurements of food intake, which reduces their impact considerably. Furthermore, almost nothing is known about the duration of action of fiber isolates and optimum timing of consumption in relation to meals although habitually fiber isolate capsules are consumed 60 minutes before eating.

Fiber-Supplemented Foods

Studies reported in the literature using dietary fiber-supplemented foods suggest that this mode of delivery produces more consistent effects on hunger and satiety. In general, less hunger was experienced after consuming high fiber meals than after the low fiber equivalents, and in some cases this also led to reductions in subsequent energy intake (Porikos and Hagamen, 1986). Probably one of the best studies using fiber-supplemented foods was conducted by Stevens et al., in 1988. In this study *ad libitum* food intakes in 12 overweight women were closely monitored for four 2-week periods, during which they consumed 12 crackers per day containing variable amounts of dietary fiber. Low fiber control crackers were consumed for one 2-week period, and during the other three 2-week periods crackers were made with either added wheat bran, psyllium gum (a water-soluble form of fiber) or a mixture of bran and gum. During the 2 weeks when gum-rich crackers were eaten there was an 11% decrease in freely chosen energy intake. Consumption of the bran-rich crackers had no impact on energy intake, and the bran-gum combination crackers gave an intermediate effect on intake. These data suggest that the addition of a fairly large quantity of soluble dietary fiber to the diet over a two-week period will significantly reduce energy intake. However, the impact of other soluble fiber supplements over a longer time period is unknown. This study was unable to reveal information about the time course of action of psyllium gum; however, we have recently completed an acute meal study using sugar beet fiber supplemented meals which suggests that this type of dietary fiber has a potency which lasts in excess of 4 hours.

In this study, 18 non-obese male and female subjects consumed a low fiber and sugar beet fiber supplemented breakfast using a repeated measures within-subjects design. Each breakfast consisted of orange juice, milk, grilled tomato, butter, jelly, breakfast cereal, bread, crispbread and English sausages. The latter four foods were prepared with and without the addition of sugar beet fiber which generated an additional non-starch polysaccharide content of 27.7 g. Sugar beet fiber (the dried residue or pulp of beets after the sugars have been extracted) contains approximately 75% non-starch polysaccharides, of which 35–40% is soluble in water. The energy and macronutrient content (obtained by chemical analysis) of each test breakfast is shown in Table 1.

Due to the low energy content of sugar beet fiber the energy and nutrient content of the high fiber breakfast was slightly lower than the control meal. Meals were of equal weight. These breakfasts were consumed by each subject, acting as his or her own control with a one week interval between test days.

Following consumption of these breakfasts subjects recorded their perceived level of hunger on an hourly basis using 100 mm visual analogue scales. Direct assessment of motivation to eat was made by the

Table 1. Energy and nutrient (g) analysis of sugar beet fiber supplemented and low fiber control breakfasts

	kcal	Fat	Protein	Carbohydrate
Fiber	677 (2830 kJ)	32	28	55
Control	714 (2984 kJ)	38	30	66

Table 2. Mean (with standard deviation (SD)) energy and nutrient intakes at the *ad libitum* test lunches following sugar beet fiber and control breakfasts

	After sugar beet fiber		After control	
	Mean	SD	Mean	SD
Energy (kcal)	896*	307	1039	256
Protein (g)	54*	19.6	62	11.8
Fat (g)	37*	16.7	44	17.6
Carbohydrate (g)	94	40.5	104	33.1

*Mean significantly different from control value (smallest $t = 2.16$ $p < 0.045$).

administration of an *ad libitum* test lunch (4½ hours after breakfast) at which subjects were free to select as much or as little food as they wished from a range of bread, cheese, sliced meats, salad, yoghurts, fruit and cookies. Further food intake for the rest of the day was weighed and recorded by the subjects in a food diary. At the *ad libitum* test lunch a 14% reduction in energy intake was observed following the high fiber breakfast (1038 vs. 998 kcal (4338 vs 4172), t=2.59 17df, p<0.01), as shown in Table 2.

Thus, following consumption of the sugar beet fiber breakfast energy, protein and fat intakes were significantly lower than after the control breakfast. At this *ad libitum* lunch subjects ate for 21.3 minutes on average after the control breakfast and for 18.5 minutes after the high fiber breakfast. The difference between these means (paired Student's t test) was statistically significant (t = 2.19 17 df, p < 0.04). Thus, after consuming a high fiber breakfast eating time at lunch was shortened by just over 2 minutes and amount consumed reduced by 14%.

Food diary analysis showed that a further 1010±578 kcal was consumed on the control day and 936±449 kcal on the high fiber day. The difference between these intakes did not reach statistical significance. There was no further *active* suppression of intake on the high fiber day, but as the subjects did not eat *more* in this phase, it suggests that the effect of the breakfast was sustained. This short term study showed a clear effect of sugar beet fiber on energy intake for at least 4½ hours after consumption.

Fiber Intact Foods

Foods naturally high in dietary fiber (or fiber intact foods) have been investigated in relatively few behavioral studies, primarily due to the difficulties involved in providing a control or placebo product. However, the few studies reported in the literature all strongly support the concept of the original 'dietary fiber hypothesis' (Burley, 1992). To determine whether high and low fiber lunches (composed of foods 'naturally' high in fiber) differ in their effects on satiety and to determine the time course of action, two studies were conducted on a group of lean, healthy females. In each study a within-subjects repeated measures design was used. High or low fiber lunches were given at midday and then satiety was monitored for the rest of the day using a combination of procedures (see Figure 2 for overall design). Subjective ratings of hunger, fullness and so on were completed using visual analogue scales. *Ad libitum* test meals were offered at different times after the lunches in order to directly assess the effects of consuming the lunches on subsequent food intake. Food diaries were also completed by all the subjects after the lunches in order to assess food intake for the whole period between lunch and bedtime on each study day. Table 3 lists the components of each lunch, and Table 4 shows their calculated nutrient and dietary fiber content.

Analysis of the motivational ratings data in study 1 showed that for 2½ hours following each lunch, there was no significant difference between the meals in terms of their effect on motivational ratings. Moreover, at the afternoon meal, consumed by half the subjects, energy intake did not differ significantly according to whether high or low fiber lunches had been consumed. However, energy intake calculated from food diaries, from 2½–3 hours after lunch until 12.0 pm was significantly lower after the high fiber lunch (967 ± 532 vs 1559 ± 930 kcal).

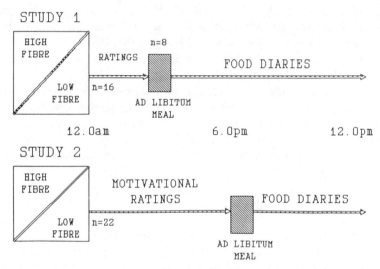

Figure 2. Experimental strategies used to assess the time course of action of dietary fibre.

Table 3. Composition of test lunches high or low in dietary fiber

High fiber	Low fiber
Lentil soup	Chicken soup
Wholemeal bread	White bread
Butter	Butter
Wholemeal pasta	White pasta
Spiced red kidney beans	Bolognese sauce
Cheddar cheese	
Tinned black currants	Fruit yogurt
Fruit yogurt	

Figure 3 illustrates cumulative energy intake following high and low fiber test lunches from food diaries (including energy intake of subjects who consumed the afternoon meal). This figure shows that until approximately 5–6 hours after lunch no effect of fiber on energy intake was apparent.

Analysis of visual analogue scale data generated in study 2 revealed a greater reduction in motivation to eat following the high fiber lunch compared to the low fiber meal, a difference which persisted from 30 minutes to 6 hours after eating. Figure 4 illustrates the mean prospective

Table 4. Energy (kcal) and nutrient content (g) of high and low fiber lunches (*Southgate values)

	High fiber	**Low fiber**
Energy kcal	795	790
Protein	33	33
Fat	28	29
Carbohydrate	106	106
Fiber*	30	3.3

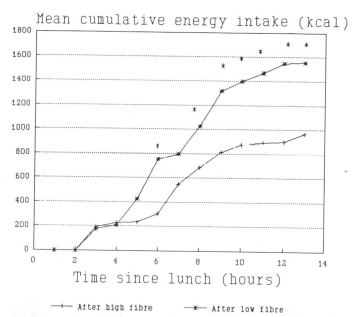

Figure 3. Effect of high and low fiber lunches on cumulative energy intake (from food diaries) for 13 hours after consumption. *Means significantly different $p < 0.03$.

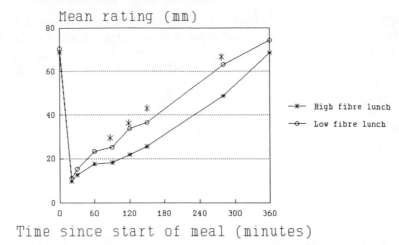

Figure 4. Effect of high and low fiber lunches on post-prandial prospective consumption ratings. *Means significantly different p<0.01.

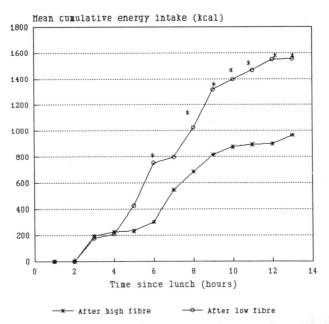

Figure 5. Effect of high and low fiber lunches on cumulative energy intake for 13 hours after consumption (from food diaries). *Means significantly different p<0.03.

consumption rating (on a scale of 0–100 mm asking the question, 'How much food do you think you could eat?' Nothing at all—A large amount) following both meals.

Energy intake at the *ad libitum* meal presented 6 hours after lunch was lower by 86±187 kcal after the high fiber meal (p<0.04), and intakeafter this meal, obtained from food diary analysis was also lower by a further 112±528 kcal after fiber, though this difference failed to reach statistical significance. These studies indicate that although there was some suggestion of increased satiety in the first 3 hours following the high fiber lunches, the primary impact of this meal was on later energy intake (5–6 hours after consumption). It is likely therefore, that dietary fiber consumed as 'whole' or fiber-intact foods reduces energy intake by an action on post-absorptive satiety, rather than via its action on early or post-ingestive satiety.

A more detailed analysis of the time course of food intake recorded in food diaries after the lunches enabled an analysis of meal patterns to be conducted. When cumulative energy intake is plotted against time since lunch it is clear that the difference in energy intake after the two meals does not appear until approximately 5 hours after lunch (see Figure 5). As total energy intake was reduced by approximately 600 kcal after the high fiber lunch, an investigation of the meal patterns after the lunches was undertaken to disclose whether this was brought about by a reduction in the size of meals or by the elimination of snacks. Figure 6

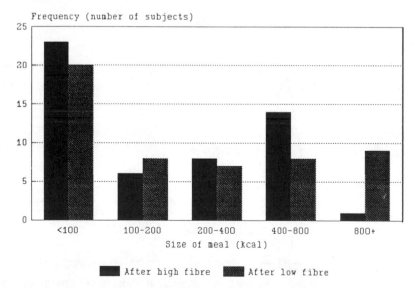

Figure 6. Effect of high and low fiber lunches on subsequent meal size (from diet diaries).

shows the number of meals consumed after the high or low fiber lunches within a range in size chosen to represent snacks (<100 kcal—400 kcal) and large meals (>400 kcal). Similar numbers of small eating events took place after both meals, but the number of larger meals consumed differed after high or low fiber lunches. This suggests that there was a general reduction in the size of the main evening meal, but no elimination of snacks after the high fiber lunch.

Analysis of variance of the energy intake per hour after high and low fiber lunches revealed a statistically significant main effect of meal type ($F(1,12)=7.36$, $p < 0.01$), but no significant time effect or meal type by time effect. This suggests that energy intake per hour is significantly reduced by the high fiber lunch but not specifically at any particular time. When mean energy intake per hour is plotted against time since lunch it suggests that the effect of consuming a high fiber lunch was to increase the time to the main evening meal by about one hour and to reduce the size of that meal by about 270 kcal (see Figure 7).

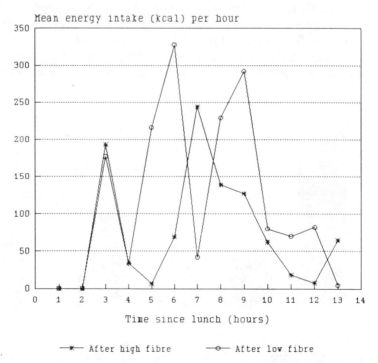

Figure 7. Effect of high and low fiber lunches on subsequent energy intake per hour, for 13 hours after eating (from food diaries). Significant main effect of meal type p<0.01.

Conclusions

How can this large effect of fiber be accounted for? There are a number of potential mechanisms of action for fiber to prolong satiety.

A number of studies, using *in vitro* and *in vivo* techniques have shown that dietary fiber added to a meal may prolong carbohydrate absorption, which is reflected in a smaller post prandial area under the curve for blood glucose (Jenkins et al., 1984; Jenkins et al., 1978). The slower rate of absorption of carbohydrate such as would occur with a high fiber meal has been suggested as a potential influence on hunger and satiety (Booth, 1981). Leathwood and Pollett (1988) demonstrated that a reduced area under the curve for blood glucose was associated with a slowing of the return of rated hunger when volunteers were fed meals based on slow-release carbohydrate (bean starch) compared with similar meals containing fast-release carbohydrate (potato starch). A similar effect may be created by the addition of certain types of dietary fiber to a meal. Sepple and Read (1989) postulated that the return of hunger after a meal is directly related to a decline in the exposure of the upper small intestine to nutrient stimuli. By reducing the rate of digestion and absorption the addition of fiber to a meal may result in a prolongation of exposure of the upper small intestine to nutrients and delay the onset of hunger sensations.

Studies implicating the role of the small intestine were conducted by Davis and Collins (1978). They showed, using mannitol, a nonabsorbable carbohydrate that food intake in the rat is suppressed for the duration of time that the small intestine remains full. They suggested that as dietary fiber sequesters water and swells it will fill the small intestine sufficiently to suppress meal size and prolong the length of inter meal intervals. Certainly the naturally high fiber lunch was slightly more bulky than the low fiber version, and took on average 2 minutes longer to consume. The increased eating time was presumably brought about by the greater chewiness of the high fiber meal. Increased chewing would have generated more saliva and may have increased the cephalic phase of gastric secretion. These effects may have contributed to greater gastric distension but, whether the high fiber lunch would have distended the small intestine longer than the low fiber meal is unknown.

An alternative mode of action would involve the ileal brake. Read and his colleagues (1984) have shown that the infusion of fat into the terminal ileum delays the movement of a labelled meal through the stomach and small intestine and also reduces energy intake at a subsequent meal by approximately 700 kcal (Read, 1986). This process may be activated if dietary fiber slows the absorption of fat, which is then carried further down the intestinal tract (Read, Sepple and Brown, 1990).

Data presented here on the short term effects of fiber-supplemented and naturally high fiber meals are in agreement with a study reported by Levine and co-workers (1989), indicating that a period of 3.5 to 4 hours can elapse and a significant effect of dietary fiber on energy intake will still be apparent. Furthermore, these investigators also found that food intake could be reduced at lunch time following consumption of a high fiber breakfast, without the perception of feeling less hungry. They suggested that, although the relationship is not a perfect one, the degree of bacterial fermentation, monitored by the production of breath H_2 is related to energy ingestion at lunch. The precise contribution of dietary fiber to food energy intakes resulting from its bacterial fermentation and the subsequent absorption of utilisable metabolites is unknown, at least in man. It appears that the energy available will depend on the degree of fermentation of the various types of dietary fiber; some types are more readily degraded than others. Livesey (1988) reviewed the estimates of apparent caloric value of unavailable carbohydrate and found that it varied from -4.7 to +2.4 kcal/g. Cummings and Branch (1986) estimated that the short-chain carboxylic acids produced contribute between 60 and 70% of the food energy that would have been available had the carbohydrate of dietary fiber been absorbed as carbohydrate. This issue requires further investigation to determine whether colonic bacterial fermentation directly reduces appetite or if the consumption of fiber is associated with some other process which reduces appetite.

Thus, it is possible that food intake was reduced in the studies reported here by an effect of fiber on slowing digestion and absorption and/or an action related to the production of fermentation products in the colon. It should be emphasized that these studies have investigated the acute effects of dietary fiber administration only, and that the results found here may not be extrapolated to the use of fiber as a long term aid to weight loss. Furthermore, although we do not have direct evidence for this, it is possible that obese subjects may respond differently to dietary fiber than lean subjects. Porikos and Hagamen (1986) found a greater suppression of food intake following a lunch prepared with methylcellulose in obese subjects compared to lean. Other studies have not revealed a clear difference between obese and lean (Duncan, Bacon and Weinsier, 1983; Stevens et al., 1987). However, the data presented here suggest that there is good potential for the use of dietary fiber as an aid to appetite control, and further research on its role in weight management is justified.

One further interpretation of the studies presented here, consistent with our previous experiments, is that one meal high in dietary fiber can exert good meal to meal control over appetite. This can be compared for example, with supplementary carbohydrate in a breakfast meal (up to

400 kcal) which exerts a control over appetite for a limited period of about 2 hours during the post-ingestive window (Cotton et al., 1992) or with additional fat (400 kcal supplement) which does not appear to exert any appreciable effect on satiety at all (Cotton et al., 1992; Blundell et al., 1992) under experimental conditions similar to those prevailing in the present study. Consequently, this meal to meal action of dietary fiber is not trivial and compares very favourably with effects of additional nutrients. The sustained effect of fiber on satiety (suppression of later meal intake and prevention of any subsequent compensatory catch-up) indicates that one high fiber meal can affect the pattern of intake over a substantial portion of the day. This sustained action on satiety is biologically intriguing and there is now an urgent need to identify the mechanisms responsible for this effect. Furthermore, there is still a pressing need for research aimed at identifying the most potent and palatable source of dietary fiber with regard to appetite suppression. This research coupled with investigations of the effectiveness of dietary fiber as a replacement for dietary fat is an area which is under active development. These possibilities show encouraging signs regarding the development of new foods to allow fiber to modulate the pattern of eating and to allow people to gain more effective control over their appetite.

References

Blundell, J. E., Burley, V. J., Cotton, J., and Lawton, C., 1992, Dietary fat and appetite control: weak effects on satiation (within meals) and satiety (following meals), in: "Determinants of Preference, Selection and Consumption of Dietary Fats," D. Mela, ed., Elsevier, Cambridge.

Booth, D. A., 1981, The physiology of appetite. Brit Med Bull. 37:135.

Burley, V. J., 1992, Dietary fibre and satiety—Experimental evidence, in: "Dietary Fibre and Obesity: Seminar Report," A. R. Leeds, ed., Smith Gordon, London (in press).

Burley, V. J., and Blundell, J. E., 1990, Time course of the effects of dietary fibre on energy intake and satiety, in: "Dietary Fibre: Chemical and biological aspects," D. A. T. Southgate, K. Waldron, I. T. Johnson & G. R. Fenwick eds., Royal Society of Chemistry, Cambridge.

Cotton, J. R., Burley, V. J., and Blundell, J. R., 1992, Fat and satiety: No additional intensification of satiety following a fat-supplemented breakfast, Int. J. Obesity. (suppl) 16:11.

Cummings, J. A., and Branch, W. J., 1986, Fermentation and the production of short chain fatty acids in the human large intestine, in: "Dietary Fiber in Health and Disease," G. V. Vahouny, D. Kritchevsky, eds., Plenum Press, New York.

Davis, J. D. and Collins, B. J., 1978, Distension of the small intestine, satiety, and the control of food intake, Am J Clin Nutr. 31:S255.

Duncan, K., Bacon, J. A. and Weinsier, R. L., 1983, The effect of high and low energy density diets on satiety, energy intake, and eating time of obese and non-obese subjects, Am J Clin Nutr., 37:763.

Gregory, J., Foster, K., Tyler, H., and Wiseman, M., 1990, "The Dietary and Nutritional Survey of British Adults," HMSO, London.

Livesey, G., 1988, Energy from food—old values and new perspectives, Nutr Bull., 13(52):9.

Jenkins, D. J. A., Wolever, T. M. S., Leeds, A. R., Gassull, M. A., Dilawari, J. B., Goff, D. V., Metz, G. L., and Alberti, K. G. M. M., 1978, Dietary fibres, fibre analogues and glucose tolerance: Importance of viscosity, Br Med J. 1:1392.

Jenkins, D. J. A., Wolever, T. M. S., Thorne, M. J., Jenkins, A. L., Wong, G. S., Josse, R. G., and Csima, A., 1984, The relationship between glycemic response, digestibility, and factors influencing the dietary habits of diabetics, Am J Clin Nutr., 40:1175.

Leathwood, P. and Pollett, P., 1988, Effects of slow release carbohydrates in the form of bean flakes on the evolution of hunger and satiety in man, Appetite 10:1.

Levine, A. S., Tallman, J. R., Grace, M. K., Parker, S. A., Billington, C. J. and Levitt, M. D., 1989, Effect of breakfast cereals on short-term food intake, Am J Clin Nutr., 50:1303.

Porikos, K. and Hagamen, S., 1986, Is fibre satiating? Effects of a high fibre preload on subsequent food intake of normal-weight and obese young men, Appetite 7:153.

Read, N. W., 1986, Dietary fiber and bowel transit, in: "Dietary Fiber: Basic and Clinical Aspects," G. V., Vahouny, D., Kritchevsky, eds., Plenum Press, New York.

Read, N. W., MacFarlane, A., Kinsman, R., Bates, T., Blackhall, N. W., Farrar, G. B. J., Hall, J. C., Moss, G., Morris, A. P., O'Neill, B., Welch, I., Lee, Y., Bloom, S. R., 1984, Effect of infusion of nutrient solutions into the ileum on gastrointestinal transit and plasma levels of neurotensin and enteroglucagon in man, Gastroenterology 86:274.

Read, N. W., Sepple, C. P., and Brown, N. J., 1990, The ileal brake. Is it relevant to the action of viscous polysaccharides, in: "Dietary Fiber. Chemistry, Physiology, and Health Effects," D. Kritchevsky, C. Bonfield, and J. W. Anderson, eds., Plenum Press, New York.

Sepple, C. P., and Read, N. W. 1989, Gastrointestinal correlates of the development of hunger in man, Appetite 13:183.

Stevens, J., Levitsky, D. A., VanSoest, P. J., Robertson, J. B., Kalkwarf, H. J., and Roe, D. A., 1987, Effect of psyllium gum and wheat bran on spontaneous energy intake, Am J Clin Nutr. 46:812.

Effect of Dietary Fiber on Intestinal Microflora and Health

A. V. Rao
Department of Nutritional Sciences,
University of Toronto, Toronto, Ontario,
Canada. M1G 3R6

Introduction

Historically, interest in intestinal microflora began in 1719 when Leeuwenhock made the first microscopic observation of fecal bacteria. In 1885, Eschenich initiated a systematic study of the intestinal microflora of bottle fed infants. Most of the subsequent studies on intestinal microflora focused on the aerobes such as the coliform and enterococcal bacteria for the simple reason that they were the easiest to grow. Over the past two decades, however, it has been recognized that a great number of intestinal bacteria can not be cultivated *in vitro* using conventional microbiological techniques. These bacteria in general are extremely sensitive to oxygen and unless strict anaerobic techniques and suitable media are used they are liable to be ignored. Recent advances in the culturing techniques have enabled us now to cultivate most of the intestinal microflora.

Composition of Intestinal Microflora and Metabolic Activity

Studies have shown that intestinal microflora represents a complex ecosystem consisting of several hundred species of bacteria that play an important role in human health and disease (1,8,11,15,16,17) (Figure 1).

Typically, the total bacterial count of an adult healthy human subject range between 10^{11} and 10^{12} per gram fecal material, accounting for over 40% of the total dry fecal mass (4). Depending on the predominance of the bacterial species their influence on the host could either be beneficial or harmful (Figure 2).

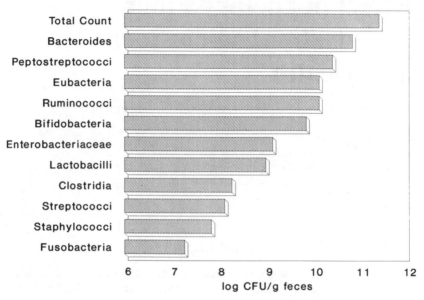

Figure 1. Typical normal fecal flora of healthy human subjects.

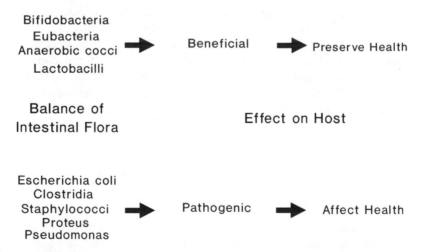

Figure 2. Interrelationship between intestinal microflora and the host.

Substrate entering the large intestine consisting of unabsorbed fat, protein, fiber and starch, together with endogenous carbohydrates is metabolized by these bacteria and their enzymes into a range of metabolic end products. Production of short chain fatty acids such as acetate, propionate, and butyrate by the bacterial fermentation of carbohydrates in the colon is increasingly being asssociated with the maintenance of a healthy colonic mucosa in humans (2,3,4,5,20) (Table 1). On the other hand, metabolic activity of other bacteria are responsible for the production of harmful products that adversely influence human health (14) (Figure 3).

Table 1. Predominant short chain fatty acid producing bacteria in the large intestine

Genus	Major fermentation products
Bacteroides	Acetate
	Propionate
	Succinate
Fusobacteria	Butyrate
	Acetate
	Formsate
Bifidobacteria	Acetate
	Lactate

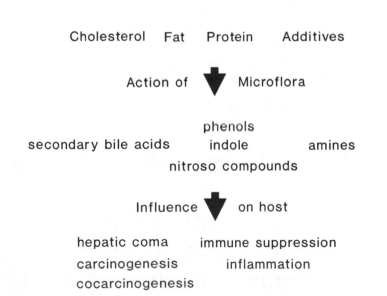

Figure 3. Harmful products from intestinal microflora and influence on the host.

In general the composition of intestinal microflora of humans is very stable. However, several factors including diet and age can influence their activity (9,10,14) (Figure 4). Dietary intake can mediate its influence directly through a change in substrate availability or indirectly through its effect on host metabolic functions. Among the food components which influence the total fermentable load entering the colon is dietary fiber (5,6).

Effect of Dietary Fiber on Intestinal Microflora

The effect of long-term dietary fiber intake on the composition of intestinal microflora has not been investigated extensively. *In vitro* incubation of various fiber sources with human fecal bacteria as inoculum showed that fiber sources are fermented differently and that it may be possible to select fiber sources capable of supporting stipulated amounts of total and individual short chain fatty acids in the human colon (12,18, 19,20).

Conflicting observations are reported on the effect of dietary fiber on fecal bacteria in humans. A recent study comparing the fecal microflora

A. External

Age, Diet, Drugs, Stress, Exogenous microorganisms

B. Internal

Host physiology, Gastric acid Redox potential, Peristalsis Microbial interactions Nutrient availability Immune mechanisms

Figure 4. Factors affecting gastrointestinal microflora in humans.

of healthy adult men consuming either polished or brown rice diets for 14 days showed the presence of similar genera of bacteria in both the groups. However, an increased percentage of Bifidobacteria, Ruminococcus and Peptostreptococcus and a reduction in Eubacteria and Eschrisia were observed after 14 days of the brown rice diet. In addition, low percentage of all clostridia and low incidences of *Cl. paraputrificum* and *Cl. perfringens* were observed for the brown rice (2).

Healthy adult urban Canadians consuming a low fiber and high fat diets showed increasing percentage of the total bacterial population of Bacillus and Clostridium and a reduction in Bifidobacteria and Euobacteria. On the other hand the dominant bacterial species in rural Japanese consuming high fiber low fat diets consisted of Bifidobacteria and Eubacterium species. The presence of the fecal clostridia in low fiber diets is of importance since they are capable of exhibiting nuclear dehydrogenation and the formation of carcinogens from bile acids (2,3). The high incidence of colon cancer in western countries may therefore be associated with the composition of intestinal microflora which in turn are influenced by dietary fiber and fat (8,22).

The effect of types of dietary fiber on fecal bacterial enzyme activities were studied in healthy female subjects by administering wheat, oat and corn bran cereals for a period of 8 weeks (16). Significant differences in the bacterial enzyme activities were observed among different fibers. During the period of wheat bran significant decrease in the activities of β-glucuronidase, 7α-dehydroxylase, azoreductase and nitroreductase were observed. Dietary oat bran on the other hand deceased the activity of azoreductase and nitroreductase only while corn bran had little or no effect on the activity of bacterial enzyme activities.

We investigated the effect of lactulose administration on the intestinal microflora in human subjects. Eight healthy human volunteers were placed on two identical 2-week metabolic diets with the exception that on one diet 1g lactulose was added per 100 kcals to a maximum of 25g per day. On the 13th day of each metabolic period end-expiratory alveolar samples were obtained before breakfast and at 1h intervals over a 14h period for determining breath hydrogen levels as a measure of colonic fermentation. Venous blood samples were also collected before breakfast and at 2h intervals over a 12h period for the measurement of serum acetate levels. Fecal samples were collected on days 0 and 14 for microbiological enumeration. Results are summarized in Table 2. A significant increase in the breath hydrogen level of 78% was observed upon the administration of lactulose, indicating increased colonic fermentation. Consumption of lactulose also resulted in significant increases in total anaerobes/total aerobes ratio and bifidobacteria. The 22% increase in seum acetate level observed in this study may be due to increased numbers of bifidobacteria which are predominantly acetate producers (14).

The effect of polydextrose, a water-soluble polysaccharide that is not absorbed from the intestine, on fecal microflora, bacterial enzyme activity and fecal putrifactive products was studied in eight healthy volunteers. A high cholesterol diet supplemented with 15 g/day polydextrose was fed for two weeks. Polydextrose supplementation was observed to increase fecal weight and decrease fecal pH and stool concentration of indole, p-cresol, iso-valeric acid and iso-butyric acid. A significant reduction of clostridium in the feces was also observed during the high-cholesterol polydextrose diet period. The frequency of occurrence and number of *Clostridium perfringence* in the feces were also found to be lower (7).

Gum arabic, a water-soluble polysaccharide, was shown to induce rapid increases in the proportion of fecal flora that are able to degrade the polysaccharide from the initial 6.5% to more than 50% in a healthy human volunteer consuming a diet supplemented with 10 g fiber per day. These levels of bacteria returned to the control levels after ingestion of fiber ceased (21). In another study dietary supplementation with 5.4 g of fiber was shown to increase the mean stool weights and fecal anaeobic counts significantly in six volunteer subjects. Although trends in bacterial genus changes were observed in this study they were not significant. Total aerobic counts remained stable throughout the study (10).

Table 2. Effect of lactulose intake on breath hydrogen, serum acetate and fecal bacteria

	Diet		
	Control	Lactulose	% change on lactulose
Breath hydrogen (ppm), n = 7	8.7 ± 1.7	16.2 ± 1.97	77.8 ± 13.3[*]
Serum acetate (mmol/L)	97.0 ± 10	110.0 ± 12	22.9 ± 17.1
Total anerobes/ aerobes ratio	1.38 ± 1.15	2.32 ± 0.89	154.08 ± 47.06[+]
Bifidobacteria (CFU/g feces)	6.65 ± 0.83	7.82 ± 0.78	22.90 ± 18.67[+]

[*]Significance of % change between control and lactulose by paired 2-tail t-test, p < 0.001.
[+]Significance of % change between control and lactulose by paired 2-tail t-test, p < 0.05.

We investigated the long term effects of ingesting soluble and insoluble fibers on intestinal microflora of human subjects. At the end of a two month American Heart Association (AHA) Step II diet 39 healthy subjects aged 57.4±9.0 (range 29–70) were randomly placed on either a high soluble fiber diet or a high insoluble fiber diet for a four month metabolic period. The macro nutrient composition of the diets was similar, with 20% of the dietary calories as fat, 20% as protein, and 60% as available carbohydrates with 2.5 to 3 g of fiber per 100 kcals. The high fiber foods in the soluble fiber diet consisted of dried peas, beans, lentils, barley, psyllium, and oat bran breakfast cereals, while those in the insoluble fiber diet consisted mainly of food high in wheat bran. Fecal samples were collected on week 0, 2 and 15 for analyses. Results are summarized in Tables 3 and 4. Significant increases in wet and dry fecal mass was observed after two weeks on the diets that lasted to 15 weeks. Fecal pH was significantly lowered on both soluble and insoluble fiber diets at the end of 15 weeks. However, the type of fiber did not have any effect on these measurements. Similarly, when bacteria were expressed as daily dry fecal output, significant time effects were observed in total aerobes, total anaerobes, and bifidobacteria but there were no differences between soluble and insoluble fibers. Insoluble fiber diet is expected to induce increased fecal bulking where as a soluble fiber diet is expected to decrease fecal pH (13). However, both an increase of fecal

Table 3. Effect of dietary fiber on total fecal mass and fecal pH

			Time		
	Fiber type	Week 0	Week 2	Week 15	p value
Mean wet fecal mass (g/day)	Soluble	171.05 ± 65.40 (39)[1] a[2]	223.04 ± 97.84 (39) b	254.31 ± 120.48 (39) b	diet = 0.6984 time = 0.0001
	Insoluble	169.48 + 64.89 (39)	244.38 ± 71.84 (39)	244.36 ± 95.16 (39)	
Mean dry fecal mass (g/day)	Soluble	40.44 ± 14.89 (39) a	45.34 ± 14.76 (39) b	50.73 ± 19.73 (39) b	diet = 0.0429 time = 0.0001 diet*time = 0.0150
	Insoluble	37.78 ± 15.56 (39)	53.70 ± 14.87 (39)	56.30 ± 20.13 (39)	
Fecal pH	Soluble	6.62 ± 0.56 (39) a	6.52 ± 0.46 (37) a	6.45 ± 0.65 (38) b	diet = 0.8968 time − 0.0046
	Insoluble	6.58 ± 0.49 (37)	6.61 ± 0.48 (39)	6.39 ± 0.41 (38)	

1. The n values are given in parentheses.
2. Values with the same letters across rows are not significantly different (p > 0.05).

Table 4. Effect of dietary fiber on fecal aerobes, anaerobes, and bifidobacteria counts expressed per daily dry fecal output

	Fiber type	Week 0	Time Week 2	Week 15	p value
Total fecal aerobes (log(CFU/ fecal output))	Soluble	9.76 ± 1.42 (38)[1] a^2	9.91 ± 1.35 (38) a	9.45 ± 1.12 (37) b	diet = 0.4909 time = 0.0001
	Insoluble	9.67 ± 1.40 (39)	10.05 ± 1.09 (38)	9.06 ± 1.24 (37)	
Total fecal anaerobes (log(CFU/ fecal output))	Soluble	11.78 ± 0.98 (38) a	12.34 ± 1.15 (38) b	11.74 ± 0.99 (37) a	diet = 0.7756 time = 0.0001
	Insoluble	11.81 ± 1.15 (39)	12.34 ± 0.87 (39)	11.58 ± 0.92 (38)	
	Soluble	9.74 ± 1.32 (38) a	10.20 ± 1.27 (38) b	9.41 ± 0.92 (37) a	diet = 0.1900 time = 0.0001
Fecal Bifidobacteria (log(CFU/ fecal output))	Insoluble	9.46 ± 1.20 (39)	10.03 ± 1.08 (39)	9.21 ± 1.16 (38)	

1. The n values are given in parentheses.
2. Values with the same letters across rows are not significantly different (p > 0.05).

bulk and decrease of pH were observed in this study with the intake of either diet. This may be attributed to the small actual difference of 4% by weight in the soluble fiber content between the two diets. Diets supplemented with pure forms of fibers may, therefore, be necessary to detect statistically and biologically significant changes in the flora between the two types of fibers. Subjects were following the AHA Step II diet for two months before entering this study, as a result the magnitude of changes in the microflora may also be lessened.

Conclusion

The effects of long-term dietary fiber intake on the composition of intestinal microflora in humans have not been investigated extensively. Results from our study, however, support the conclusion that human intestinal microflora can be altered as early as two weeks of increased intake of dietary fiber. Although the composition of microflora returned back to the baseline pattern at week 15, enhanced intestinal fermentation activity was still evidenced by the significant reduction in fecal pH. This may have important human health implications.

References

1. Attebery H R, Sutter V L and Finegold S M. 1972. Noraml human intestinal flora, p. 81-97. In: Balows A, Dettaan R M, Dowell V R and Guze L B. (Eds.), Anaerobic Bacteria: Role in disease, Charles C. Thomas, Springfield.
2. Benno Y and Mitsuoka T. 1991. Effect of diet and aging on human fecal microflora. Bifidobacteria Microflora. 10:89-96.
3. Benno Y, Suzuki K, Suzuki K, Narisawa K, Bruce W R and Mitsuoka T. 1986. Comparison of the fecal microflora in rural Japanese and urban Canadians. Microbiol. Immunol. 30:521-532.
4. Borriello S P. 1986. Microbial flora of the gastrointestinal tract, p.1-20. In: Hill M J. (Ed.), Microbial Metabolism in the Digestive Tract. CRC Press Inc., Boca Raton.
5. Cummings J H. Shortchain fatty acids in the human colon. 1981. Gut 22:763-779.
6. Drasar B S, Jenkins D J A and Cummings J H. 1976. The influence of diet rich in wheat fiber on the human fecal flora. J. Med. Microbiol. 9:423-431.
7. Endok K, Kumemura M, Nakamura K, Fujisawa T, Suzuki K, Benno Y and Mitsuoka T. 1991. Effect of high cholesterol diet and polydextrose supplementation on the microflora, bacterial enzyme activity, putrifactive products, volatile fatty acid (VFA) profile, weight and pH of the feces in healthy volunteers. Bifidobacteria Microflora. 10:53-64.
8. Finegold S M, Flora D J, Atterbery H R and Sutter V L. 1974. Effect of diet on human fecal flora: Comparison of Japanese and American diets. Am. J. Clin. Nutr. 27:1456-1469.
9. Finegold S M and Sutter V L. 1978. Fecal flora in different populations with special reference to diet. Am. J. Clin. Nutr. 31:S116-S122.
10. Fuchs H M, Dorfman S and Floch M H. 1976. The effect of dietary fiber supplementation in man. II. Alterations in fecal physiology and bacterial flora. Am. J. Clin. Nutr. 29:1443-1447.
11. Hill M J. 1987. The role of bacteria in human carcinogenesis. Anticancer Research 7:1079-1084.
12. Jenkins D J, Jenkins A L, Rao A V and Thompson L U. 1987. Starchy foods: Types of fiber and cancer risk. Preven. Med. 76:545-553.
13. McCarthy R E and Salyers A A. 1988. The effect of dietary fiber utilization on the colonic microflora, p. 295-314. In: Rowland IR (Ed.), Role of the gut flora in toxicity and cancer, Academic Press, New York.
14. Mitsuoka T. 1982. Recent trends in research on intestinal flora. Bifidobacteria Microflora 1:3-24.
15. Moore W E C and Holdeman L V. 1974. Human fecal flora: The normal flora of 20 Japanese-Hawaiians. Appl. Microbiol. 27:961-979.
16. Reddy B S. 1990. Intestinal microflora and carcinogenesis. Bifidobacteria and Microflora 9:65-76.
17. Reddy B S, Weisburger J H and Wynder E L. 1975. Effect of high risk and low risk diets for colon carcinogensis on fecal microflora and steroids in man. J. Nutr. 105:878-884.
18. Roediger W E W. 1980. Role of anaerobic bacteria in the metabolic welfare of

the colonic mucosa in man. Gut 21:793- 798.

19. Salyers A A and Leedle J A Z. 1983. Carbohydrate metabolism in human colon, p. 129-146. In: Hentges D J (Ed.), The human intestinal microflora in health and disease, Academic Press, New York.

20. Titgemeyer E C, Bourquin L D, Fahey G C Jr., and Garleb K A. 1991. Fermentability of various fiber sources by human fecal bacteria in vitro. Am. J. Clin. Nutr. 53:1418-1424.

21. Wyall G M, Bayliss C E and Holeroft J D. 1986. A change in human faecal flora in response to inclusion of gum arabic in the diet. Br. J. Nutr. 55:261-266.

22. Wynder E L and Reddy B S. 1983. Dietary fat and fiber and colon cancer. Semin. Oncol. 10:264-272.

Dietary Fiber and Mineral Nutrition

Dennis T. Gordon, Dan Stoops, and Vicki Ratliff
Department of Food Science and Human Nutrition
University of Missouri
Columbia, Missouri 65211

Introduction

There remains strong controversy regarding the possible adverse effects of dietary fiber (DF) on mineral absorption. This negative opinion has been continually perpetuated in reviews on DF (Kritchevsky, 1988; Torre, et al., 1991), and nutrition advisory publications (Life Sciences Research Office, 1987; Dietary Fiber, 1989). Continued scientific reports on the in vitro mineral binding capacity of DF (Persson et al., 1987; Nair et al., 1987; Ward and Reichert, 1986) and metabolic studies in animals and humans have had the tendency to maintain this issue as a viable nutritional problem. With any potentially harmful nutritional issue, once introduced, it remains difficult to dispel.

We are of the strong conviction and can find no convincing scientific evidence that any DF, even when consumed in large amounts (i.e., 50g total dietary fiber per day), has or should have any adverse effect on mineral absorption or nutrition in humans. This position was originally presented at the last Vahouny Symposium on Dietary Fiber (Gordon, 1990) along with a comprehensive review of the literature up to that time and substantiated with additional experimental data. To further support our hypothesis that no DF has any negative effect on mineral nutrition, we report on two additional studies from our laboratory. In these experiments, we have developed new methodology and employed a new technology to address this issue. We present the threshold concept of mineral utilization and the simultaneous use and measurement of

267

multiple radionuclides to test DF effects on mineral absorption and retention using a rat model.

Minerals and Dietary Fiber

The Recommended Dietary Allowances (1989) for minerals in humans are reported in Table 1. Significant changes have been approved and these new values are generally lower compared to previous recommendations (Recommended Dietary Allowances, 1980). This latest guideline publication, along with other reports (Life Sciences Research Office, 1987; National Research Council, 1989; American Diabetes Association, 1987; American Dietetic Association, 1988), has also recommended that dietary fiber intakes be increased to 25 or more g per day. If a negative effect of DF on mineral nutrition does occur, these two recommendations would appear to be in conflict. Low mineral intakes can result in lower net mineral availability, which could be further reduced with increasing amounts of DF. This problem could be more serious in developing and under-developed countries, where mineral intakes have been reported to be marginal and DF intakes may exceed by a factor of two to three the amounts consumed in developed countries. Fortunately for all populations associated with these recommendations or dietary intakes, there has been no evidence of mineral deficiencies found to be caused by or resulting from DF consumption (Walker, 1987).

Table 1. Essential minerals for humans with their highest recommended dietary allowance (RDA) or estimated safe and adequate daily dietary intake (ESADDI)

	RDA[1]		ESADDI		Minimum requirement	No exact requirement intake established
	mg/day		mg/day		mg/day	
Ca	1,200	Mg	2.0–5.0	Na	500[2]	Ni
P	1,200	F	1.5–4.0	K	2,000[2,3]	As[4]
Mg	400	Cu	1.5–3.0	Cl	750[2]	Co
Fe	15	Mn	2.0–5.0			Si
Zn	15		μg/day			Sn
	μg/day	Cr	50–200			V
I	150	Mo	75–200			
Se	70		75–250			

[1] Maximum RDA (Recommended Dietary Allowances 1989).
[2] No evidence that higher amounts confer any health benefits.
[3] Desirable intakes for adults may reach 3,500 mg/day.
[4] Considered essential in trace amounts but toxic in higher amounts.

These recommendations regarding requirements for all minerals and DF intakes present at least two special problems or questions. Do specific DF affect specific minerals, or are there non-specific effects of DF on all minerals that alter their absorption and utilization? Most scientific reports are limited in the number of minerals and sources of DF evaluated. In the experiments briefly presented in this report, an extensive number of minerals and sources of dietary fiber were evaluated.

Mineral Bioavailability

Mineral bioavailability is defined as the ratio of the amount of a mineral absorbed and utilized compared to the total amount ingested (O'Dell, 1985). The determination of mineral bioavailability and factors that affect mineral bioavailability still remains an area of extensive research activity. When working to determine a nutrient's bioavailability, the researchers in this area are plagued with a recurring set of related problems. First, no reliable method has been developed to accurately measure the bioavailability of an ingested mineral and to separate this exogenous intake and its associated biological response from the amount of endogenous mineral in the body being reabsorbed and reutilized. Secondly, it has remained a challenge to find a biological response or index sufficiently sensitive to measure a change in the body's storage or use of a mineral that reflects the true amount of a specific dietary mineral absorbed and utilized. These problems are further complicated when the bioavailability of more than one mineral and the interactions among minerals are considered (Gordon, 1987). Without newer methodology or technology to address these problems, it remains a difficult challenge to measure mineral bioavailability and accurately determine the effects of dietary factors such as DF on mineral utilization. Previous data and especially the results of balance studies must be critically reexamined, and more modern tools must be employed to address these problems.

A Classic Study

The original study by McCance and Widdowson (1942) may have been the report to initiate the negative hypothesis regarding DF and mineral nutrition. The work by Reinhold et al. (1976) may have been the second most significant scientific report relative to creating the belief that DF impairs mineral balance and adversely affects mineral nutrition. This report also came at a time when interest in DF was at a peak. Recently this publication was given classic citation status in *Nutrition Re-*

views (1991). The work of Reinhold et al. (1976) is worth reviewing, and some of the most important observations from this study are reported in Table 2.

Only two subjects were used in this study, but they were maintained for two 20 day periods to determine mineral balance. To the authors' credit, the two subjects were placed on a hospital diet for one week prior to the start of the experiment, to have both become acclimated to the type of food to be used in this study. However, it must be questioned whether this was sufficient time to allow the subjects to achieve a uni-

Table 2. Summary of data presented by J. G. Reinhold *et al.*[1] on effect of dietary fiber on mineral balance in two human subjects

Subject	Diet/bread	Nutrient intake	Urine[3]	Feces[3]	Balance[3]
RAH					
	White				
	Dietary fiber, g/day[2]	21.9	...	4.6	...
	Zinc, mg/day	18.1	0.7	15.8	1.6
	Calcium, mg/day	733	154	522	57
	Magnesium, mg/day	348	170	188	10
	Phosphorus, mg/day	1288	764	346	178
	Bazari				
	Dietary fiber, g/day[2]	29.7	...	10.0	...
	Zinc, mg/day	19.0	0.7	20.7[b]	−2.4[a]
	Calcium, mg/day	784	99[a]	846[a]	−161[a]
	Magnesium, mg/day	650	210[a]	484[a]	−44[a]
	Phosphorus, mg/day	1740	654[b]	1118[a]	−32[b]
MOR					
	White				
	Dietary fiber, g/day[2]	21.9	...	4.0	...
	Zinc, mg/day	19.0	0.7	18.3	−0.0
	Calcium, mg/day	772	187	625	−40
	Magnesium, mg/day	380	185	191	+4
	Phosphorus, mg/day	1400	887	287	+226
	Bazari				
	Dietary fiber, g/day[2]	34.0	...	12.3	...
	Zinc, mg/day	19.4	0.8	20.1[b]	−1.5[b]
	Calcium, mg/day	841	128[a]	835[a]	−122[a]
	Magnesium, mg/day	724	235[a]	618[a]	−129[a]
	Phosphorus, mg/day	1940	1240[a]	948[a]	−248[a]

[a] Reinhold, J. G., *et al.* (1976).
[2] Dietary fiber determined by acid detergent method (van Soest 1963 and 1967).
[3] Mean values for each subject not followed by the same superscript letter are significantly different between white and Bazari bread diets; [a] P ≤0.001; [b] P ≤ 0.01.

form mineral balance. Both subjects were maintained in a metabolic ward during the study, but were allowed to leave the hospital one afternoon a week. During the first 20 day period, both subjects were fed meals supplemented with white bread. One subject required additional energy to maintain body weight and was given an additional 100 g of bread per day. This created large differences between the two subjects in regards to mineral intake. The subjects occasionally did not eat all meals provided and only calculated amounts of nutrients from food not consumed were deducted from intake values. Drinking water was reported to be rich in Zn, Ca and Mg and was freely available to both subjects. Because water intakes could not be reliably measured, its consumption was estimated. In reviewing the protocol of this experiment, it is suggested that mineral intake values were moderately to grossly underestimated, which resulted in inaccurate mineral balance calculations (Table 2).

The subject's DF intake was determined to be 21 g per day in the first period. Dietary fiber was measured by the acid detergent fiber (ADF; Van Soest, 1963; Van Soest and Wise, 1967) method. Since the ADF method for DF determination does not include hemicellulose or soluble dietary fiber components, it can be assumed that the two individuals were consuming in excess of 40 g of total dietary fiber (TDF; insoluble and soluble) per day in the first period. During the second 20 day period, the subjects received Bazari bread in place of white bread and their ADF intake increased to 31 g or approximately 60 g of TDF per day. Phytate contents of the breads/diets were reported to have been determined, but no data on these amounts were provided in the report. Phytic acid is a known chelator of Zn (Mills, et al., 1988) and could be the primary cause of the negative Zn balance observed when the subjects consumed the Bazari bread. The P in phytic acid is not available and, since a large amount of P was supplied by phytic acid in the Bazari bread during the second period, this could have contributed to the negative P balance observed in both subjects. Mineral intake values were not similar between periods, with mineral intakes being much higher in the second period. This difference could have been the primary reason for the negative mineral balances observed in the second period.

Because of the many variables in the design of this experiment and the many differences in nutrient intake values for the two individuals, we feel it is impossible to factor out or imply that increased DF intake was the cause of, or contributed to, the negative mineral balances observed in this study. Our brief review of this now classic paper has been intended as an initial and constructive way of trying to diffuse the belief that DF has a negative effects on mineral utilization. We encourage all readers to review this paper.

Dietary Fiber Effects on Minerals: Scientific Citations

Prior to the Third Vahouny Symposium on Dietary Fiber in 1988, numerous reviews citing many original studies suggested a negative effect of DF on mineral nutrition (Gordon, 1990). It must be noted that all reviews and original research publications have not been negative. During the intervening years, continuing research has further addressed this issue. A partial listing of original research reports and a brief summary of the results obtained from these studies are provided in Table 3. There have also been recent reviews on the interaction between minerals and DF (Harland, 1989; Torre et al., 1991). There still remains a great deal of concern that phytate, associated in the chemical matrix described as DF, is primarily responsible for impaired mineral utilization (Mills, et al., 1988; Brune et al., 1992).

New Methodology: Dietary Mineral Thresholds Concentrations—Experiment #1

To unequivocally determine the effect of DF on mineral bioavailability in humans remains a formidable challenge as previously mentioned. Many variables exist, and it is extremely difficult to control and monitor the status of all minerals in the body. As is so often the case, the use of animal models is required to more rigorously investigate a problem of this nature.

In theory, use of the balance technique is practical, and should provide acceptable results especially in the area of mineral nutrition. In practice, it has limitations as previously reviewed (Gordon, 1990), and is equally difficult in humans and animals. Among other problems associated with the balance technique, mineral concentrations in diets usually exceed the minimum amounts required by the body. This in turn leads to balance values that reflect the body's inability to store more minerals and does not assess mineral status or true balance. The storage capacity for any mineral in the body is not accurately known. The balance technique lacks the ability to accurately reflect any change in nutrient status.

As with current dietary mineral recommendations for the human, mineral intake recommendations for the rat exceed minimum requirements (American Institute of Nutrition, 1977). Based on previous studies in our laboratory, we have been able to determine the minimum or threshold requirements for certain minerals (i.e., Fe, Zn, Cu and Mn) in the rat (Gordon and Chao, 1984; Lee et al., 1988; Gordon, 1987). Ad-

Table 3. Summary of selected reports on the effects of dietary fiber on mineral status in human subjects since 1989

1. Oat porridge/oat bran inhibits iron absorption.

    A. AUTHORS: Rossander-Hulthen *et al.* 1990.

    B. EXPERIMENTAL DESIGN: Nineteen subjects were divided into two groups, and each group was fed breakfast meals with added: 1) oat porridge and milk; or 2) oat bran in bread. Subjects served as their own controls by eating the same meals without added oat porridge or oat bran. Iron absorption was measured by the amount of Fe-55 and Fe-59 consumed with the meals and retained after two weeks. Retention of a reference dose of Fe was also independently determined in all subjects given 10 mL of 0.01M HCL/L containing 3 mg Fe (with Fe-59) and 30 mg ascorbic acid. Retention of the reference dose was also measured after two weeks and values for reference dose were used to standardize retention values for Fe in test meals among subjects.

    C. RESULTS: In subjects consuming a breakfast meal, Fe-59 retention was 9.6% without and 3.6% with oat porridge. Retention of the Fe-59 reference dose among these individuals was 26.9%. Retentions of Fe-59 in subjects consuming a breakfast meal without and with oat bran in the bread were 12.3 and 6.6%, respectively. Retention of the Fe-59 reference dose among these individuals was 32.1%. The authors stated that phytate (120 mg) in the oat products was responsible for the significantly reduced Fe-59 retention observed in this study.

2. Guar gum did not reduce Fe, Cu Zn, Ca, Mn or Mg balance in human NIDDM subjects.

    A. AUTHORS: Behall *et al.* 1989.

    B. EXPERIMENTAL DESIGN: Humans with non-insulin dependent diabetes (NIDDM) were allowed to self-select diets for 6 months. Average daily dietary fiber intakes from meals were not provided. Eight subjects consumed an additional 32 g guar gum per day; 8 subjects served as controls with no additional dietary fiber. Mineral balances were conducted for one week prior to and one week after the end of the 6 month period.

    C. RESULTS: Apparent retention for 6 minerals are listed in the following order: prestudy placebo; prestudy guar; poststudy placebo; and poststudy guar. The minerals evaluated in this study were: Ca: 4.7, 6.5, 7.7 and 9.7 mg/day; Zn: 7.1, 4.6, 4.6 and 6.6 mg/day; Cu: 0.22, 0.15, 0.19 and 0.53 mg/day/ Ca: 281, 54, 595 and 492 mg/day; Mg: 2, -33, -45 and 9 mg/day; and Mn: 0.9, 0.5, -2.4 and -0.2 mg/day. Guar gum had no effect on apparent mineral balance.

(*continued on next page*)

Table 3 (continued)

3. Wheat bran reduces plasma zinc

A. AUTHORS: Hall *et al.* 1989.

B. EXPERIMENTAL DESIGN: Twenty six human subjects were given 50 mg elemental Zn (Zn SO_4 · $7H_2O$) after an overnight fast and their basal plasma Zn concentrations were determined every hour over a 6 hr period. These values were used to calculate a curve representing the magnitude of the serum response over the 6 hrs and the area under the curve (AUC). After 7 days, subjects were divided into 3 groups and given 50 mg Zn with test meals containing: 17 g wheat bran; 17 g reduced phytate wheat bran; or 17 g Rice Krispies. Plasma Zn concentrations were measured and AUC values calculated.

C. RESULTS: Percent reduction in plasma Zn concentration compared to AUC values determined with basal diet in the three meals were: wheat bran, 106; dephytanized wheat bran, 76; and Rice Krispies, 46. The authors concluded that: "Standard raw wheat bran totally abolished the plasma zinc response that was obtained when zinc was given alone, suggesting little, if any absorption, of zinc."

4. Fruit and vegetable dietary fiber did not reduce plasma Cu, Zn, P, Mg and Ca concentrations

A. AUTHORS: Scholfield, *et al.* 1990. (Also see Kelsay et al., 1988).

B. EXPERIMENTAL DESIGN: Twelve men were divided into two groups and fed diets with 5 or 25 g of neutral detergent fiber as fruits, vegetables and their juice for 6 weeks each in a crossover design. All meals were supplemented with 450 mg oxalic acid/day; spinach supplied the oxolic acid. Plasma mineral concentrations were measured at the start of the experiment, after 6 weeks and after 12 weeks.

C. RESULTS: Plasma mineral concentrations at the start of the experiment, after 6 weeks and after 12 weeks were: Cu: 16.4[a,b], 15.3[a] and 17.9[b] $\mu mol/L$; Zn: 15.0, 15.0 and 14.8 $\mu mol/L$; P: 1.75[a], 1.55[b] and 1.30[b] $\mu mol/L$; Mg: 0.98[a], 1.05[b] and 1.04[b] mmol/L and; Ca: 2.34[a]; 2.52[b] mmol/L. Neither dietary fiber not oxylate affected plasma mineral concentrations.

5. Oat bran did not impair Ca, P, Mg or Zn balance.

A. AUTHORS: Spencer *et al.* 1991.

B. EXPERIMENTAL DESIGN: Eleven subjects participated in a metabolic balance study in which the first 40 days served as the control period, which was followed by a 32 day balance test period. During the control period, dietary fiber intake was 22.6 g/day. In the test period, subject consumed 4 oat bran muffins providing an additional 21.8 g of oat

(*continued on next page*)

Table 3 (continued)

bran. The total daily dietary fiber consumed during test period was 43.2 g. Intestinal absorption (i.e., retention) and fecal excretion of Ca-47 were also measured.

C. RESULTS: Mineral balance for 4 elements during the control and test periods, respectively, were: Ca: -31 and -32 mg/day; P: 26[b] and 144[a] mg/day; Mg: -6 and 15 mg/day; Zn: 0.8 and 0.4 mg/day. Calcium-47 retention, reported as percent of original dose for control and test periods, respectively, were: 41.3 and 39.9%; fecal Ca-47 for control and test periods as percent of original dose were: 12.2 and 14.5%. Oat bran did not impair mineral balance. Phosphorus balance increased in human subjects consuming large amounts, 21.8 g, of oat bran per day.

6. Barley fiber concentrate caused negative balance for Ca, Mg, Zn and Fe with reduced dietary protein

A. AUTHORS: Wisker *et al.* 1991.

B. EXPERIMENTAL DESIGN: Twelve females participated in three 22 day test periods in which they were fed diets providing low fiber, (22.5 g/day) and high protein (71.8 g/day); high fiber (38.6 g/day; 23 g barley-fiber concentrate) and high protein (73.8 g/day); high fiber (38.6 g/day; 23 g barley-fiber concentrate) and low protein (55.7 g/day). Each 22 day period was separated by a 2 day period.

C. RESULTS: Mineral balance was conducted for the last 7 days of each test period. Daily apparent balance values for subjects on 3 diets, 1) low fiber, 2) high fiber - high protein and 3) high fiber - low protein, respectively, were: Ca: 0.2, 1.9 and -0.8 mmol/day; Mg: 0.3, 0.2 and -0.5 mmol/day; Zn: 3.0, -4.6 and -18.4 μmol/day; and Fe: 16.1, 5.4 and -23.3 μmol/day. A high fiber diet with lower protein content compared to a diet of the same amount of dietary fiber with higher protein content can significantly reduce Ca, Mg, Zn and Fe balance in females.

7. Wheat bran caused a negative effect on Ca-47 retention

A. AUTHORS: Knox *et al.* 1991.

B. EXPERIMENTAL DESIGN: Calcium-47 retention (absorption) was determined in 9 normal elderly subjects and 8 elderly subjects with achlorhydria after consuming the isotope with 3 types of meals. The meals were: low fiber, (0.5 g dietary fiber, 0.035 g phytate and 245 mg Ca), high fiber (10.5 g dietary fiber from 23.7 g wheat bran, 0.35 g phytate and 275 mg Ca); and high fiber with 120 mL of 0.1 mL HCl/L.

C. RESULTS: Calcium-47 retention, as percent of dose, measured by whole body counting was 25.7 percent with a low fiber meal, 19.1 percent with a high fiber meal and 18.9 percent with a high fiber meal and acid in normal subjects. Similar values were observed in achlorhydria subjects. High fiber meals significantly reduced Ca-47 retention by 20 percent in the elderly.

ditional work is in progress to determine the more exact threshold requirements for Ca, P and Mg. This concept is illustrated in Figure 1 and briefly described. When diets which contain recommended mineral requirements are fed to rats, growth and other physiological/biochemical functions will proceed in a normal manner, but with excess dietary mineral concentrations. We theorize and have partially demonstrated, that there exists for minerals, a minimum or threshold dietary concentration sufficient to permit the animal to grow properly and maintain normal physiological and biochemical functions. An amount less than minimal or threshold value in the diet would cause the animal to fail to grow or to have lower measurable physiological and biochemical parameters. The model also assumes that any dietary factor (i.e., DF) able to adversely affect mineral utilization would cause the animal to fail to thrive.

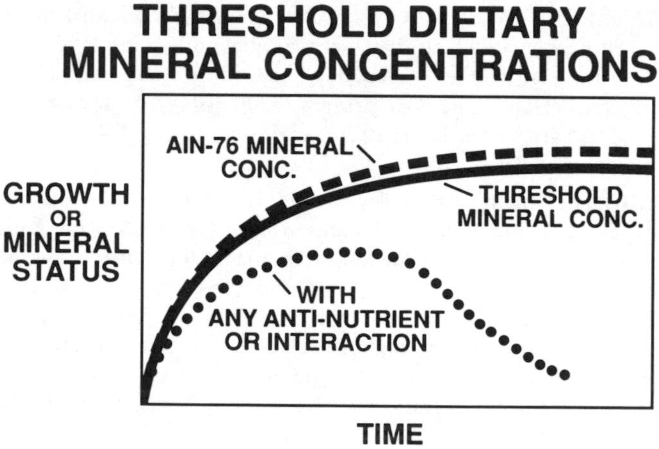

THRESHOLD DIETARY MINERAL CONCENTRATIONS

TIME

Figure 1. Recommended mineral requirements for the rat provide for a sufficient margin of safety to insure adequate growth and maintenance with a wide variety of dietary components. Growth and all physiological and biochemical parameters in animals consuming diets with mineral concentrations as recommended by the American Institute of Nutrition (AIN, 1976) have optimum and reproducible values. The threshold theory of dietary mineral concentrations assumes there is a lowest dietary concentration for each mineral which will support growth and indices of mineral status identical to values observed with recommended dietary mineral concentrations. Using threshold dietary mineral concentrations, it is also theorized that any antinutrient or negative interaction between or among minerals will cause the animal to first have a decrease in one or more physiological or biochemical parameters and finally growth. The threshold concept of mineral requirements is proposed for use in determining: 1) the effects of dietary components on mineral availability; 2) mineral bioavailability; and 3) mineral interaction studies.

This threshold hypothesis has been tested using a number of different DF and a summary of our results is provided (Stoops, et al., 1991). In this experiment, 9 dietary fibers were compared as to their effects on mineral status in the rat. The experimental design for Experiment #1 is presented in Figure 2. The DF used in this experiment and their TDF content and mineral concentrations are reported in Table 4. Recommended mineral requirements (AIN-76; American Institute of Nutrition, 1977) and threshold mineral requirements for the rat are reported in Table 5. Using the American Institute of Nutrition diet formulation, diets were produced after determining the amount of each mineral provided by each dietary component and adding additional minerals to achieve threshold concentrations if necessary. The primary control group of animals in this experiment was fed a diet containing mineral concen-

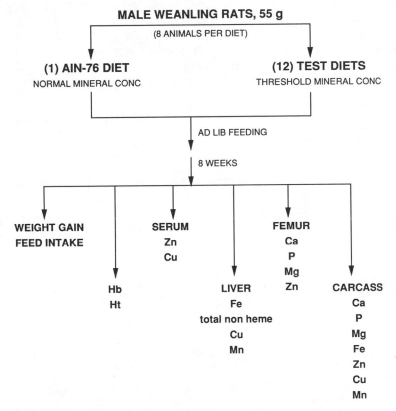

Figure 2. Experiment #1–The experimental design used to test the effects of different dietary fibers on growth and mineral retention in rats among various organs using the threshold mineral concept is illustrated. See Table 8 for the amount of TDF in each diet.

trations as recommended by the AIN and containing 5% cellulose (Table 5). Two additional control groups of animals were fed diets containing 5% cellulose or no fiber, but prepared to contain threshold mineral concentrations.

Male, weanling Sprague Dawley rats were individually housed and provided diets and distilled water ad libitum for 8 weeks. The animals

Table 4. Total dietary fiber and mineral content of dietary fibers — Experiment #1.

Dietary fiber	TDF %[1]	Ca	P	Mg	Fe	Zn	Cu	Mn
				μg/g[2]				
Cellulose	96.4	<3	10	0.4	0.3	0.1	0.1	0.1
Agar	79.0	1,910	430	506	127.0	2.1	0.4	24.6
Gellan	72.8	2.660	3,460	749	292.0	54.7	8.4	35.8
Locust bean	86.5	930	440	297	5.3	6.4	3.6	3.0
Guar gum	85.1	910	550	456	90.0	5.1	1.6	3.0
Carrageen	72.2	4,150	620	3,990	61.0	1.8	0.5	17.0
Pectin, low methoxy	83.1	1,030	160	24.3	88.7	2.7	2.7	0.8
Wheat bran	42.7	1,010	13,600	5,910	125.0	77.3	10.7	136
Oat bran	47.7	3,720	19,100	7,750	272.0	104.0	6.0	148

[1] Mean of duplicate determinations; value on dietary fibers added to diets and not corrected for moisture content.
[2] Mean of duplicate determinations.

Table 5. Mineral requirement for the rat and mean mineral concentrations of diets — Experiment #1

	Recommended AIN-76[1]	Threshold	Diet AIN-76[4]	Threshold diets[5,6]
		(μg/g)		
Calcium	5,200	3,640[2]	5,680	3,707 ± 182
Phosphorus	4,000	2,800[2]	5,410	4,408 ± 524
Magnesium	500	350[2]	530	487 ± 222
Iron	35	22–25[3]	31	23.1 ± 0.9
Copper	6	2–3[3]	6.5	2.7 ± 0.1
Zinc	30	9–11[3]	30	11.2 ± 6
Manganese	54	3–4[3]	53	5.0 ± 3.1

[1] J. Nutr. 1977. 107.1340–1348.
[2] Not absolute threshold, but 70% of amount recommended by AIN-76; see footnote 1.
[3] Threshold amount range.
[4] Actual dietary concentration of one control diet prepared to meet AIN-76 specifications; see footnote 1.
[5] Mean ± SD; concentration of 12 test diets.
[6] Oat bran and wheat bran diets exceeded threshold values of Mg, Mn, P and Zn because of high endogenous concentrations; See Table 4.

were killed and tissues analyzed for: serum Cu and Zn concentrations; liver Fe, Mn, and Cu concentrations; femur Ca, P, Mg, and Zn concentrations and the remaining carcass Ca, P, Mg, Fe, Zn, Cu and Mn content.

Weight gain, feed consumption, hemoglobin concentration and hematocrit (percent) for the control group of animals fed the diet with recommended mineral requirements and the mean values for the combined 12 groups of rats fed diets with threshold mineral concentrations are reported in Table 6. For these four parameters, there was no significant difference between the control group of animals fed the diet with AIN-76 recommended amounts of minerals and the 12 groups fed diets with threshold mineral concentrations. Nor were there any significant differences in the mean values for these four parameters among the 12 groups of fed rats diets with threshold mineral concentrations.

Mean serum, liver, femur and carcass mineral concentrations in rats fed diets with recommended and threshold mineral concentrations are reported in Table 7. Among the 16 mineral parameters examined, 5 were found to differ significantly among treatments. Mean values observed among the 13 treatments for these 5 parameters are reported in Table 8.

Three of the 5 parameters found to have significant differences among mean values were serum Cu, liver Cu and carcass Cu concentrations. Although these data initially suggested that some DF might have adversely affected Cu utilization, two sets of data do not support this theory. First, the mean dietary Cu concentrations among the 12 threshold test diets was 2.7 µg/g compared to 6.5 µg/g Cu in the AIN-76 control diet. Eleven of the 12 groups of rats fed diets with threshold mineral

Table 6. Weight gain, feed consumption, hemoglobin concentration and hematocrit in rats fed threshold dietary mineral concentrations with different dietary fibers–Experiment #1 [1]

	AIN-76 cellulose control diet [2,4]	Threshold diets [3,4]
Weight gain, g	228 ± 23	231 ± 36
Feed consumption, g	916 ± 89	933 ± 86
Hemoglobin, g/DL	17.0 ± 0.9	15.9 ± 1.7
Hematocrit, %	51.7 ± 3.4	50.4 ± 4.1

[1] Experiment used weanling male rats 23 days old, 55 g starting weight; animals were fed diets ad libitum for 8 weks.
[2] Mean ± SD, n = 7; control group was fed a diet with mineral concentrations as recommended by AIN; See Table 5.
[3] Mean ± SD of 12 groups, 8 animals per group unless noted.
[4] No significant difference in mean values observed among 13 groups of animals.

concentrations had serum Cu concentrations that were lower compared to the group of rats fed the AIN-76 diet with adequate Cu, and 8 of these mean serum Cu concentrations were significantly lower. We suggest these low serum Cu values are the result of a slightly lower than threshold dietary Cu concentration used in this experiment. Since serum Cu is most sensitive to inadequate dietary Cu or impaired Cu absorption, we attribute these low Cu concentrations to slightly lower than threshold dietary Cu intake and not any adverse action of DF. The second set of data, hepatic Cu concentrations, suggests that the DF did not impair Cu utilization because animals having low serum Cu did not have correspondingly low liver nor low carcass Cu concentrations. If Cu status was impaired by any dietary fiber, all parameters examined should have been lowered. There were two exceptions. Two groups of rats having

Table 7. Pooled mean serum, liver, femur and carcass mineral concentrations in groups of rats fed with AIN recommended and threshold dietary mineral concentrations with different dietary fibers—Experiment #1

	AIN-76 cellulose control diet[1]	Threshold diets[2,3]
Serum		
Zinc, μg/ml	1.8 ± 0.3	1.6 ± 0.3[3]
Copper, μg/ml	1.1 ± 0.4	0.7 ± 0.4[b]
Liver[4]		
Iron, μg/g	312 ± 51	321 ± 79
Copper, μg/g	12 ± 0.6	11.7 ± 2.5[a]
Manganese, μg/g	7.8 ± 1.0	7.0 ± 1.0
Femur[4]		
Calcium, mg/g	223 ± 13	219 ± 11
Phosphorus, mg/g	109 ± 7	107 ± 5
Magnesium, mg/g	4.1 ± 0.3	3.9 ± 0.3[a]
Zinc, μg/g	189 ± 25	185 ± 15
Carcass[4]		
Calcium, mg/g	25.1 ± 5.6	25.3 ± 4.3
Phosphorus, mg/g	16.4 ± 2.6	16.6 ± 2.4
Magnesium, mg/g	0.96 ± 0.10	0.96 ± 0.13
Iron, μg/g	97 ± 8	113 ± 48
Znc, μg/g	62 ± 4	62 ± 5
Copper, μg/g	3.9 ± 1.8	5.1 ± 2.9[b]
Manganese, μg/g	1.3 ± 1.1	1.1 ± 0.6

[1] Mean ± SD, n ± 7.
[2] Mean ± SD, 13 groups of rats, 8 animals per group unless noted in Table 8.
[3] Subscript letters indicate significant differences exist among 13 groups of rats; [a]P ≤ 0.05; [b] P ≤ 0.01; See Table 8 for mean values in each group of rats.
[4] Dry weight.

the lowest serum Cu concentration also had the lowest liver Cu concentrations. Rats fed diets with carrageen and no fiber had identical serum Cu concentrations of 0.3 µg/ml and liver Cu concentrations of 10.1 and 9.6 µg/g, respectively. However, these liver Cu concentrations were not significantly different compared to the mean value of 12.0 µg/g, determined in the control group of animals fed the diet with 6 µg Cu/g diet. The three lowest carcass Cu concentrations were observed in groups of rats fed diets with threshold mineral concentrations and no fiber (3.8 µg Cu/g), oat bran (3.6 µg Cu/g), and 2.5% (1.82% TDF) gellan gum (3.5 µg Cu/g). These mean values were not significantly different compared to the mean carcass Cu concentrations observed in the group of animals fed the recommended amount of dietary Cu (3.9 µg/g). In conclusion, these data for Cu retention in this study verify the sensitivity of the threshold concept. They suggest that dietary Cu concentrations were slightly below threshold, but these lower Cu retention values are not to be attributed to DF.

Table 8. Mean serum zinc and copper, liver copper, femur magnesium and carcass copper concentrations among groups of rats fed AIN recommended and threshold dietary mineral concentrations with different dietary fibers and having significant differences among treatments—Experiment #1

Diet	Dietary fiber[1] % TDF	n	Serum[2] Zn	Serum[2] Cu (μg/ml)	Liver[2] Cu (μg/g[3])	Femur[2] Mg (mg/g[3])	Carcass[2] Cu (μg/g[3])
AIN-76[4]							
Cellulose	4.82	7	1.8[a]	1.1[a,b]	12.0[a,b,c]	4.1[a,b,c]	3.9[b,c]
Threshold[4]							
Cellulose	4.82	8	1.4[a,b,c]	0.9[a,b]	11.2[a,b,c]	3.9[a,b,c,d]	8.6[a]
Agar	3.64	8	1.7[a]	1.2[a]	14.2[a]	3.8[b,c,d]	3.8[c]
Gellan gum	3.64	8	1.7[a,b]	0.9[a,b]	13.0[a,b]	3.6[d]	4.5[b,c]
Gellan gum	1.82	8	1.6[a,b]	0.6[b,c]	12.0[a,b,c]	4.0[a,b,c]	3.5[c]
Gellan gum	0.91	7	1.6[b,c]	0.6[b,c]	11.7[a,b,c]	3.9[a,b,c,d]	4.8[b,c]
No fiber	...	8	1.7[a]	0.3[c]	9.6[c]	3.8[c,d]	3.8[c]
Locust bean	3.64	8	1.7[a]	0.7[b]	12.0[a,b,c]	3.9[b,c,d]	7.5[a,b]
Guar gum	3.64	8	1.7[a]	0.7[b]	13.0[a,b]	4.0[a,b,c]	6.6[a,b,c]
Carrageen	1.82	8	1.7[a]	0.3[c]	10.1[b,c]	4.2[a,b]	4.1[b,c]
Pectin, LM	3.64	7	1.3[b,c]	0.9[a,b]	12.1[a,b,c]	3.9[a,b,c,d]	3.9[c]
Wheat bran	3.64	7	1.4[a,b,c]	0.6[b,c]	11.5[a,b,c]	4.2[a]	5.6[a,b,c]
Oat bran	3.64	7	1.2[a]	0.6[b,c]	10.4[b,c]	4.1[a,b,c]	3.6[c]

[1] Total dietary fiber (TDF) in diet.
[2] Mean values among 13 groups not having the same superscript letter are significantly different at the $P \leq 0.05$ level or lower.
[3] Dry weight.
[4] See table 5 for dietary mineral concentrations.

The lowest serum Zn concentrations were observed in groups of animals fed diets containing pectin (1.3 µg Zn/ml) and oat bran (1.2 µg Zn/ml). These values were significantly lower compared to the mean value of 1.8 µg Zn/ml observed in the group of animals fed the diet containing 30 µg Zn/g diet as recommended by the AIN. But these two mean values were not significantly different compared to the mean value of 1.4 µg Zn/ml observed in the group of animals fed the diet with a threshold concentration of Zn (9.5 µg Zn/g) and 5% cellulose.

The Mg concentration in the femur of animals consuming a diet with 1.25% (0.91% TDF) gellan gum and a threshold Mg concentration (380 µg Mg/g diet) was 3.6 mg Mg/g and was significantly lower compared to the mean value of 4.1 mg Mg/g observed in animals fed a diet with 5% cellulose and the recommended dietary amount of Mg (530 µg Mg/g). The mean value of 3.6 mg Mg/g was not significantly different compared to the mean value of 3.9 mg Mg/g determined in animals fed a diet with a threshold Mg concentration (360 µg Mg/g) and 5% (4.92% TDF) cellulose. There was very little variation among all 13 groups of animals in their femur Mg concentrations (3.9 ± 0.3 mg Mg/g).

The results of this study suggest no uniform nor negative effects of any DF evaluated on mineral nutrition or status in the rat. The threshold method appears to be sensitive to possible adverse effects of diet on mineral utilization. The authors acknowledge that additional work will be required to use this sensitive methodology, but it appears highly satisfactory for its reported use.

New Technology—High Resolution Gamma Ray Spectroscopy—Experiment #2

Radioisotopes have played a vital role in determining mineral absorption, utilization and requirements. In the past, these studies have usually centered on measuring the absorption of a single radionuclide.

Colleagues at the University of Missouri (Zinn and Morris, 1988; Zinn et al., 1992) have developed the hardware and software for a high resolution gamma-ray spectrometer which allows for the simultaneous resolution of a multitude of radionuclides. High resolution gamma-ray spectroscopy utilizes a solid state germanium-lithium (Ge-Li) detector, and can accurately resolve gamma-ray peaks that differ by as little as a few KeV in energy. Using this new technology, we have built upon the knowledge obtained in our previous experiment employing dietary mineral thresholds (Gordon et al., 1992). In this second experiment, we determined the effect of different DF, at different dietary concentrations, on the retention of Se-75, Mn-54, Fe-59, Zn-65 and Ca-47 in rats. These radionuclides have a number of gamma ray energies which are reported in Table 9. The energy spectrum associated with these 5 radionuclides is illustrated in Figure 3.

Nine dietary treatments were used for this second experiment (Experiment #2). One control diet with no cellulose had mineral concentrations as recommended by the AIN and identical to values used and reported in Experiment #1 (Table 5). The second control diet also with no DF, had threshold mineral concentrations as used and reported in Experiment #1 (Table 5). The other 7 test diets were prepared to achieve threshold mineral concentrations (Table 5). But this was not always feasible for every mineral because of endogenous minerals provided by the different dietary fibers. This was especially the case when DF were evaluated at increasing concentrations in diets. No attempt has been made to measure the Se content of the diets and all diets had 0.1 µg Se/g added as sodium selenite in the mineral premix. Diets were formulated and prepared to contain 5, 10 and 15 percent TDF from cellulose (Soy cellulose; Fibred, Cumberland MD) and 5 and 10 percent TDF from

Table 9. Gamma ray energies and abundance associated with the radionuclides selenium-75, manganese-54, iron-59, zinc-65 and calcium-47

Element	Half life t 1/2 (days)	Gamma ray energy (Kev[1])	Gamma ray abundance (%[2])
Selenium-75	119.8	121.12	16.4
		136.00	56.0
		246.65[3]	58.6
		1,279.53	27.4
		400.65	11.1
Manganese-54	312.1	834.8[3]	99.98
Iron-59	44.5	142.65	1.02
		192.35	3.08
		1,099.25[3]	56.50
		1,291.60	43.20
Zinc-65	243.9	1,115.55[3]	50.70
Calcium-47	4.5	489.2	6.7
		807.8	6.9
		1,297.1[3]	75.0
Scandium-47[4]	3.34	159.4	68.0

[1] Photons, Kev thousand electron volts.
[2] Indicates how fast different energy gamma-rays are produced.
[2] Principal energy value used to detect and quantify radionuclide retention by high resolution (Ge-Li) gamma-ray spectroscopy.
[2] Calcium-47 will decay to scandium-47 and this latter radionuclide is present in animals when administered calcium 47.

wheat bran (AACC Certified Wheat Bran-Hard Red; AACC, St Paul, MN). The TDF content of the soy derived cellulose and wheat bran were 87 and 42.7 percent, respectively, as determined by the Association Official Analytical Chemists (AOAC) method (Prosky, et al., 1988). Of the two remaining diets, one contained 1.5 percent chitosan (Protan, Seattle, WA) and the second contained 1.5 percent BioRad AG 50W-X12 cation exchange resin (BioRad, Richmond, CA). Chitosan is the deacylated product of chitin which we have previously shown to adversely affect Fe absorption in the rat (Gordon and Besch-Williford, 1983). We had no record of research in which cation exchange resin was evaluated as to its effects on mineral retention in animals. If DF can be suspected of impairing mineral nutrition because of its ion binding capacity, a cation exchange resin would also cause a negative response.

A summary of the experimental design for Experiment #2 is illustrated in Figure 4. Rats were fed diets and distilled water ad libitum for 11 days. On the morning of day 11, and with free access to their diets during the previous night, animals were administered a mixture of the 5 radionuclides in solution by stomach gavage. Animals were counted in a whole body counter with the Ge-Li detector (Figure 5) 5 hrs after dosing

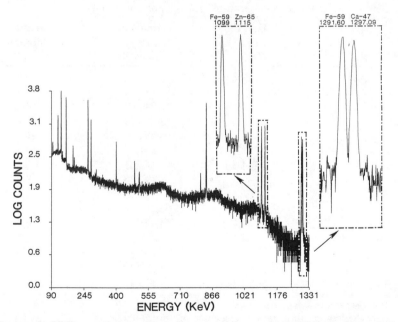

Figure 3. High resolution gamma-ray spectrum obtained from the whole body counting of a rat given a mixture of Se-75, Mn-54, Fe-59, Zn-65 and Ca-47 by stomach gavage. Each peak corresponds to the gamma-ray energy values for the 5 radionuclides reported in Table 9.

and at 4 additional periods during the remaining 10 days of the experiment. Animals were weighed on the last day of the experiment, counted and killed. We present the results of animal weight gain and radionuclide retention measured on the last day of the experiment. Percent final radionuclide retention was determined as the ratio of the final count in each animal divided by the whole body count measured 5 hrs after dosing.

Weight gain among the 7 groups of animals consuming diets containing cellulose, weight bran or no fiber with AIN recommended mineral or threshold mineral concentrations were not significantly different (Table 10). Weight gain for the two groups of rats consuming diets with chitosan and cation exchange resin were significantly lower compared to the 7 other groups of animals in this experiment. Two of the animals consuming the diet with the cation exchange resin and three of the animals consuming the diet with chitosan died during the experiment. The

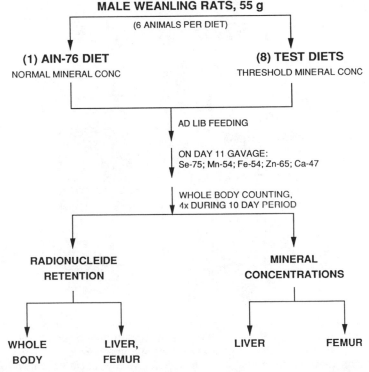

Figure 4. Experiment #2—The experimental design used to determine the effects of wheat bran, cellulose, chitosan and cation exchange resin on whole body retention of 5 radionuclides is illustrated. Retention of non-radionuclides in liver and femurs are not provided in this report.

cause of death in animals consuming chitosan was attributed to septicemia. Necropsy of the animals that died on the cation exchange resin diet indicated the animals were severely malnourished at the time of death, but no exact cause of death could be diagnosed.

The percent retentions of the 5 radionuclides determined on the last day of the experiment among the 9 dietary treatments are reported in Table 11. The use of Se-75 in this experiment accomplished two objectives. First, it was an additional mineral evaluated, but not at a dietary threshold concentration. Secondly, it was provided as an anion. The average Se-75 retention among the 9 groups of animals was 43%. The only group of animals having a significantly different and lower Se-75 retention was for the animals fed 10% TDF provided as wheat bran. This lower retention is attributed to the higher amount of Se provided by the wheat bran which subsequently decreased the amount of Se required and retained by this group of animals.

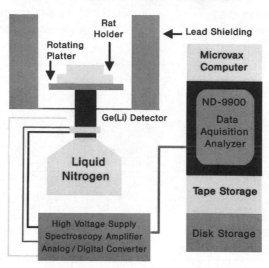

Figure 5. In-vivo whole body small animal counter. Animals are restrained in a holder which is secured to a 360° continuously rotating platter (20 rpm). This rotation insures uniform geometry of the gamma rays for the Ge-Li high resolution gamma-ray detector. This detector with associated software instrumentation is capable of accurately resolving gamma-ray peaks that differ by as little as a few KeV in energy. For example, the last major peak in Figure 3 is a doublet consisting of Ca and Fe gamma ray energies of 1291.6 and 1297.1 KeV, respectively.

Table 10. Weight gain in rats fed diets with AIN recommended and threshold dietary mineral concentrations, different dietary fibers and gavaged with radionuclides—Experiment #2

Diet	Dietary fiber[1] (%)	n	Weight gain[2,3] (g)
AIN-76			
Cellulose	5	6/6	149 ± 13[a]
Threshold			
No fiber	...	6/6	149 ± 21[a]
Wheat bran	5	6/6	145 ± 19[a]
Wheat bran	10	6/6	147 ± 19[a]
Cellulose	5	6/6	160 ± 16[a]
Cellulose	10	6/6	166 ± 10[a]
Cellulose	15	6/6	165 ± 17[a]
Chitosan	1.5	3/6	90 ± 47[b]
Cation exchange resin[4]	1.5	4/6	132 ± 23[b]

[1] Amount of total dietary fiber added to diets.
[2] Mean ± SD weight gain after 21 days; starting weight 54.9 ± 2.9 g.
[2] Mean values not followed by the same letter superscript are significantly different at the $P \leq 0.01$ level.

Table 11. Radionuclide retention in rats fed diets with AIN recommended and threshold dietary mineral concentrations and cellulose, wheat bran, chitosan or cation exchange resin—Experiment 2

Diet	Dietary fiber (%)	Se-75	Mn-54	Fe-59 %[1,2]	Zn-65	Ca-47
AIN-76						
No fiber	0	47.9±2.4[a,b]	3.2±1.0[b]	45.3±3.6[c]	27.1±2.4[d]	50.1±4.0[d]
Threshold						
No fiber	0	48.1±1.0[a]	8.5±1.5[a,b]	73.4±5.1[b,c]	66.5±2.2[a]	72.6±4.1[c]
Wheat bran	5	42.9±1.9[a,b]	3.7±2.1[b]	82.6±5.8[a,b]	61.2±4.0[a,b,c]	76.8±2.5[b,c]
Wheat bran	10	29.3±1.1[c]	1.9±0.8[b]	81.2±5.8[a,b]	55.0±3.9[b,c]	76.6±3.5[b,c]
Cellulose	5	46.3±1.7[a,b]	6.3±0.2[a,b]	88.4±3.8[a]	61.5±2.8[a,b,c]	72.5±1.5[c]
Cellulose	10	42.4±2.7[b]	12.2±6.3[a]	66.7±5.8[d,e]	62.2±2.3[a,b]	79.8±1.1[a,b,c]
Cellulose	15	42.9±2.8[a,b]	5.9±0.3[a,b]	56.6±5.8[d,e]	52.4±1.9[c]	81.9±2.0[a,b]
Chitosan	1.5	44.1±1.9[a,b]	10.9±2.0[a,b]	89.4±2.7[a,b]	61.6±3.1[a,b,c]	87.3±4.2[a]
Cation exchange resin	1.5	42.3±1.6[b]	4.3±0.7[a,b]	59.0±4.9[d,e]	55.1±3.1[b,c]	56.1±3.3[d]

[1] Mean±S.E. determined on the 10th days after administration of radionuclides.
[2] Mean values not followed by the same superscript letter are significantly different at least at the $P \leq$ level.

Higher amounts of a dietary mineral provided to an animal will result in adequacy within the body and subsequently lower absorption and retention. This was clearly observed among the 4 other radionuclides and especially comparing percent retention values between the two diets having no fiber and either AIN recommended dietary mineral concentrations or threshold mineral concentrations. Retention of the radionuclides, Mn-54, Fe-59, Zn-65 and Ca-47 were significantly lower in animals having higher dietary mineral concentrations compared to lower mineral concentrations (Table 11).

Significantly lower retention of all radionuclides except Se-75 was observed in the group of animals fed the diet containing cation exchange resin with threshold mineral concentrations compared to the group of animals fed a diet with no fiber and threshold mineral concentrations. Selenium, provided as the anion, was not expected to be bound by the cation-exchange resin.

The impaired retention of the four cations by the cation exchange resin supports our contention that a material of this nature will bind minerals in vivo. Dietary fiber in the intestine is not an ion exchange resin and does not impair mineral absorption and retention.

Percent retention of the 4 radionuclides, Mn-54, Fe-59, Zn-65 and Ca-47 was high in the remaining 3 animals consuming the diet containing chitosan was generally the highest among all groups of animals. Because these animals were not eating properly and were not growing, they failed to properly digest and pass their intestinal waste products. We theorize these animals did not thoroughly pass the radionuclides they failed to absorb.

The retention of Mn-54 was generally decreased in the groups of rats fed diets with increasing amounts of cellulose or wheat bran. This lower retention was attributed to the higher amount of the Mn provided by the higher amounts of DF added to the diets, therefore exceeding the threshold concentrations. A satisfactory explanation is not available to account for the 12.2% Mn-54 retention observed in the group of rats fed a diet containing 10% TDF from cellulose. This value was twice the percent retention values observed in rats fed diets with 5 and 15% TDF provided as cellulose. With the radionuclides, Fe-59 and Zn-65, percent retention in rats decreased with increasing amounts of wheat bran and cellulose in their diets. Percent Ca-47 retention values in rats fed diets with cellulose were directly related to dietary cellulose concentrations. Higher Ca-47 retention was observed in animals with higher dietary cellulose content. A satisfactory explanation for this observation is not available.

These data provide no evidence that wheat bran or cellulose adversely affect mineral retention in the rat. Furthermore, the technology used in this experiment provided more convincing evidence that there is no negative effect caused by increasing the DF concentration on minerals retention.

Conclusion

Fourteen minerals are considered to be essential for humans and animals. A far greater number of different DF are available for consumption. Because DF do bind minerals in vitro, plus the numerous balance studies that have been conducted showing negative mineral balance with different types and amounts of DF, this anti-nutritional aspect regarding DF has been difficult to dispel.

Continued use of balance trails cannot adequately indicate the effect of DF on mineral status or nutrition. Using a threshold nutrient concept and employing the use of multiple radionuclides, stronger experimental

---

FACTORS AFFECTING MINERAL BIOAVAILABILITY

INTRINSIC	EXTRINSIC
MINERAL STATUS	MINERALS
AGE	PROTEIN
GENDER	ASCORBIC ACID
HEALTH/DISEASE	PHYTIC ACID
PREGNANCY	~~FAT~~
	~~CARBOHYDRATE~~
	~~TOTAL DIETARY FIBER~~
	~~MAILLARD PRODUCTS~~

Figure 6. Both intrinsic (i.e., within the body) and extrinsic (i.e., of dietary origin) factors can effect mineral absorption and utilization. Dietary factors such as fat, carbohydrate, Maillard products and total dietary fiber are strongly believed not to effect mineral bioavailability. Animal protein appears to have an enhancing effect on Fe. Ascorbic acid enhances Fe bioavailability, but is reported to impair Cu bioavailability. Phytic acid is a strong chelator of Zn, and has been shown to inhibit Zn bioavailability when its concentration is very high in the diet and dietary Zn is low. Those factors that are considered to have the most significant effects on mineral absorption and utilization (i.e. bioavailability) are the mineral status of the host and dietary mineral concentrations.

evidence has been obtained to support the contention that no DF impairs mineral absorption and retention. It is acknowledged that these studies have been conducted in animals, but it is argued that animal models can and do provide the necessary information to make important contributions and decisions regarding human metabolism and nutrition. It is important to determine the safety of DF as increased intakes are recommended. Although there is no information to suggest this problem occurs in the very young, the elderly, the pregnant or lactating women, these groups are vulnerable to nutritional inadequacies and are of concern to us. We cannot state equivocally that no effect on mineral absorption occurs among these special groups of the population with DF consumption, but there is no evidence to suggest that a problem exists nor will DF interfere with mineral nutrition.

The effect of dietary components on mineral bioavailability remains an important and interesting area of nutrition research. Based on other studies in our laboratories, we suggest the hypothesis that dietary mineral concentrations and the mineral status of the host control mineral bioavailability. Dietary fiber has no effect on mineral utilization (Figure 6). A diet too high in foods rich in DF may case a reduction in mineral and other nutrient density, but not a reduction in mineral bioavailability.

Acknowledgment

The authors acknowledge the pioneering work of Reinhold and his colleagues who suggested an important area of nutrition and research regarding DF. These early studies have allowed for the initiation and accomplishmet of research that has benefitted everyone in the areas of DF and mineral nutrition. We appreciate our other colleagues and students who have been very helpful and contributed directly or indirectly to this work. Our special thanks are extended to Kurt Zinn, Dan Trokey, and Mike Peluso. Portions of this work have been supported by the University of Missouri Agricultural Station.

References

American Diabetes Association, 1987, Position statement. Nutritional recommendations and principles for individuals with diabetes mellitus: 1986. Diabetes Care, 10:126-132.

American Dietetic Association, 1988, Health implications of dietary fiber-technical support paper, J. Am. Diet. Assoc. 88:217.

American Institute of Nutrition, 1977, Report of the AIN Ad Hoc Committee on Standards for Nutritional Studies, J. Nutr. 107:1340-1348.

Behall, K. M., Scholfield, D. J., McIvor, M. E., Van Duyn, M. S., Leo, T. A., Michnowski, J. E., Cummings, C. C., and Mendeloff, A. I., 1989, Effect of guar gum on mineral balances in NIDDM adults, Diabetes Care 12:357-364.

Brune, M., Rossander-Hulten, L., Hallberg, L., Gleerup, A., and Sandberg, A. S., 1992, Iron absorption from bread in humans: Inhibiting effects of cereal fiber, phytate and inositol phosphates with different numbers of phosphate groups, J. Nutr. 122:442-449.

Dietary Fiber, 1989, A Scientific Status Summary by the Institute of Food Technologists' Expert Panel on Food Safety and Nutrition, Food Tech. 43:133-139.

Gordon, D. T., and Besch-Williford, C., 1983, Chitin and chitosan: Influence on element absorption in rats, in: "Unconventional sources of dietary fiber," I. Furda, ed., American Chemical Society, Washington, DC. pp. 155-184.

Gordon, D. T., and Chao, L. S., 1984, Relationship of components in wheat bran and spinach to iron bioavailability in the anemic rat, J. Nutr. 114:526-535.

Gordon, D. T., 1987, Interactions among iron, zinc and copper, in: "AIN Symposium Proceedings. Nutrition '87," O. A. Levander, ed., The American Institute of Nutrition, Bethesda, MD. pp. 27-31.

Gordon, D. T., 1990, Total dietary fiber and mineral absorption in: "Dietary Fiber," D. Kritchevsky, C. Bonfield and J. W. Anderson, eds., Plenum Publ. pp. 105-127.

Gordon, D. T., Pelluso, M., Zinn, K., Stoops, D., Ratliff, V., and Trokey, D., 1992, Retention of Ca-47, Mn-54, Fe-59, Zn-65 and Se-75 in rats fed diets containing different types and amounts of dietary fiber, 1992 IFT Ann. Meeting/Book of Abstracts #415. p. 107.

Hall, M. J., Downs, L., Ene, M. D., and Farah, D., 1989, Effect of reduced phytate wheat bran on zinc absorption, European J. Clin. Nutr. 43:431-440.

Harland, B. F., 1989, Dietary fibre and mineral bioavailability, Nutr. Res. Revs. 2:133-147.

Kelsay, J. L., Clark, W. M., Prather, E. S., Canary, J. J., 1988, Mineral balances of men fed a diet containing fiber in fruits and vegetables and oxalic acid in spinach for six weeks, J. Nutr. 118:1197-1204.

Knox, T. A., Kassarjian, Z., Dawson-Hughes, B., Golner, B. B., Dallal, G. E., Arora, S., and Russell, R. M., 1991, Calcium absorption in elderly subjects on high- and low-fiber diets: effect of gastric acidity. Am. J. Clin. Nutr. 53:1480-1486.

Kritchevsky, D., 1988, Dietary fiber, in: Ann. Rev. Nutr. 8:301-328.

Lee, D., Schroeder, J. III, and Gordon, D. T., 1988, Enhancement of Cu bioavailability in the rat by phytic acid, J. Nutr. 118:712-717.

Life Sciences Research Office, Federation of American Societies of Experimental Biology, 1987, Physiological effects and health consequences of dietary fiber, prepared for Center for Food Safety and Applied Nutrition, Food and Drug Administration, Department of Health Services, Washington, D.C.

McCance, R. A., and Widdowson, E. M., 1942, Mineral metabolism of healthy adults on white and brown bread dietaries, J. Physiol. (London), 101:44-85.

Mills, C. F., Davies, N. T., Aggett, P. J., Drakenberg, T., Blakeborough, P., Frolich, W., Ratcliffe, R. G., Sandberg, A. S., Sandstrom, B., and Wise, A., 1988, Report of a study group on the significance of dietary phytate, its analogues and other dietary factors on trace element availability to man, Nutrition Abstracts and Reviews, 58:501-516.

Nair, B. M., Asp, N. G., Nyman, M., and Persson, H., 1987, Binding of mineral elements by some dietary fibre components—in vitro (I), Food Chem. 23:295-303.

National Research Council, 1989, "Diet and Health: Implications for Reducing Chronic Disease Risks." National Academy of Sciences, Washington, D.C.

Nutrition Reviews, 1991, Nutrition Classic, 49:204-206.

O'Dell, B. L., 1984, Bioavailability of and interactions among trace elements. in: Trace Elements in Nutrition of Children, R. K. Chandra, Ed. Vevey/Raven Press, New York, pp. 41-62.

Persson, H., Nair, B. M., Frolich, W., Nyman, M., and Asp, N. G., 1987, Binding of mineral elements by some dietary fibre components—in vitro (II), Food Chem. 26:139-148.

Prosky, L., Asp, N-G., Schweizer, T. F., DeVries J., and Furda, I., 1988, Determination of insoluble, soluble and total dietary fiber in foods and food products: Interlaboratory study, JAOAC, 71:1017-1023.

Recommended Dietary Allowances, National Academy of Sciences, 1980, 9th rev. ed., National Academy Press, Washington, D.C.

Recommended Dietary Allowances, National Academy of Sciences, 1989, 10th ed. National Academy Press, Washington, D.C.

Reinhold, J. G., Faradji, B., Abadi, P., and Ismail-Beigi, F., 1976, Decrease absorption of calcium, magnesium, zinc and phosphorus by humans due to increased fiber and phosphorus consumption as wheat bread, J. Nutr. 106:493-503.

Rossander-Hulthen, L., Gleerup, A., and Hallberg, L., 1990, Inhibitory effect of oat products on non-haem iron absorption in man, European J. Clin. Nutr. 44:783-791.

Scholfield, D. J., Behall, K. M., Kelsay, J. L., Prather, E. S., Clark, W. M., Reiser, S., and Canary, J. J., 1990, The effects of natural dietary fiber from fruit and vegetables with oxalate from spinach on plasma minerals, lipids and other metabolites in men, Nutr. Res. 10:367-378.

Spencer, H., Norris, C., Derler, J., and Osis, D., 1991, Effect of oat bran muffins on calcium absorption and calcium, phosphorus, magnesium and zinc balance in men, J. Nutr. 121:1976-1983.

Stoops, J. D., Ratliff, V., Hindenberger, E., and Gordon, D. T., 1991, Mineral retention in rats fed diets containing dietary fibers with restricted dietary mineral concentration, The FASEB J. 5:A568(1147).

Torre, M., and Rodriguez, A. R., and Saura-Calixto, F., 1991, Effects of dietary fiber and phytic acid on mineral availability. Critical Reviews in Food Sci. and Nutr. 30:1-22.

Van Soest, P. J., 1963, Use of detergents in the analyses of fibrous feeds, JAOAC, 46:829-835.

Van Soest, P. J., and Wise, R. H., 1967, Use of detergents in the analyses of fibrous feeds. IV. Determination of plant cell-wall constituents. JAOAC, 50:50-55.

Walker, A. R. P., 1987, Dietary fibre and mineral metabolism, Molec. Aspects Med. 9:69-87.

Ward, A. T., and Reichert, R. D., 1986, Comparison of the effect of cell wall and hull fiber from canola and soybean on the bioavailability for rats of minerals, protein and lipid, J. Nutr. 116:233-241.

Wisker, E., Nagel, R., Tanudjaja, T. K., and Feldheim, W., 1991, Calcium, magnesium, zinc, and iron balances in young women: effects of a low-phytate barley-fiber concentrate. Am. J. Clin. Nutr. 54:553-559.

Zinn, K. R., and Morris, J. S., 1988, High resolution gamma-ray spectroscopy as an *in vivo* tool for following the zinc-selenium interaction. in: "Trace Elements in Man and Animals," L. Hurley, C. L. Keen, B. Lonnerdal, and R. B. Rucker, eds., Plenum Press, New York. p. 591.

Zinn, K. R., Morris, J. S., Fairfax, C. A., Berlinger, R. R., Lui, H. B., and Brugger, R. M., 1992, The development of a rectilinear scanner utilizing high resolution gamma-ray detection. J. Radioanalytical and Nuclear Chem. 1:15-24.

Effects of Lignans and Other Dietary Estrogens

Kenneth D. R. Setchell

Clinical Mass Spectrometry
Children's Hospital Medical Center
Cincinnati, Ohio 45229-2899

Introduction

Some two thousand years ago it became recognized that plants contained substances with estrogenic potential that were capable of influencing heredity. However, it was not until the last fifty years that scientific evidence accrued linking diet with compounds having estrogenic activity, and this was highlighted by several well documented examples of the way in which the dietary intake of phytoestrogens can influence reproductive physiology of animals.[1,2]

While the mammalian estrogens, estrone and estradiol have been shown to occur in only a few plants, the major classes of plant estrogens are the isoflavones, lignans, coumestrans and resorcylic lactones.[3-7] The striking feature of the chemical structures of all of these compounds is the presence of a phenolic ring (Fig 1) which is an essential moiety for binding to the estrogen receptor.[8] Consequently, all of these compounds possess weak estrogenic activity but also behave as partial estrogen antagonists. Although the concentration of many of these compounds is relatively low, they are widely distributed in foods commonly consumed by man[6,7] (Table 1). In particular, legumes have relatively high concentrations of isoflavones,[9-11] while flaxseed (linseed) is a rich source of precursors to the mammalian lignans.[12]

Current interest in this field appears to have been stimulated by the independent discovery by two groups that several novel lignans were present in biological fluids from man and animals at concentrations exceeding the levels of the major endogenous steroids[13,14] and the speculation that these may be natural anticancer agents.[15,16] The first and principal mammalian lignans to be identified by mass spectrometry were 2,3-bis(3-hydroxybenzyl-γ-butyrolactone and 2,3-bis(3-hydroxybenzyl)-1,4-diol to which we coined the trivial names enterolactone and enterodiol, respectively.[17] These unique compounds were shown to be derived from precursors of more complex plant lignans by the action of intestinal microflora; secoisolariciresinol was identified in relatively high concentrations in flaxseed.[12] During the course of these studies, equol, an additional non-steroidal dietary estrogen, was identified[18] and was shown to increase markedly in the urine following soy protein ingestion by humans and animals.[19] Interestingly, equol, which belongs to the isoflavone class, was first identified in pregnant mares' urine[20] and was the estrogenic agent responsible for "Clover disease" in sheep.[1,21] Subsequent studies established the importance of intestinal bacteria for the synthesis of both lignans and equol[15,22–24] and showed that in common

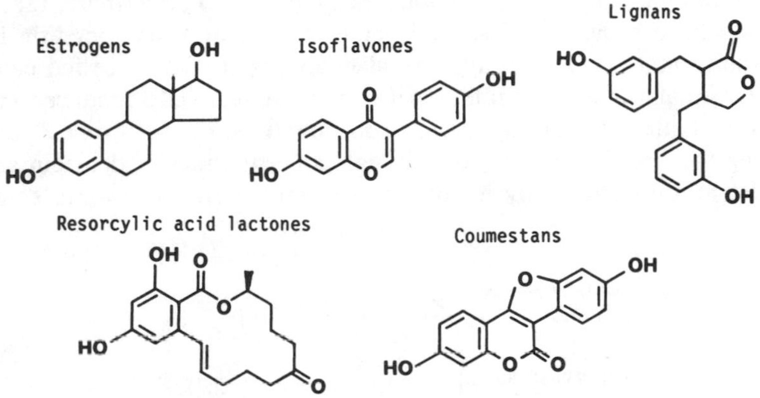

Figure 1. Common classes of phytoestrogens.

Table 1. Edible plants with recognized estrogenically active compounds

Estrogens	Isoflavones	Lignans	Coumestans	Resorcylic acid lactones	Others
Licorice	Soybean	Flaxseed	Alfalfa	Oat	Fennel
French bean	Chickpea	Wheat bran	Soy sprouts	Barley	Carrot
Date palm	Cherry	Rye meal	Cowpea	Rye	Anise
Pomegranate		Buckwheat	Green bean	Sesame	Hops
Apple		Oatmeal	Red bean	Wheat	
		Barley	Split pea	Corn	

with endogenous estrogens all of these nonsteroidal dietary estrogens undergo an enterohepatic circulation (Fig 2).

Equol was shown to be a specific intestinal bacterial metabolite of daidzein and genistein (Fig 3), isoflavones that are found in high concentrations as sugar conjugates (daidzin and genistin) in all soy protein products.[25,26]

When soy protein was ingested acutely (40g/day) the level of equol was found to exceed the levels of endogenous estrogens by several orders of magnitude.[19,24] In early studies, equol was considered to be a major and specific metabolite of daidzein and genistein but more recent studies have established that in addition to equol, daidzein and genistein are also absorbed efficiently from the gastrointestinal tract and are excreted in urine. In most individuals, equol accounts for <30% of the total isoflavones in biological fluids.

The role of microflora in the metabolism of isoflavones and lignans is well illustrated from the fact that germ-free animals do not produce these compounds despite challenge by food containing the precursors,[22] and antibiotic administration abolishes synthesis.[15] Furthermore, recent studies have shown significant differences in isoflavone excretion by newborn infants fed soy-milk formulae compared with those fed cows milk formula or human milk.[27] All of the commercially produced soy milk formulae contain significant concentrations of isoflavones[25] and during the first four months of life high concentrations of daidzein and genistein are excreted by infants fed soy milk formulae[27] while equol

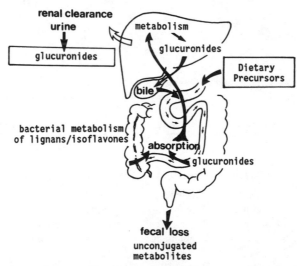

Figure 2. Schematic of the enterohepatic circulation of dietary estrogens.

cannot be detected in urine. The lack of synthesis of equol from precursor isoflavones may be explained by the developmental lack of necessary microflora, while the urinary equol found in cows milk formula-fed and human milk-fed infants can be explained by the presence of low concentrations of this isoflavone in these milks.[28]

The fact that such high levels of dietary estrogens can be attained when soy protein products are ingested led to our speculation[24] that "soy protein may be beneficial in the prevention and/or treatment of hormone dependent diseases such as breast cancer because of the presence of non-steroidal dietary estrogens which may behave as partial estrogen antagonists and which we subsequently have shown to have anti-cancer activity."[12]

Breast cancer is one of the so-called hormone dependent cancers[29] and has a significantly higher incidence in the Western World compared to the Third World and Oriental countries.[30-32]

Epidemiological studies clearly show that the incidence of breast cancer in countries of the Western World is significantly greater than, for example, in the Orient where the lifetime risk for developing breast cancer is 5–8 fold less. On the other hand, the incidence of breast cancer in Asian migrants and their offspring is no different from indigent Westerners.[33-35] Taken together with case control and population studies, these data suggest that rather than genetic differences, the susceptibility

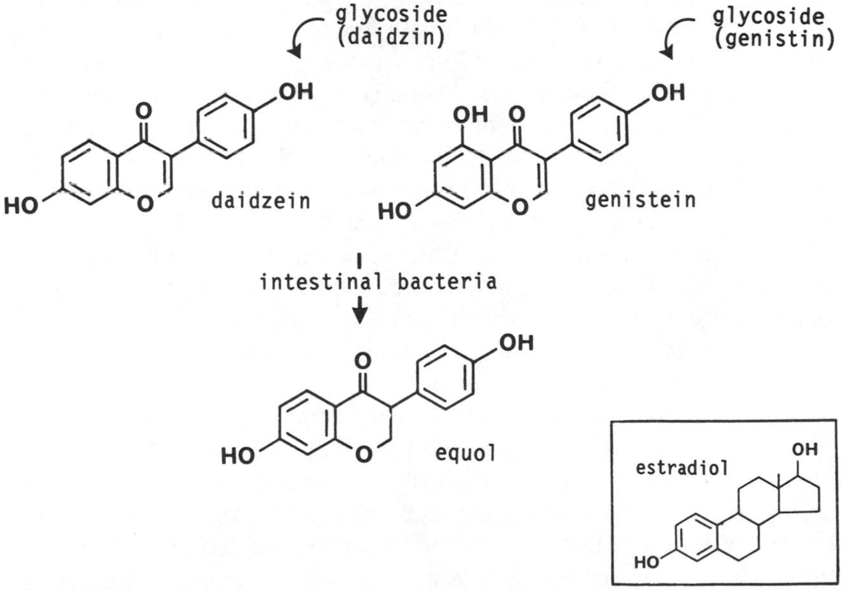

Figure 3. Structures of the principal isoflavones of soy and their metabolism.

to breast cancer is the result of environmental differences between these populations, and that diet is a particularly important factor.

Most of the studies relating to diet and breast cancer have focused on the potential carcinogenic role of the diet and have proven inconclusive, but it is very difficult to evaluate the potential of individual components because of the problems of accurately evaluating dietary intake over extended periods of time.[34]

For some years now we have concentrated our attention on the hypothesis that differences in breast cancer incidence between Oriental and Western populations may be attributed to the presence of protective (anticarcinogenic) agents in the diet[16,24] and specifically have suggested that dietary estrogens should be considered important.[24] This is an area that has received little attention save the concerns over the contamination of meat products by synthetic estrogens such as diethylstilbestrol (DES) that were used as anabolic agents in the agricultural industry.[36]

Circumstantial data supporting a role for non-steroidal dietary estrogens as possible anti-cancer agents include: (i) the finding that vegetarians, who also have a low incidence of breast cancer, and Orientals excrete relatively high concentrations of dietary estrogens[37-39]; (ii) the recent epidemiological data indicating that a high soy protein intake is associated with a lower risk for breast cancer in women in Hong Kong and Singapore.[40]

Furthermore, we have demonstrated that the long-term ingestion of soy protein can significantly modify the length of the menstrual cycle in women.[41] Specifically, follicular phase length was increased and a significant suppression in the mid-cycle surge of circulating gonadotrophins, follicle stimulating hormone (FSH) and luteinizing hormone (LH) occurred. The cycle length increased by an average of 2.5 ± 1.6 days in the six women studied. These effects clearly indicate how diet can modify hormonal status in normal women and these responses are similar to reported effects of the synthetic antiestrogen tamoxifen,[42] which is used in the treatment of breast cancer.[14,43-45] Furthermore, it is interesting that tamoxifen has been proposed as a candidate for the prophylactic treatment of women at high risk for breast cancer, i.e., first degree relatives of breast cancer victims, and clinical trials have been carried out.[45]

Since metastatic breast cancer is rarely curable, prevention is an important and challenging goal. In most instances it is difficult to identify factors responsible for initiation of the disease and, therefore, emphasis has been placed on limiting the promotion and progression of tumor growth and metastatic disease.[46] The importance of diet and nutrition in breast cancer is unequivocal. In Asia where the incidence of breast cancer is low, soy protein is consumed in large quantities and this led us to suggest that isoflavones present in soy may play a role in protecting against breast cancer.[24,47]

Furthermore, the possibility that soy protein may be protective in breast cancer is suggested from experiments by Troll *et al.,*[48] where a 50% reduction in experimentally induced mammary tumors was observed in rats exposed to X-rays and consuming a powdered soybean diet. This effect was attributed to the presence of trypsin or protease inhibitors present in the soybean,[49] and a large literature has been published on the role of trypsin inhibitors in cancer. Our own studies would refute some of this evidence. We have shown that commercial trypsin inhibitors contain large concentrations of the isoflavones, daidzein and genistein, while autoclaved soy protein, in which the trypsin inhibitor was inactivated, was found to be as effective as non-autoclaved soy in reducing the number of tumors in experimental models of breast cancer.[47]

Animal Studies of Isoflavones and Breast Cancer

To test the thesis that isoflavones present in soy protein are active in protecting against breast cancer, Barnes and Setchell used two standard experimental animal models of breast cancer in which mammary tumors

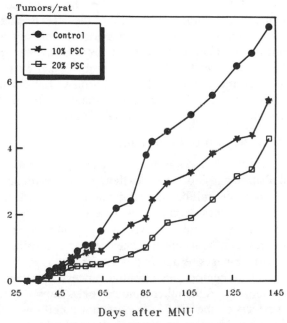

Figure 4. Effect of powdered soybean chips on mammary tumors in the MNU rat model of chemically induced mammary carcinoma.

were induced by the chemical carcinogens, MNU and DMBA. Animals were maintained on standard diets that were isocaloric and isonitrogenous and where the protein (casein) was replaced by various forms of soybean protein containing differing levels of isoflavones, including one preparation that was devoid of isoflavones.

In all of our experiments a dose dependent reduction in the number of histologically proven mammary tumors was observed with soy protein (Fig 4), and there were no significant differences between autoclaved and non-autoclaved soy protein diets.[47] These studies confirm that soy protein ingestion leads to a reduction in mammary tumors and would suggest that the trypsin or protease inhibitor does not play a role in the observed effect.[47] While these studies do not conclusively prove that isoflavones are responsible for the protective effect, the fact that a soy protein product with no detectable isoflavones (Arcon F) gave no significant difference in the number of tumors/rat compared with controls lends strong support for a role for these compounds. In addition to lower numbers of tumors in the soy fed animals, estrogen receptor concentrations were reduced and the mean tumor estrogen receptor concentration was positively correlated with the average number of tumors per animal, but there were no differences in the progesterone receptor concentrations between groups.[47] Contrary to the effects of these isoflavones on the reproductive tract in other animals[20,21,26] there was no deleterious effect on the uterus or the menstrual cycle of the experimental rats.

These animal studies provide strong evidence that soy protein containing significantly high concentrations of isoflavones will protect against tumor development and that they probably act by inhibiting the promotion of mammary tumors. The reduction in tumors was linearly correlated with the total isoflavone concentration of the diet, and most strongly correlated with the dietary genistein content.

Mechanism of Action of Isoflavones

While our initial thesis was that the isoflavones may act as anti-estrogens in a similar fashion to tamoxifen, it must be realized that there are several other possibilities based upon recent evidence for non-hormonal actions of these compounds. One exciting possibility is that they may act directly on tumor growth by regulating protein phosphorylation. In this respect, genistein has been recognized to be a potent inhibitor of tyrosine kinases[50,51] and in this way it may regulate phosphorylation of estrogen receptors, an essential process in estrogen receptor activation.[52] Daidzein on the other hand has been shown to possess anti-proliferative effects on the ZR-75-1 breast cancer cell line.[53] Other interesting potential mechanisms of action that are worthy of consideration involve the inhibition of topoisomerases I and II by genistein in a similar manner to the action of the anticancer agent and complex plant lignan etoposide.[54]

Conclusions

All of these circumstantial pieces of evidence lend support for the notion that a diet of soy protein may be beneficial to women in the protection against, or treatment of, breast cancer. However, before implementing clinical studies, much additional work is necessary to investigate aspects of the metabolism and absorption of these isoflavones in man, and there is a critical need for evaluating the dietary composition of isoflavones in soy based foods.

In general, the amounts of dietary estrogens ingested by Asians calculated from the daily intake of soy protein products is 150–200 mg/day and this exceeds the dosage that we have shown will inhibit the appearance of mammary tumors in the experimental model of breast cancer in rats.[47] Dietary modification by the inclusion of foods containing isoflavones may therefore prove to be beneficial in the prevention and treatment of breast cancer in the Western World.

References

1. H. J. Bennetts, E. J. Underwood, and F. L. Shier, A specific breeding problem of sheep on subterranean clover pastures in Western Australia, *Aust. Vet. J.* 12:22 (1946).
2. K. D. R. Setchell, S. J. Gosselin, M. B. Welsh, J. O. Johnston, W. F. Balistreri, L. W. Kramer, B. L. Dresser, and M. J. Tarr, Dietary Estrogens—A probable cause of infertility and liver disease in captive cheetahs, *Gastroenterology* 93:225 (1987).
03. K. D. R. Setchell, and H. Adlercreutz, Mammalian lignans and phytooestrogens: recent studies on their formation, metabolism and biological role in health and disease, *in:* "The Role of Gut Microflora in Toxicity and Cancer," I. A. Rowland, ed. BIBRA (1988).
4. B. B. Bradbury and D. E. White, Oestrogens and related substances in plants, *Vitam. Horm. (NY).* 12:207 (1954).
5. N. R. Farnsworth, A. S. Bingel, G. A. Cordell, F. A. Crane, and H. H. S. Fong, Potential value of plants as sources of new antifertility agents II, *J. Pharm. Sci.* 64:717 (1975).
6. K. D. R. Setchell, Naturally occurring non-steroidal estrogens of dietary origin, *in:* "Estrogens in the Environment: Influence on Development," J. McLachlan, ed. Elsevier, New York, (1985).
7. K. R. Price and G. R. Fenwick, Naturally occurring oestrogens in food—a review, *Food Addit Contam.* 2:73 (1985).
8 G. Leclercq and J. C. Heuson, Physiological and pharmacological effects of estrogens in breast cancer, *Biochim. Biophys. Acta* 560:427 (1979).

9. E. Walz, Isoflavon-und Saponin-glucoside in Soja hispida, *Justus. Liebigs. Annin. Chem.* 489:118 (1931).

10. P. A. Murphy, Phytoestrogen content of processed soybean products, *Food Technology (Champaign).* 60-64 (1982).

11. A. C. Eldridge and W. F. Kwolek, Soybean isoflavones: effect of environment and variety on composition, *J. Agri. Food Chem.* 31:394 (1983).

12. M. Axelson, J. Sjovall, B. E. Gustafsson, and K. D. R. Setchell, Origin of lignans in mammals and identification of a precursor from plants, *Nature* 298:659 (1982).

13. S. R. Stitch, J. K. Toumba, M. B. Groen, C. W. Funke, J. Leemhuis, J. Vink, and G. F. Woods, Excretion, isolation and structure of a new phenolic constituent of female urine, *Nature* 287:738 (1980).

14. K. D. R. Setchell, A. M. Lawson, F. L. Mitchell, H. Adlercreutz, D. N. Kirk, and M. Axelson, Lignans in man and animal species. *Nautre* 287:740 (1980).

15. K. D. R. Setchell, A. M. Lawson, S. P. Borriello, R. Harkness, H. Gordon, D. M. L. Morgan, D. N. Kirk, H. Adlercreutz, and M. Axelson, Lignan formation in man—microbial involvement and possible roles in relation to cancer, *Lancet* 2:4 (1981).

16. H. Adlercreutz, Does fiber-rich food containing animal lignan precursors protect against both colon and breast cancer? An extension of "Fiber Hypothesis," *Gastroenterology* 86:761 (1984).

17. K. D. R. Setchell, A. M. Lawon, E. Conway, N. F. Taylor, D. N. Kirk, G. Cooley, R. D. Farrant, S. Wynn, and M. Axelson, The definitive identification of the lignans trans-2,3-bis(3-hydroxybenzyl)-γ-butyrolactone and 2,3-bis(3-hydroxybenzyl)-butane-1,4-diol in human and animal urine, *Biochem. J.* 197:447 (1981).

18. M. Axelson, D. N. Kirk, R. D. Farrant, C. Cooley, A. M. Lawson, and K. D. R. Setchell, The identification of the weak oestrogen equol[7-hydroxy-3-(4'-hydroxyphenyl)chroman] in human urine, *Biochem. J.* 201:353 (1982).

19. M. Axelson, J. Sjovall, B. E. Gustafsson, and K. D. R. Setchell, Soya—A dietary source of non-steroidal oestrogen equol in humans and animals, *J. Endocr.* 102:49 (1984).

20. G. F. Marrian and G. A. D. Haslewood, Equol, a new inactive phenol isolated from the ketohydroxyoestrin fraction of mares' urine, *Biochem. J.* 26:1227 (1932).

21. D. A. Shutt, The effects of plant oestrogens of dietary origin, *Endeavour* 35:110 (1980).

22. M. Axelson and K. D. R. Setchell, The excretion of lignans in rats—Evidence for an intestinal bacterial source for this new group of compounds, *FEBS Letts.* 123:337 (1981).

23. K. D. R. Setchell, A. M. Lawson, S. P. Borriello, H. Adlercreutz, and M. Axelson, Formation of lignans by intestinal microflora, *Proceedings of the 31st Falk Symposium.* pp. 93-99 (1981).

24. K. D. R. Setchell, S. P. Borriello, P. Hulme, D. N. Kirk, and M. Axelson, Nonsteroidal oestrogens of dietary origin: possible roles in hormone dependent disease, *Am. J. Clin. Nutr.* 40:569 (1984).

25. K. D. R. Setchell, M. B. Welsh, and C. K. Lim, HPLC analysis of phyto-

estrogens in soy protein preparations using ultraviolet, electrochemical and thermospray mass spectrometric detection, *J. Chromatogr.* 368:315 (1986).

26. L. Umble, N. C. Barnes, K. D. R. Setchell, J. Carlson, and S. Barnes, The phytoestrogens, isoflavones, in soybean food of the American and Asian diets, *Am. J. Clin. Nutr.* (submitted) (1991).

27. M. L. A. Cruz, W. W. Wong, F. Mimouni, D. L. Hachey, K. D. R. Setchell, P. K. Klein, and R. C. Tsang, Effects of infant nutrition on cholesterol synthesis rates, *Am. J. Clin. Nutr.* (in press) (1992).

28. C. Bannwart, H. Adlercreutz, K. Wahala, T. Kotiaho, A. Hesso, G. Brunow, and T. Hase, Identification of the phyto-oestrogen 3',7-dihydroxyisoflavan, an isomer of equol, in human urine and cow's milk, *Biomed. Environ. Mass Spectrom.* 17:1 (1988).

29. G. T. Beatson, On the treatment of inoperable cases of carcinoma of the mammary. Suggestion for a new method of treatment with illustrative cases, *Lancet* 2:104 (1896).

30. B. Armstrong and R. Doll, Environmental factors and cancer incidence and mortality in different countries with special reference to dietary practices, *Int. J. Cancer* 15:617 (1975).

31. D. P. Rose, A. P. Boyar, and E. L. Wynder, International comparison of mortality rates for cancer of the breast, ovary, prostate, and colon, and per capita fat consumption, *Cancer* 58:2363 (1986).

32. Diet, Nutrition, and Cancer. Committee on Diet, Nutrition and Cancer, National Academy Press, Washington, D.C. (1982).

33. R. L. Smith, Recorded and expected mortality among the Japanese of the United States and Hawaii, with special reference to cancer, *J. Natl. Cancer Inst.* 17:459 (1965).

34. D. P. Rose, Dietary factors and breast cancer, *Cancer Surveys* 5:671 (1986).

35. W. Haenzel and M. Kurihara, Studies of Japanese migrants: I. Mortality from cancer and other diseases among Japanese in the United States, *J. Natl. Cancer Inst.* 40:43 (1968).

36. J. McLachlan. "Estrogens in the Environment: Influence on Development," Elsevier, New York (1985).

37. H. Adlercreutz, T. Fotsis, R. Heikkinen, J. T. Dwyer, B. R. Goldin, S. L. Gorbach, A. M. Lawson, and K. D. R. Setchell, Diet and urinary excretion of lignans in female subjects, *Med. Biol.* 59:259 (1981).

38. H. Adlercreutz, T. Fotsis, R. Heikkinen, J. T. Dwyer, M. Woods, B. R. Goldin, and S. L. Borbach, Excretion of the lignans enterolactone and enterodiol and of equol in omnivorous and vegetarian post-menopausal women and in women with breast cancer, *Lancet* 2:1295 (1982).

39. H. Adlercruetz, H. Honjo, A. Hagashi, T. Fotsis, E. Hamalainen, T. Hasegawa, and H. Okada, Urinary excretion of lignans and isoflavonoid phytoestrogens in Japanese men and women consuming a traditional Japanese diet, *Am. J. Clin. Nutr.* 54:1093 (1991).

40. H. P. Lee, L. Gourley, S. W. Duffy, J. Esteve, L. Lee, and N. E. Day, Dietary effects on breast cancer risk in Singapore, *Lancet* 337:1197 (1991).

41. A. Cassidy, S. A. Bingham, and K. D. R. Setchell, Suppression of human ovulation by soya protein, *N. Engl. J. Med.* (submitted) (1991).

42. M. P. Golder, E. A. Phillips, D. R. Fahmy, P. E. Preece, V. Jones, J. M. Henk, and K. Griffith, Plasma hormones in patients with advanced breast cancer treated with Tamoxifen, *Eur. J. Cancer* 12:719 (1976).

43. Early breast cancer treatment collaborative group: Effects of adjuvant Tamoxifen and of cytotoxic therapy on mortality in early breast cancer—overview of 61 randomized trials among 28,896 women. *New Engl. J. Med.* 319:1681 (1988).

44. B. J. A. Furr and V. C. Jordan, The pharmacology and clinical use of Tamoxifen, *Pharmac. Ther.* 25:127 (1984).

45. R. L. Prentice, Tamoxifen as a potential preventative agent in healthy postmenopausal women, *J. Natl. Cancer Inst.* 82:1310 (1990).

46. W. R. Miller, Endocrine treatment for breast cancer. Biological rationale and current progress, *J. Steroid Biochem.* 37:467 (1990).

47. S. Barnes, C. Grubbs, K. D. R. Setchell, and J. Carlson, Soybeans inhibit mammary tumors in models of breast cancer, *Proceedings Mutagens and Carcinogens in the Diet.* Wiley-Liss, Inc. pp. 239-253 (1990).

48. W. Troll, R. Wiesner, C. J. Shellabarger, S. Holtzmann, and J. P. Stone, Soybean diet lowers breast tumor incidence in irradiated rats, *Carcinogenesis* 1:469 (1980).

49. W. Troll, K. Frenkel, and R. Wiesner, Protease inhibitors as anticarcinogens, *J. Natl. Cancer Inst.* 73:1245 (1984).

50. H. Ogawara, T. Akiyama, S. Watanabe, N. Ito, M. Koboti, and Y. Seoda, Inhibition of tyrosine protein kinase activity by synthetic isoflavones and flavones, *J. Anitbiotics* XLII:340 (1989).

51. T. Akiyama, J. Ishida, S. Nakagawa, H. Ogawara, S. Watanabe, N. Itoh, M. Shibuya, and Y. Fukami, Genistein, a specific inhibitor of tyrosine-specific protein kinases, *J. Biol. Chem.* 262:5592 (1987).

52. F. Auricchio, Phosphorylation of steroid receptors, *J. Steroid Biochem.* 32:613 (1989).

53. R. Hirano, K. Oka, and M. Akiba, Antiproliferative effects of synthetic and naturally occurring flavonoids on tumor cells of the human breast carcinoma cell line, ZR-75-1, *Res. Comm. Chem. Path. Pharm.* 64:69 (1989).

54. A. Okura, H. Arakawa, H. Oka, T. Yoshinari, and Y. Monden, Effect of genistein on topoisomerase activity and on the growth of [val 12]Ha-ras-transformed NIH 3T3 cells, *Biochem. Biophys. Res. Comm.* 157:183 (1988).

Phytic Acid and Other Nutrients: Are They Partly Responsible for Health Benefits of High Fiber Foods?

Lilian U. Thompson

Department of Nutritional Sciences
Faculty of Medicine
University of Toronto
Toronto, Ontario, Canada M5S 1A8

Introduction

There is substantial evidence that diets rich in high fiber foods such as cereals, legumes, fruits and vegetables are associated with lower risk for chronic diseases. Because these diets differ not only in the types of dietary fiber but also in the content of nutritive and non-nutritive substances, however, it remains uncertain whether the benefits of high fiber diets are due to the total dietary fiber or a specific type of dietary fiber, nutrient or non-nutrient. High fiber foods are rich in antinutrients, e.g., protease and amylase inhibitors, saponins, lectins, phenolic compounds, phytoestrogens, lignans and phytic acid (PA), and it has been hypothesized that they are in part responsible for the effects of high fiber foods (Setchell and Adlercreutz, 1988; Thompson, 1988, 1989, 1992; Troll and Kennedy, 1989; Adlercreutz, 1990; Oakenful and Sidhu, 1990; Messina and Barnes, 1991).

The health benefits associated with the intake of high fiber foods include (a) delaying nutrient absorption, (b) decreasing cancer risk, (c) lowering blood lipids, and (d) increasing fecal bulk. This paper describes some studies from our laboratory and others suggesting that antinutrients, specifically phytic acid (PA), can also produce these same effects. The role of the other antinutrients has been reviewed (Thompson, 1992).

Delay Nutrient Absorption

A delay in the digestion and absorption of starchy foods and consequently the flattening of blood glucose and endocrine responses has been suggested to be beneficial to healthy, diabetic, hyperlipidemic and cirrhotic individuals (Wolever, 1990). Thus, factors contributing to this effect may be considered desirable, and antinutrients appear to be one of them. The antinutrient-rich legumes produced the lowest blood glucose response when compared to other starchy foods with lower content of antinutrients, e.g., white bread, potatoes (Jenkins et al., 1980, 1986). A significant negative relationship was observed between the concentration or intake of PA (Figure 1) (Yoon et al., 1983; Thompson, 1988), lectins (Rea et al., 1985) or polyphenol (Thompson et al., 1984) and the glycemic response of normal or diabetic individuals as well as the in-vitro rate of starch digestion. Fractionation of the navy beans into starch, hull, protein, starch, fiber and soluble whey, followed by the measurement of in-vitro digestibility of the starch fraction with or without the other fractions alone or in combination, showed the maximum lowering of starch digestibility when digestion was done in the presence of the soluble whey, the fraction richest in the antinutrients, e.g., PA, tannins and lectins (Thompson, 1988). Dephytinization of navy bean flour caused increases in the in-vitro rate of starch digestion and the blood glucose response while the readdition of PA back to the dephytinized bean flour produced the opposite effect (Thompson et al., 1987). The addition of PA (2% starch basis) to unleavened bread prepared from white flour reduced the starch digestibility rate and blood glucose response (Yoon et al., 1983). We also observed significant reductions in blood glucose and insulin responses upon addition of 0.8 g PA to 50 g glucose solutions.

Phytic acid is a highly negatively charged molecule capable of binding with positively charged groups such as mineral ions and proteins, and with starch either directly or indirectly through the protein it is associated (Thompson, 1988). Thus, PA may reduce starch digestion either by binding and inactivating the amylase, which is a protein, by binding with the calcium needed for the amylase stability and activity, or by binding with the starch and influencing its solubility and accessibility to the digestive enzymes, or its degree of gelatinization. Other mechanisms such as effect on gastric emptying may likewise be involved, since PA also influenced the glycemic response to glucose; cal-

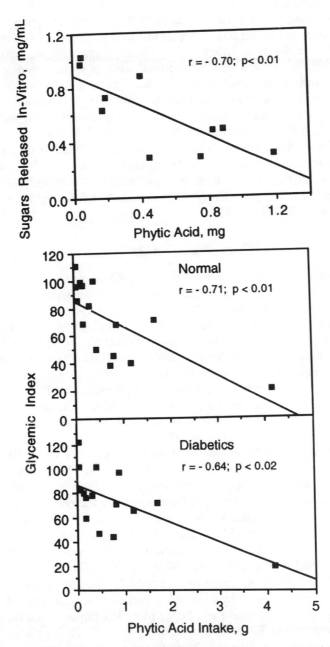

Figure 1. Relationship between phytic acid concentration or intake and glycemic index or in-vitro rate of starch digestion.

cium binding substances have been shown to prolong gastric emptying (Sognen, 1965a, 1965b).

The slowing down of rate of starch digestion and absorption by PA caused some malabsorption although not to a large extent (Thompson, 1988). While 43–75% difference in glycemic response was seen between the high GI, low antinutrient food such as white bread and low GI, high antinutrient food such as boiled legumes, there was only 2–17% difference in carbohydrate malabsorption. Dephytinization of navy bean flour caused an increase in glycemic response by 54%, while the decrease in carbohydrate malabsorbed was 7.8%. Likewise, the addition of 1% PA to dephytinized bean flour caused a reduction in glycemic response by 29%, while the increase in carbohydrate malabsorbed was only 5.3%. In any case, some starch malabsorption is thought to be desirable in the colon particularly when the intake of dietary fiber is low (Thornton et al., 1986, 1987).

Decrease Cancer Risk

Ileostomate studies suggest that up to 4 g PA may reach the colon per day (Thompson, 1989), an amount which may be sufficient to influence colonic health. A negative relationship was observed between the dietary PA concentration and the rate of cell proliferation in both the ascending and descending colon of rats (Nielsen et al., 1987). Since cancer initiation involves the alteration of DNA molecules by carcinogens and this oncogenic response is greater in highly than slowly proliferating cells, this suggests protective effect. The provision of 1% PA in the drinking water of rats one week before up to 12 months after the injection of the carcinogen azoxymethane, caused a 34.7% reduction in number of tumors and at least 63% lower tumor volume in the colon (Shamsuddin et al., 1988). When provided two weeks before up to 30 weeks after the last dose of carcinogen, the reduction was 52.2% in the tumor prevalence, 55.8% in the tumor frequency and 62.3% in the tumor size (Ullah and Shamsuddin, 1990). A similar effect was seen with 0.1% PA except for a smaller reduction in tumor prevalence (21%) and a greater reduction in tumor size (71%). These effects appear to be unrelated to the high pH (10.8–11.4) of the PA solutions since neutralization of the pH of the 1% PA solutions caused no significant effect on tumor prevalence and frequency. Although neutralized PA solution caused a reduction in the tumor volume by 65%, this effect may be more related to the slightly greater water intake and hence more PA intake in the rat group fed the neutralized PA solution. In rats given 2% PA in the drinking water two weeks after the last dose of carcinogen, the tumor incidence was 10% compared to 43% in the control (Shamsuddin et al., 1988). The

provision of 2% PA in the drinking water 5 months after the last carcinogen dose, caused a 27.2% fewer tumor/rat, 64.9% smaller tumor
volume and 43.3% less tumor load/unit area of the colon than the control (Shamsuddin and Ullah, 1989). The percentage mitotic rate was also
reduced by over 50%. The large incidence and number of colon tumors
in rats caused by high levels of iron (580 ppm) was also reduced by PA
(Nelson et al., 1989).

PA has also been suggested to reduce the risk for mammary carcinogenesis particularly when the level of dietary minerals such as calcium
and iron is high (Thompson and Zhang, 1991). A 29–30% reduction in
mammary epithelial cell proliferation (as labelling index) and in nuclear
aberration after carcinogen injection, was seen when 1.2% PA was provided in the diet of mice. The reduction in cell proliferation, nuclear aberration, and intraductal proliferation was even greater (25–53%) when
the 1.2% PA was added to the diet supplemented by high levels of iron
(535 ppm) and calcium (1.5%). A significant relationship was observed
between the cell proliferation in the mammary gland and in the colon,
suggesting that both tissues can be influenced similarly by PA (Thompson and Zhang, 1991).

In the above studies, PA was tested as sodium phytate. However,
pentapotassium dimagnesium phytate, a form commonly found in grains
(Reddy et al., 1982), also was found, at 12% concentration, to reduce
the tumor growth promoting effect of 1.4% MgO (Jariwalla et al.,
1988). Since in this case, tumor was induced by injection of the tu-
morigenic cell line capable of forming palpable fibrosarcomas after
subcutaneous injection, the result also suggests that tumorigenesis in
tissues other than the colon and mammary gland may also be influenced
by PA.

In a wide-spectrum organ carcinogenesis model, however, PA caused
both anticarcinogenic and carcinogenc effects (Hirose et al., 1991). In
this model, tumor was initiated in rats by injections of 2,2-dihydroxy-
di-n-propylnitrosamine followed by N-ethyl-N-hydroxy-ethylnitrose-
amine, and then 3,2-dimethyl-4-aminobiphenyl; the 2% PA was fed for
32 weeks starting 1 week after the last injection. No significant effect of
PA was seen on the lung, colon, esophagus, forestomach, small intestine, kidney, and thyroid gland of the rats. However, the incidence of
liver hyperplastic nodule and hepatocellular carcinoma as well as the
eosinophilic focus in the pancreas tended to be lower while the incidence and number per rat of urinary bladder papillomas were signicantly
increased in the PA-fed rats. PA is thought to have altered the urinary
pH and sodium concentration to levels which have been shown to enhance bladder carcinogenesis. It is unknown whether salts of PA other
than sodium would produce the same effect.

Several mechanisms have been suggested for the effect of PA on carcinogenesis (Graf and Eaton, 1985, 1990; Baten et al., 1989; Shamsuddin et al., 1989; Thompson, 1989; Ullah and Shamsuddin 1990; Thompson and Zhang, 1991).

(a) Since PA can increase the amount of starch that is malabsorbed in the small intestine (Thompson et al., 1987, 1989; Thompson, 1988, 1989), fermentation of this starch to short chain fatty acids in the colon may lower the pH to a protective level. We have observed, in rats, significant reductions in cecal pH with increasing levels of PA (Nielsen, 1987) and, in humans, significant relationships between PA intake, the amount of malabsorbed carbohydrate and the production of short chain fatty acids (Thompson et al., 1989).

(b) PA may influence carcinogenesis through its ability to inhibit iron-mediated production of hydroxy radical (.OH) and lipid peroxidation (Graf et al., 1984; Graf et al., 1987; Graf and Eaton,1990). Hydroxy radicals are genotoxic and thus are involved in the initiation of cancer (Halliwell and Gutteridge, 1984). They likewise are thought to be involved in tumor promotion (Ames, 1983). PA may exert its antioxidative function in three ways (Graf and Eaton, 1990): (i) by occluding all reactive coordination position, thereby making the iron catalytically inert; (ii) by acting as a potent ferroxidase and accelerating the oxidation of Fe^{2+} to Fe^{3+}; this will block the redox cyling of the iron and its catalytic activity; and (iii) since some iron reactions such as the scission of DNA may require juxtaposition of the reactive iron with the substrate, by preventing the binding of iron to the host molecule. The chelating and antioxidative functions of PA have been demonstrated in-vitro (Graf et al., 1984, 1987; Shamsuddin et al., 1988; Graf and Eaton, 1990). The augmented cell proliferation (Thompson and Zhang, 1991), tumor yield and incidence (Siegers et al., 1988; Nelson et al., 1989) caused by high levels of iron (535–580 ppm) and the reversal of this effect by the addition of PA (0.25–1.2%), are indications, in vivo, that PA may be acting as an iron chelating agent and antioxidant.

(c) The ability of PA to reduce the bioavailability of minerals is well-documented (Spivey-Fox and Tao, 1989; Torre et al., 1991). Chelation by PA of minerals that are involved in DNA synthesis such as Zn can reduce cell proliferation (Prasad and Oberleas, 1974; Nielsen et al., 1987). Zn deficient rats have lower cell proliferation in the small intestine (Southon et al, 1985) and the reduced cell proliferation in the colonic epithelium caused by PA has been reversed by zinc supplementation (Nielsen et al, 1987; Thompson and Nielsen, 1988).

(d) PA may cause reductions in bacterial enzymes such as B-glucuronidase and mucinase, which have been associated with increased carcinogenesis (Reddy and Wynder, 1973; Reddy et al., 1974, 1977;

Goldin and Gorbach, 1976; Goldin et al., 1980). We have observed some reduction in the activities of these enzymes in the presence of increasing levels of PA, although the mechanism for this remains to be elucidated (Nielsen, 1987; Thompson and Nielsen, 1988).

(e) Calcium has been hypothesized to be cancer protective, based on epidemiological data, its ability to form insoluble soaps with bile and free fatty acids, to induce cell differentiation, and to reduce cell proliferation and colon tumor incidence (Durham, 1982; Appleton et al., 1987; Pence and Buddingh, 1988; Sorenson et al., 1988; Wargovich et al., 1988, 1990; Reshef et al., 1990), although the contrary has also been suggested particularly when the level of calcium is > 1.0% (McSherry et al., 1989; Kaup et al., 1989; Behling et al., 1990; Bull et al., 1987; Gregoire et al., 1989; Thompson and Zhang, 1991). If calcium is protective, then the binding of PA with Ca may cause adverse effect as the Ca will no longer be able to bind to the bile acids or free fatty acids. On the other hand, if excessive calcium has adverse effect, then the binding of PA with calcium may produce a beneficial effect.

(f) In mice, PA enhanced the natural killer (NK) cell activity which was depressed by a colon carcinogen (Baten et al., 1989). The enhancement correlated negatively with tumor incidence. The in-vitro treatment of spleen cells and NK-enriched fraction with PA also enhanced the NK cytoxicity. Thus the enhancement of NK activity may be another mechanism whereby PA may have antitumor effects. How PA increases the NK activity, however, is not clear. It has been hypothesized (Baten et al., 1989) that it may involve the formation of inositol triphosphate, a product of PA hydrolysis, since inositol triphosphate appears to be generated in activated NK cells (Seaman et al., 1987). Since physical contact between the NK cells and the target cells, e.g., tumor cells, is necessary for cytoxicity, the inositol triphosphate could influence the membrane phosphatidyl inositol proteins which may be important in attachment and fusion with the target cells (Baten et al., 1989).

(g) Inositol, which alone has been shown to stimulate the growth of malignant human cells in tissue culture (Eagle et al., 1957), has been shown in mice to potentiate the antineoplastic effects of PA (Shamsuddin et al., 1989). Hence it has been hypothesized (Shamsuddin et al., 1989) that the free phosphate formed from the breakdown of PA to lower phosphorylated forms in the gut may react with the inositol to produce excess inositol triphosphate. As inositol triphosphate is a second messenger in cellular signal transduction (Berridge and Irvine, 1984; Osborne et al., 1988), its excessive amount may cause a negative feedback inhibition and decreased cell proliferation. However, as yet, there is no concrete evidence that this mechanism does take place.

Lower Serum Lipids

The high intake of legumes has been linked to lower blood lipid levels in man (Jenkins et al., 1983; Sharma, 1986; Erdman and Fordyce, 1989). Several components may be responsible for this effect, but PA may be one of them. In 1977, Klevay et al. demonstrated that PA in the diet of rats can lower the plasma blood lipid levels. Since then, others have demonstrated similar effects (Sharma, 1980, 1984; Jariwalla et al, 1991). In hypercholesterolemic rats, both serum cholesterol and triglycerides were significantly reduced by the addition of 0.2% PA (Table 1) (Sharma,1980), an amount equivalent to that present in the bengal gram diet which also produced a hypolipidemic effect. In normocholesterolemic rats, significant reductions were also observed (Jariwalla et al., 1991); however, the PA level used in this case was high (9%) and it is unknown whether similar effects can be seen at lower levels of intake. Furthermore, PA as a hypolipidemic agent may be effective only when added in the purified form or when present in certain food systems such as the legumes. Wheat bran, a PA-rich food, does not have a hypolipidemic effect. The effect of PA on blood lipid levels is thought to be related to the ability of PA to bind to zinc and thus lower the plasma zinc to copper ratio; lower ratios have been suggested to predispose humans to cardiovascular disease (Klevay et al., 1977). In addition, the effect may be related to the ability of PA to lower the plasma glucose and insulin concentrations which, in turn, may lead to reduced stimulus for hepatic lipid synthesis (Thompson, 1988; Wolever, 1990).

Increase Fecal Bulk

The fecal bulking effect of dietary fiber is well established. On the other hand, little work has been done to demonstrate the effect of PA on stool weight. The addition of 1–2% PA to a basal diet containing 5% cellulose caused significant increases in fecal weight (Table 2). Like

Table 1. Effect of phytic acid on serum cholesterol and triglyceride

Diet group[1]	Phytic acid level	Serum cholesterol	Serum triglyceride	Reference
Basal + Chol + CA	0	564 ± 16.7	182 ± 13.7	Sharma
Basal + Chol + CA + PA	0.2%	477 ± 23.1*	128 ± 10.7*	1980
Basal + Chol	0	126 ± 10	235 ± 53	Jariwalla
Basal + Chol + PA	9.0%	86 ± 6*	85 ± 22*	*et al.* 1991

[1] Chol = cholesterol; CA = cholic acid; PA = phytic acid.
* Significantly different from the control.

fiber, malabsorbed starch gets fermented by the bacteria in the colon and contributes to the production of short chain fatty acids, gas and bacterial cells. Thus since PA can cause some starch malabsorption, the increased bacterial mass and hence fecal weight may not be unexpected. The increase in fecal bulk due to PA, however, is small compared to that caused by fiber from dephytinized wheat bran (Table 2).

Conclusion

Phytic acid and other antinutrients have physiological effects which are similar to those seen with high fiber diets. Thus it is likely that they are responsible in part for some of the health benefits of high fiber foods. The same mechanism that is responsible for the antinutritive effects of PA, i.e., mineral, protein and starch binding, appears to be also responsible for its health beneficial effects.

Whether PA has adverse or health effects undoubtedly depends on its level of intake, the conditions they are taken, and the type of individuals involved. Thus the decision to remove PA or other antinutrients in foods should take into consideration the target population for its use. In infants and young children where the nutrient requirement is high and the risk for cancer and cardiovascular disease is low, the tip of the balance should be towards increased nutrient availability and very low PA concentration. On the other hand, in mature individuals with high caloric and nutrient intakes and predisposition to chronic diseases, a certain level of PA may be tolerated. Dose-response studies to determine the level that will best benefit the individual need to be conducted in the future. In addition, the "antinutrient" label connotes only adverse effect and probably should be reevaluated considering the potential health benefits.

Table 2. Effects of phytic acid on fecal weight of rats

Diet	Phytic acid, %	Fecal weight, g/day
Basal	0	1.19 ± 0.12 a
Basal + PA	0.6	1.19 ± 0.10 a
Basal + 1.2 PA	1.2	1.48 ± 0.14 b
Basal + 2.0 PA	2.0	1.47 ± 0.15 b
Basal	0	2.49 ± 0.09 a
Basal + DWB	0.1	7.04 ± 0.31 b
Basal + DWB + PA	1.2	7.79 ± 0.35 b

* Means with different letters are significantly different.
Adapted from Nielsen, 1987 and Shih, 1991.

Acknowledgment

The work of the author was financially supported by Natural Sciences and Engineering Research Council and Health and Welfare Canada.

References

Adlercreutz, H., 1990, Western diet and Western diseases: some hormonal and bio-chemical mechanisms and associations, Acad. J. Clin. Lab. Invest., 50 (Suppl. 201):3.

Ames, B. N., 1983, Dietary carcinogens and anticarcinogens, *Science* 221:1256.

Appleton, G. V. N., Davies, P. W., Bristol, J. B., and Williamson, R. C. N. 1987, Inhibition of intestinal carcinogenesis by dietary supplementation with calcium, *Br. J. Surg.* 74:523.

Baten, A., Ullah, A., Tomazic, V. J., and Shamsuddin, A. M., 1989, Inositol phosphate induced enhancement of natural killer cell activity correlates with tumor suppression, *Carcinogenesis* 10:1595.

Bjorck, I. M., and Nyman, M. E., 1987, In-vitro effects of PA and polyphenols on starch digestibility and fiber digestion, *J. Food Sci.* 52:1588.

Bull, A., Bird, R. P., Bruce W. R., Nigro N., and Medline, A., 1987, Effect of calcium on azoxymethane induced tumors in rats, *Gastroenterology* 92:1332.

Durham, A. C. H., and Walton, J. M., 1982, Calcium ions and the control of proliferation in normal and cancer cells, *Biochem Soc.* 10:15.

Eagle, H., Oyama, V. I., Levy, M., and Freeman, A., 1957, Myoinositol as an essential growth factor for normal and malignant human cells in tissue culture, *J. Biol. Chem.* 266: 191.

Erdman, J. W., and Fordyce, E. J., 1989, Soy products and the human diet, *Am. J. Clin. Nutr.* 49: 725- 37.

Goldin, B. R., and Gorbach, S. L., 1976, The relationship between diet and rat fecal bacterial enzymes implicated in colon cancer, *J. Natl. Cancer Inst.* 57:371.

Goldin, B. R., Swenson, L., Dwyer, J., Sexton, M., and Gorbach, S. L., 1980, Effect of diet and Lactobacillus acidophilous supplements on human fecal bacterial enzymes, *J. Natl. Cancer Inst.* 64: 255.

Graf, E., and Eaton, J.W., 1990, Antioxidant functions of phytic acid. *Free Rad. Biol. Med.* 8:61.

Graf, E., and Eaton, J.W., 1985, Dietary suppression of colonic cancer: fiber or pytate? *Cancer* 36:717.

Graf, E., Mahoney, J. R., Bryant, R. G., and Eaton, J. W., 1984, Iron catalyzed hydroxyl radical formation. Stringent requirements for free iron coordination site, *J. Biol.Chem.* 259:3620.

Graf, E., Empson, K., and Eaton, J. W., 1987, Phytic acid. A natural antioxidant, *J. Biol. Chem.* 262:11647.

Gregoire, R. C., Stern H. S., Yeung, K. S., Stadler, J., Langley, S., Furrer, R., and Bruce, W. R., 1989, Effect of calcium supplementation on mucosal cell proliferation in high risk patients for colon cancer, *Gut* 30:376.

Halliwell, B., and Gutteridge, J. M. S., 1984, Oxygen toxicity, oxygen radicals, transition metals and disease, *Biochem. J.* 219:1.

Hirose, M., Ozaki, K., Takaba, K., Fukushima, S., Shirai, T., and Ito, N., 1991, Modifying effects of the naturally occuring antioxidants gamma oryzanol, phytic acid, tannic acid and n-tritriacontane-16, 18-dione in a rat wide-spectrum organ carcinogenesis model, *Carcinogenesis* 12:1917.

Jariwalla, R. J., Sabin, R., Lawson, S., Bloch, D. A, Prender, M., Andrews, V. and Herman, Z. S., 1988, Effects of dietary phytic acid (phytate) on the incidence and growth rate of tumors promoted in Fisher rats by magnesium supplement. *Nutr. Res.* 8:813.

Jariwalla, R. J., Sabin, R., Lawson, S., and Herman, Z. S., 1990, Lowering of serum cholesterol and triglycerides and modulation of divalent cation by dietary phytate, *J. Applied Nutr.* 42:18.

Jenkins, D. J. A., Wolever, T. M. S., Jenkins, A. L., Thompson, L. U., Rao, A. V., and Francis, T., 1986, The glycemic index. Blood glucose response to foods, in: "Basic and Chemical Aspects of Dietary Fiber," G. V. Vahouny and D. Kritchevsky, ed., Alan R. Liss, Inc. , New York.

Jenkins, D. J. A., Wolever, T. M. S., Taylor, R. H., Barker, H. M., Fielden, H.,1980, Exceptionally low blood glucose response to dried beans: comparison with other carbohydrate foods, *Br. Med. J.* 2:578.

Jenkins, D. J. A., Wong, G. S., Patten, R. P., Bird, J., Hall, M., Buckley, G., McGuire, V., Reichert, R., and Little, J. A., 1983, Leguminous seeds in the dietary management of hyperlipidemia, *Am. J. Clin . Nutr.* 38:567.

Klevay, L. M., 1977, Hypocholesterolemia due to sodium phytate, *Nutr. Rep. Int.* 15:587.

Messina, M., and Barnes, S., 1991, The role of soy products in reducing risk of cancer. *J. Nat. Cancer Inst.* 83:541.

Nelson, R. L., Yoo, S. J., Tanure, J. C., Andrianopoulos, G., and Misumi, A., 1989, The effect of iron on experimental colorectal carcinogenesis, *AntiCancer Res.* 9:1477.

Nielsen, B. K.,1987, Effect of phytic acid on colonic bacterial enzymes and epithelial cell proliferation, M. Sc. Thesis, Univ. of Toronto, Toronto.

Nielsen, B. K., Thompson, L. U. and Bird, R. P., 1987, Effect of phytic acid on colonic epithelial cell proliferation. *Cancer Lett.* 37:317.

Oakenful, D., and Sidhu, G. S., 1990, Could saponins be a useful treatment for hypercholesterolemia? *Eur. J. of Clin. Nutr.* 44:79.

Pence, B. C., and Buddingh, F., 1988, Inhibition of dietary fat promoted colon carcinogenesis in rats by supplemental calcium or vitamin D3, *Carcinogenesis* 91:187.

Prasad, A., and Oberleas, D., 1974, Thymidine kinase activity and incorporation of thymidine into DNA in zinc deficient tissue, *J. Lab. Clin. Med.* 83:634.

Rea, R., Thompson, L. U. and Jenkins, D. J. A., 1985, Lectins in foods and their relation to starch digestibility, *Nutr. Res.*, 5:919.

Reddy, N. R., Sathe, S. K., and Salunkhe, D. K., 1982, Phytates in legumes and cereals, *Adv. Food Res.* 28:1.

Reddy, B. S., and Wynder, E. L., 1973, Large bowel carcinogenesis: fecal constituents of populations with diverse incidence rates of colon cancer, *J. Natl.Cancer Inst.* 50:1437.

Reddy, B. S., Weisberger, J. H., and Wynder, E. L., 1974, Fecal bacterial beta glucuronidase: control by diet, *Science* 183:416.

Reddy B. S. Mangat, S., Weisberger, J., and Wynder, E. 1977, Effect of high-risk diets for colon carcinogenesis on intestinal mucosa and bacterial beta glucuronidase activity in F344 rats, *Cancer Res.* 37:3533.

Reshef, R., Rozen P., Fireman, Z., Fine, W., Barzilai, M., Shasha, S. M., and Shkolnik, T., 1990, Effect of calcium enriched diet on the colonic epithelium hyperproliferation induced by N- methyl N'nitrosoguanidine in rats in a low calcium and fat diet, *Cancer Res.* 50:1764.

Seaman, W. E., Erickson, E., Dobrwo, R., and Imeoden, J. B., 1987, Inositol triphosphate is generated by rat natural killer cell tumor in response to target cells or to cross-linked monoclonal antibody OX-34: possible signalling role for the OX-34 determinant during activation by target cells, *Proc. Natl. Acad. Sci. U.S.A.* 84:4239.

Setchell, K. D. R., and Adlercreutz, H., 1988, Mammalian lignans and phytoestrogens. Recent studies on the formation, metabolism and biological role in health and disease, in: "Role of the Gut Flora in Toxicity and Cancer," I. R. Rowland, ed., Academic Press, London.

Shamsuddin, A. M., Elsayed, A. M., and Ullah, A., 1988, Suppression of large intestinal cancer in F-344 rats by inositol hexaphosphate, *Carcinogenesis* 9:577.

Shamsuddin, A. M., and Ullah, A., 1989, Inositol hexaphosphate inhibits large intestinal cancer in F-344 rats 5 months following induction by azoxymethane. *Carcinogenesis* 10:625.

Shamsuddin, A. M., Ullah, A., and Chakvarthy, A., 1989, Inositol and inositol hexaphosphate suppress cell proliferation and tumor formation in CD-1 mice, *Carcinogenesis* 10:1461.

Sharma, R. D., 1980, Effect of hydroxy acids on hypocholesterolemia in rats, *Atherosclerosis* 37:463.

Sharma, R. D., 1984, Hypocholesterolemic effect of hydroxy acid components of Bengal gram. *Nutr. Rep. Int.* 29:1315-1322.

Sharma, R. D., 1986, Phytate and the epidemiology of heart disease, renal calculi and colon cancer, in: "Phytic Acid: Chemistry and Applications," E. Graf, ed., Pilatus Press, MN.

Shih, J., 1991, Phytic Acid and Wheat Bran Fiber: Influence on Colonic Fermentation, Mineral Availability and Risk for Colon Carcinogenesis in Carcinogen-Treated Rats, M. Sc. Thesis, Univ. of Toronto, Toronto.

Siegers, C. P., Buman, D., Baretton, G., and Younes, M., 1988, Dietary iron enhances tumor rate in dimethylhydrazine-induced colon carcinogenesis in mice, *Cancer Lett.* 41:251.

Sognen, E., 1965a, Apparent depression in the absorption of strychnine, alcohol, sulpanilamide after oral adminisration of sodium fluoride, sodium oxalate, tetracemin and sodium phytate, *Acta Pharmacol et Toxicol.* 22:8.

Sognen, E., 1965b, Effects of calcium binding substances on gastric emptying as well as intestinal transit and absorption in intact rats. *Acta Pharmacol et Toxicol.* 22:31.

Sorenson, A. W., Slattery, M. L., and Ford, M. H., 1988, Calcium and colon cancer. A review, *Nutr. Cancer* 11:135.

Southon, S., Livesey, G., Gee, J., and Johnson, I., 1985, Intestinal cellular proliferation and protein synthesis in zinc-deficient rats, *Br. J. Nutr.* 53: 595.

Spivey-Fox, M. R., and Tao, S.-H., 1989, Antinutritive effects of phytate and other phosphorylated derivatives, *Nutr. Toxicol.* 3:59.

Thompson L. U., 1988, Antinutrients and blood glucose, *Food Technol.* 42:123.

Thompson, L. U., 1989, Nutritional and physiological effects of phytic acid, in: "Food Proteins," J. E. Kinsella and W. G. Soucie, eds., AOCS, Champaign, IL.

Thompson, L. U., 1992, Benefits and problems associated with antinutrients in foods, *Food Res. Internat.* (in press)

Thompson, L. U., Button, C. L. and Jenkins, D. J. A., 1987, Phytic acid and calcium effect on starch digestibility and glucose response to navy bean flour, *Am. J. Clin. Nutr.* 38:481.

Thompson, L. U., McBurney, M., and Jenkins, D. J. A., 1989, Effect of phytic acid on the absorption and colonic fermentation of carbohydrates, *FASEB J.* 3:A759.

Thompson, L. U., and Nielsen, B. K. 1988, Effect of phytic acid in the colon, *FASEB J.* 2:A1084

Thompson, L. U., Yoon, J. H., Jenkins, D. J. A., Wolever, T. M. S., and Jenkins, A. L., 1984, Relationship between polphenol intake and blood glucose response of normal and diabetic individuals, *Am. J. Clin. Nutr.* 39:745.

Thompson, L. U., and Zhang, L., 1991, Phytic acid and minerals: effect on early markers of risk for mammary and colon carcinogenesis. *Carcinogenesis* 12:2041.

Thornton, J. R., Dryden, A., Kelleher, J., and Losowsky, M. S., 1986, Does super-efficient starch absorption promote diverticular disease? *Brit. Med. J.* 292:1708.

Thornton, J. R., Dryden, A., Kelleher, J. and Losowsky M. S., 1987, Super-efficient starch absorption: A risk factor for colonic neoplasia?, *Dig. Dis. Sci.* 32: 1088.

Torre, M., Rodriguez, A. R. , and Saura-Calixto, F., 1991, Effects of dietary fiber and phytic acid on mineral availability, *Crit. Rev. Food Sci.* Nutr. 1:1.

Troll, W., and Kennedy, A. R., 1989, Workshop report for the Division of Cancer Etiology, National Cancer Institute, National Institute of Health. Protein inhibitors as cancer chemipreventive agents, *Cancer Res.* 49:499.

Ullah, A., and Shamsuddin, A. M., 1990, Dose dependent inhibition of large intestinal cancer by inositol hexaphosphate in F344 rats. *Carcinogenesis* 11:2219.

Wargovich, M. J., 1988, Calcium and colon cancer, *J. Am Coll. Nutr.* 7:295.

Wargovich, M J., Allnutt, D., Palmer, C., Anaya, P., and Stephens, L. C., 1990, Inhibition of the promotional phase of azoxymethane induced colon carcinogenesis in the F344 rat by calcium lactate: effect of simulating two human nutrient density levels, *Cancer Lett.* 53:17.

Wolever, T. M. S.,1990, The glycemic index. *World Rev. Nutr. Diet.* 62:120.

Yoon, J. H., Thompson, L. U., and Jenkins, D. J. A., 1983, The effect of phytic acid on in vitro rate of starch digestibility and blood glucose response, *Am. J. Clin. Nutr.* 38:835.

V. Fiber Effects/In Vivo & In Vitro Laboratory Models

Comparative Aspects of Animal Models

P. J. Van Soest

Cornell University
324 Morrison Hall
Ithaca, NY 14853

Introduction

Many problems related to human nutrition and physiology require animal models for their study, because of the difficulties and expense of intrusive studies on humans. The adequacy of an animal species as a model is relevant to the kind of question being asked and the comparative physiologies of the respective species. The case of dietary fiber involves the digestive tract, particularly the lower tract and its microbial fermentation.

Animal species that eat plants have evolved various strategies for achieving their dietary energy with concomitant adaptations of their mouths, teeth (Janis and Ehrhardt, 1988; Janis and Fortelius, 1988) and gastrointestinal anatomies for the respective purpose (Moir, 1968; Stevens, 1988). The various strategies are evolutionary and show a considerable degree of parallelism among evolutionary lines. Many herbivores have evolved feeding and digestive strategies that ensure them a dietary niche, minimizing competition from other herbivorous species. Hence there is much complementary diversity. However, all mammalian species that derive energy from fibrous carbohydrates do so through the symbiotic association with gut microorganisms, that in turn convey benefits beyond the supply of energy. These benefits include the maintenance of rumen, cecal or colonic mucosa by the volatile acid (VFA) products of fermentation (Stevens, 1988). Many animal species derive balancing of amino acids and B vitamins, often deficient in herbivorous diets (Banta et al., 1975). The means by which these nutrients are obtained are either pregastric fermentation or coprophagy.

Gastrointestinal Anatomies and Feeding Behavior

Mammalian species can be classified into several groups based on the characteristics of their respective digestive tracts (Table 1). This classification may be compared with that based on dietary specializations. Nonruminants comprise a variety of adaptations relative to herbivore specializations and gut architecture (Moir, 1968). The grazing ruminants represent the most developed and specialized class in view of their ability to use fiber and other carbohydrates unavailable to animal digestion.

These specializations include animals without much gut fermentation, but with diverse feeding behaviors, such as carnivores including cats, tigers and lions, but also some omnivorous birds like chickens and turkeys, and the entirely herbivorous grazing pandas (Holmgren, 1972; Schaller et al., 1985). Cats and dogs are known to eat some grass. Also, a balance study utilizing cereal bran fed to dogs indicated about 20% digestibility of cereal fiber (Visek and Robinson, 1973). It is apparent

Table 1. Classification of some mammals based on gastrointestinal anatomy

Class	Species	Dietary habit
Colonic digesters		
Sacculated	Horse, zebra	Grazer
	new world monkeys	Folivore
	pig, man and	Omnivores
	other primates	
Unsacculated	Panda	Herbivore, grazer
	Dog	Carnivore
	Cat	Carnivore
Pregastric fermentors		
Ruminants	Cattle, sheep,	Grazing herbivores
	deer, antelope	Selective herbivores
	camel	
Nonruminants	Colobine monkey	Selective herbivore
	Langur monkey	Selective herbivore
	Hamster, Vole	Selective herbivores
	Kangaroo,	Grazing and
	Hippopotamus	selective herbivores
	Hoatzin (bird)	Folivore
Cecal fermentors	Capybara	Grazer
	Rabbit (Lemming)	Selective herbivore
	Rat, mouse	Omnivore

that some fermentation can occur, provided the substrates are rapidly degradable. Animals with significant fermentation in the colon without much cecal capacity include man, other primates, and canids.

Colonic fermentors with a cecum include large nonruminant herbivores, the perissodactyls (horse, rhinoceros) and other large herbivores (elephant, etc.), in all of which fiber digestion is more important in the sacculated large bowel as compared with the cecum. In contrast, the rodents and lagomorphs are special in that herbivorous members generally exhibit large ceca and unsacculated colons.

The comparative importance of fermentation as a means of digestion is demonstrated by the proportion of digesta residing in fermentive compartments relative to the whole digestive tract (Table 2). Ruminants are not the only animals with a large proportion of the digestive tract devoted to fermentation. The capybara, a large South American rodent, has the digestive capacity of a sheep and is a true grazer (Parra, 1978). The pig, rabbit and rat have a lesser capacity. The latter two are actually inferior to the pig in fiber digestive capacity because of their small size. Man and dog have substantially smaller proportions of their tracts adapted to microbial fermentation. This feature is generally characteristic of omnivores and carnivores.

Table 2. Fermentive capacity expressed as percentage of the total digestive tract for the respective animal (Parra 1978)

Species	Body wt. kg	Reticulo-rumen	Cecum	Colon and rectum	Total fermentive
Cattle	500	64	5	5–8	75
Sheep	50	71	8	4	83
Horse	400	...	15	54	69
Pig	100	...	15	33	48
Capybara	40	...	71	9	80
Guinea pig	0.5	...	46	20	66
Rabbit	3	...	43	8	51
Rat	0.2	...	32	29	61
Man	70	...	...	17	17
Cat	3	...	...	16	16
Dog	10	...	1	13	14
Gorilla	51[a]	...	...	56	56
Chimpanzee	33	...	...	60	60
Orangutang	11[a]	...	...	52	52
Siamang	8	...	...	54	54
Piliated gibbon	5.4	...	...	61	61
White handed gibbon	5.0	...	...	37	37

[a] Small specimen.

Fibrous carbohydrates must be digested symbiotically by gut micro-organisms in all higher animals, as they have not evolved any cellulases, hemicellulases or pectinases. If the fermentive chamber is postgastric, the animal host has first chance at the available carbohydrates and protein in the food, but loses the chance to capture microbially synthesized proteins and vitamins, important if the dietary sources are poor in these nutrients.

The simplest sequence is that exemplified by man, dog and carnivores, in which a cecum as a separate compartment is essentially lacking. Most herbivorous animals, including man, have sacculated colons. The colons of dogs, cats and pandas are unsacculated. Sacculation probably helps retain fiber and represents an herbivorous evolutionary ancestry (Stevens, 1988). Nonruminants like the pig and horse possess a sizeable cecum (though smaller than the colon), in contrast to rodents and lagomorphs, where the cecum is proportionally larger than the colon.

The main site of fermentation in many rodents lies in the cecum, which is dominant over the colon. Many of these animals practice coprophagy. Within this group there are even more specialized species such as rabbits and lemmings, where the cecum selectively admits only fine matter, coarse fiber being excluded and excreted in day feces. Night feces are reingested allowing utilization of microbial protein and vitamins derived from the most fermentable carbohydrates. Because the coarse fiber is rejected, fiber utilization is very low in these animals. These animals probably exploit vegetative tissues containing pectin and other rapidly fermentable unlignified carbohydrates. Coprophagy can be viewed as an adaptation of small herbivores, where the limiting effect of rate of passage, due to high energy demand relative to size of gastrointestinal tract, is a special problem. This strategy allows these small herbivores to consume fiber without penalty of energy intake restriction, although many potentially fermentable cellulosic carbohydrates are lost in the feces.

There are also animals that possess pregastric fermentation without rumination. These comprise a wide spectrum of mammals, including kangaroos (Hume, 1982), hamsters (Banta et al., 1975; Ehle and Warner, 1978), voles (Keys and Van Soest, 1970), colobine (Stevens, 1988) and langur monkeys (Bauchop and Martucci, 1968), hippopotamus (Moir, 1968) and most recently the hoatzin, a South American bird (Grajal et al., 1989). Probably other species remain to be discovered and described. The definition of dietary fiber for these animals would follow that of the ruminant rather than the nonruminant, because dietary fiber would ferment along with other available carbohydrates in the pregastric fermentation. It is speculated that the large herbivorous dinosaurs had a pregastric fermentation in the crop (Farlow, 1987). Apparently the dinosaurs were warm blooded and much closer to contemporary birds than has been generally realized (Bakker, 1986). The problem of evolution of gut fermentation of mammals in relation to feeding strategies has been discussed by Janis (1976).

Thus, the classification of mammals into ruminants and nonruminants is an oversimplification. Ruminant-like capacities (e.g., pregastric fermentation) exist in combination with grazing and selector types of feeding and in true ruminant and nonruminant groups. Such specializations occur even in the primates. Furthermore, there are small African ruminants that dietarily compete with higher primates (Hoffman, 1988).

Gut Fermentation in Nonruminants

Fermentation in the gut of nonruminants parallels the range occurring in ruminants. There are pregastric nonruminant fermentors as well as hindgut fermentors. As expected from the anatomies, the hindgut fermentors are subdivided into colonic and cecal fermentors. The fermentations in all of these animals have many similarities to that of the rumen in respect to microbial species and microbial products.

The volatile acid products (VFA) of gut fermentation are important sources of dietary energy for most herbivores. The VFA are normally absorbed directly across the colon wall to the blood in the form of free acids, thus relieving the acidity and maintaining the pH of the colon above 6, which is required by the normal fiber-digesting bacteria. The VFA are absorbed across the gut wall via the same mechanisms as in the rumen. This process has also been shown to occur in humans, pigs, horses and dogs (McNeil et al., 1978; Argenzio et al., 1974; Argenzio and Southworth, 1974; Stevens, 1988). Some of these acids are metabolized by the colonic wall as a maintenance source of energy. Butyrate is the most extensively metabolized followed by propionate. In all mammals, any propionate and butyrate passing to the blood is captured and metabolized by the liver. Acetate on the other hand is largely metabolized by peripheral tissues. Volatile acid concentrations vary in human feces (Ehle et al., 1982) and probably reflect the balance between rate of production and absorption as they have been shown in the rumen of ruminants (Leng, 1970). Estimates of the energy contribution of VFA in nonruminant species indicate the amounts can be a significant part of their dietary energy (Van Soest, 1982). Estimates are dependent upon the diet, and are related to the fermentation capacities. For grazing ruminants and some grazing nonruminants the contribution is about 70% of calories. Values for monogastrics are less and may be about 30% for the pig (Parra, 1978).

One way to evaluate net fermentation is to measure the microbial mass contributing to the metabolic fecal nitrogen increment in response to added dietary fiber. Such a response can be compared to microbial yields from fermented carbohydrate (Mason, 1984; Van Soest, 1982; Wolin, 1975). The expected bowel loss of microbial cell mass is about equal to that expected from fermentation balance if dietary sources are the only substrate. Some utilization could be argued on the basis that endogenous mucopolysaccharides contribute significantly to the fermentation (Vercellotti et al., 1977; Salyers et al., 1977) and that observed microbial yields in feces are higher than expected from fermentation balance (Van Soest, 1981).

The microbial fermentation is an important facet of nitrogen balance in all animals possessing a gut fermentation, ruminants and nonruminants alike. The feeding of fermentable fibrous carbohydrate raises the ammonia requirement of the microorganisms to support their cellular growth. This is supplied to a major degree by urea secreted across the gut wall, whether colon, cecum or rumen. This increases fecal loss of microbial matter at the expense of urinary urea, and is the reason that amino acid balances are of little meaning. The overall effect of fermentation on nitrogen balance is greatest in those species with capacity for larger fermentation, and is less important in species of lower capacity and with faster transits. This is relevant to the choice of animal model for humans and places emphasis on the capacity to digest fibrous carbohydrates.

Comparative Digestion

While nonruminant digestibilities of fibrous feeds are often lower than is the case with ruminants, there is considerably more variation in the capacity to utilize fibrous carbohydrates among animal species than is ordinarily realized. The factor responsible for this variation is retention time, which is in turn determined by intake and size of fermentation in the gut (Figure 1). Note that humans are about midway in the distribution. The question of retention time and digestive capacity is an important one for human nutrition, because it addresses the problems concerning which animal species are suitable models for dietary studies of the human situation and the implications of dietary fiber and disease, and also which animal species will convert feed and forage resources into human food most efficiently.

The data of Foose (1982) present digestibilities and retention times on grass and alfalfa diets for 36 species of ruminants and nonruminants. Additional data are provided by Hackenberger (1987) for elephants; Keys et al. (1970), voles; Uden and Van Soest (1982), for horses and rabbits; Ehle et al. (1982) for pigs; Dierenfeld et al. (1982) the large panda; and Milton and Demment (1988) chimpanzees. Other literature reporting digestibilities or feeding behavior, but lacking transit measurements, are various zoo animals (Hintz et al., 1976); horses (Hoffman et al., 1987); the lesser panda (Holmgren, 1972); the beaver (Hoover and Clarke, 1972). The results are particularly interesting in regard to use of cellulose from grass and legume, and also of hemicellulose (Figure 2).

These results indicate that the slower digesting cellulose from grass is limiting in all species, while the more easily digested hemicellulose is utilized in most species above the weight limit of about 90–100 kg. Retention time, while associated with body size in both ruminants and nonruminants, shows that ruminants of a smaller size achieve more fiber digestion than nonruminants of similar size. This is most apparent for the slower digesting grass cellulose (Figure 2C). This effect is less apparent in the digestibility of grass hemicellulose and in alfalfa cellulose

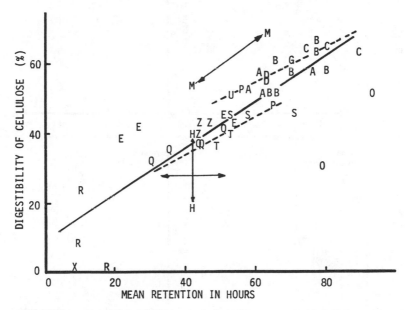

Figure 1. The relationship brtween cellulose digestion and mean retention in various species of herbivorous mammals fed grass-type fiber. Species shown ruminants (Antelope A, Grazing bovoids B, Camelids C, Deer D, Giraffe G, Sheep and goats S). The ranges of values for man (H) are shown in the figure by the vertical arrows or baboons (M), and are somewhat less than the figure for pigs (U), but more than that for rodents (R). Some large animals (Hippo O, Rhino P) may approach the capacity of ruminants, but Elephants (E), Equids (Q,Z) and Tapirs (T) are less efficients. Very small animals (Rodents and Lagomorphs R) have very low digestibilities. Panda (X) is lowest of all.

which are generally faster digesting (Figure 2AB). These carbohydrates seem to be more limiting to animals below 100 kg, arguing for a critical size cutoff for general use of structural carbohydrates (Demment and Van Soest 1985). Alfalfa hemicellulose is likely be an even more digestible fraction (Figure 2D). Its quality is such that ruminants and non-ruminants are not distinguished.

The apparent inferior ability of smaller and selector animals to digest cellulosic carbohydrates might be related to inability to retain or inability of cellulolytic microbes to adapt to their gut environments. Limits of retention at small size will require higher relative intake, though the strategy of consuming a lignified diet to a higher level in order to obtain

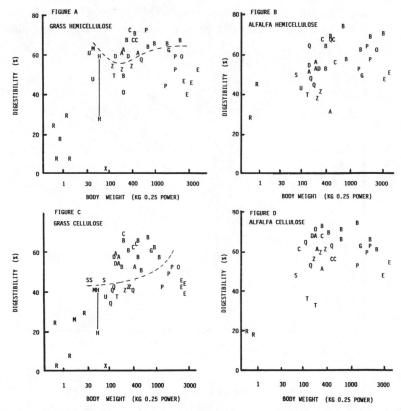

Figure 2. The relationship between digestion of hemicellulose and cellulose of alfalfa and grass-based diets and body weight for diverse species of ruminants and nonruminants. Data of Keys et al., 1969, Keys et al., 1970; Uden and Van Soest, 1982a; ehle et al., 1982 and Foose, 1982; Hackenberger, 1987; Milton and Demments, 1988. See Figure 1 for identity of species. Dashed lines in Figures A and C show separation between ruminants and nonruminants. This is not discernible in Figures B and D.

highly digestible cellular contents will preclude exhaustive cellulose digestion. A final hypothesis is that there is a level of total diet digestibility which limits animal function because of the requirement for digestible energy, and that this point occurs at higher digestibilities for small animals and most selective feeders as well.

Humans fall into this class of selective herbivory, and appear to utilize well the more easily fermentable carbohydrates. Slower digesting cellulosic fibers tend to be rejected, and are not a normal component of the ancestral diet. This factor needs to be taken into account when evaluating and choosing supplementary dietary fibers.

Cellulolytic capacity can be measured by placing animals on the same diet and conducting digestion balances. However, interpretation of results is difficult when species being compared are adapted to different food habits (Van Soest, 1982). Another way of studying the problem is to compare the in vitro (or cecal) digestion of standard substrates using inocula from the various animals.

Nonruminant digestibilities of cellulose and hemicellulose indicate varying capacities to digest these carbohydrates. Generally, the digestion of grasses is more sensitive to depression in digestibility than is the

Table 3. Comparative passage rates of liquid and particles in some animal species* (Uden 1978; Van Soest *et al.* 1978)

Species	Body wt. kg	Whole tract retention[a] Particles[c]	Liquid	Reten. in ferment. compart.[b] Particles	Liquid
		(h)			
Ruminants					
lg heifers	555	79	29	47	15
sm heifers	243	62	30	38	16
sheep	30	70	38	35	19
goats	29	52	39	28	19
Nonruminants					
horses	388	29	29	10	11
ponies	132	34	26	10	9
man	70	41	39	12	12
rabbit	3	9	193+	4	180+

[a] Mean retention according to Faichney (1975).
[b] First pool turnover (K_1) according to Grovum and Williams (1973). Compartment represents rumen in the case of ruminants and cecum and large bowel in nonruminants (Grovum and Williams, 1977).
[c] Particulate passage based on chromium mordant of the dietary fiber.
*Heifers, sheep, goats, horses, ponies and rabbits were fed on a standard timothy diet. Human subjects fed a standard diet including 20 g of dietary fiber from wheat bran.
+Due to coprophagy and recycling of indicator.

case with legumes such as alfalfa, and there is a tendency for smaller animals to show an inadequacy in handling cellulose. Somewhat higher digestibilities (as compared with the rat) occur with certain of the small rodents, for example, the hamster (Ehle and Warner, 1978) and the vole (Keys and Van Soest, 1970). This exceptional capability might be the result of the ability to select feed, or of the special adaptation of the abomasum for pregastric fermentation. Human digestion of wheat bran fibers are only slightly less than in ruminants. Most animals including humans digest the more rapidly fermentable vegetables to a high degree.

The relative passage of liquid and particles varies among animal species. In general, ruminants tend to have the slowest rates of particulate passage relative to that of liquid (Table 3). Nonruminants present varying situations. The rabbit passes particles selectively faster than liquid, while there is little separation of liquid and particles in man and other nonruminants. There is a trend toward longer retention in larger animals.

Transit also varies among animal species relative to the proportions of the digestive tract. For example, carnivores have typically short intestines and very reduced fermentive capacity. Length of tract is proportionally larger relative to volume in many herbivores. Thus, transits through the stomach, intestines, cecum, and colon can vary relative to the mean retention time. Detailed flow characteristics can be obtained by radio-opaque markers (Clemens and Stevens, 1980) or by slaughter and measurement of fill and marker in each segment of the digestive tract (Vidal et al., 1969).

Transit: Particles and Liquid

As in the rumen, other factors affect the ecology of the lower tract, such as particle size of fiber, which influences passage rate and microbial turnover. In contrast to the rumen, more rapid turnover is promoted by coarse fiber with a consequent increment in fecal nitrogen due to enhanced microbial yield. Fine particle size reduces bulk of ingesta, thereby slowing passage rate. Equal intakes of coarse and fine bran induce disparate fecal nitrogen excretion (Van Soest, 1981). Unlike the rumen, the lower tracts of the nonruminant and many other species have no filters, so that fine grinding of the diet increases density of the ingesta and retention, opposite to that of the ruminants. Sorting mechanisms are not important in the human and other species that have relatively equal passage of liquid and fiber in the lower tract.

Particulate passage of finely ground diets is affected differently in the digestive tracts of ruminants and nonruminants. Fine grinding promotes more rapid passage of fiber from the rumen, but slower passage in the lower tract of man (Van Soest, 1982; Van Dokkum et al., 1982). However in all animals including the human, the water content of feces from finely ground diets is reduced; this points out the failure of finely ground fiber to alleviate constipation (Heller et al., 1980). Fine grinding of insoluble fiber generally reduces the effectiveness of the fiber in all herbivores and may be the result of several common factors. Coarse fiber delays gastric emptying in most species (Cherbut and Ruckebusch, 1985). Coarse insoluble fiber may also stimulate gut motility (Stevens, 1988). Fine particles may also affect the ecology of the microbial fermentation, because celluloytic bacteria tend to digest plant cells from the inside out. Grinding tends to expose interior cellular space and increasing the possibility of predatory behavior among microorganisms. Generally microbial mass is reduced and VFA production increased.

The cecum has fermentive characteristics similar to the colon but differs in that ingesta must pass out of the blind sac by the route of entry. This provides the possibility of the cecum being a special environment with unique retention of selected feed fractions. The cecum tends to empty pulsatively every day or two, leading it to be more characteristic of a batch culture. Passage rate is difficult to calculate under these conditions, since the cecal emptying can prevent kinetic marker calculation and because the distribution of marker in fecal output tends to be biphasal (Van Soest et al., 1983).

Even more extreme are the cecotrophs (rabbit and lemming) that selectively retain fine ingesta in the cecum that is passed out at night to be reingested, the day feces being passed directly out and not recycled (Bjornhag, 1972, Uden et al., 1982). These animals, as exemplified by the rabbit, retain liquid for very long periods of time. Because of the selective reingestion it is not possible to calculate accurately the actual rate of turnover.

Primates and Ruminants

The mammalian order of primates is of interest in the discussion of ruminants because it contains parallel evolutionary developments in herbivory to the ungulates. The feeding strategies of primates range from insectivory, omnivory, frugivory to folivory. Setting aside the insectivores, omnivores like humans clearly have an herbivorous ancestry. Human social evolution has proceeded faster than that of the digestive tract and metabolism, and may have led to the dietary epidemiology of low fiber, high meat and fat diets in modern civilization.

Man's closest relatives, the pongid apes, have diverged in dietary habits. In primates the cecum is much reduced, but the colon is sacculated. The sacculation of the colon and a relatively smaller cecum may represent a special adaptation of the lower bowel to fermentations and, therefore, a history of evolutionary adaptation to some degree of fibrousness of the diet (Stevens, 1980). Nevertheless, there has been evolutionary diversification within the primates. Gorillas are exclusively vegetarian and lean toward folivory. Orangotangs are largely frugivorous, while chimps are more versatile, leaning toward frugivory but also catching an antelope now and then. Other groups like baboons (cercopithoid) are omnivorous and eat a wide variety of plant foods. Much of their natural diet is highly fibrous, male baboons eating a composition of 50% or more of NDF. However, there is a difference between sexes, females eating a more selected diet, as well as being smaller in size (Demment and Van Soest, 1985). Other groups, such as new world monkeys and colobines, are folivores. Colobines in Africa (Stevens, 1988) and langurs (Bauchop and Martucci, 1968) in India and SE Asia have rumen-like pregastric fermentation. Fermentation capacity may supply most of their energy in the form of VFA. Unfortunately no passage or digestion balances are available.

Thus it seems that small ruminants and some of the more advanced primates have converged in their feeding strategies. Small antelope also have diversified as concentrate selectors into frugivory and folivory (Figure 3), but they are at present less well described.

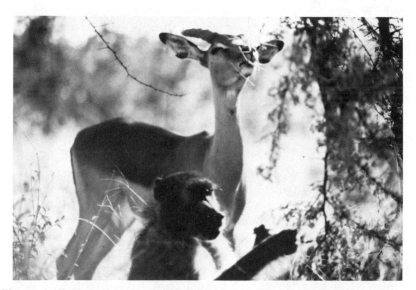

Figure 3. Baboon and gerenuk feeding off the same Acacia tree in Kruger National Park, South Africa. Photo courtesy of BDH van Niekerk and D. E. Hogue. This is an example of convergent evolution in feeding behavior.

The Relevance of Ruminants

Although ruminants have disparate anatomies, the understanding of gut fermentation in humans and other nonruminant animals owes a great deal to studies on ruminants that were the pioneering efforts in understanding the gut microorganisms and their relationship to the host. The large bowel can be regarded as a supplementary rumen (Argenzio and Stevens, 1984). Discoveries that have been later found to be important in humans include stimulation of the gut wall by VFA—found by Warner and Flatt (1965) in preruminant calves; the role of propionate in bovine ketosis (analogous in some respects to diabetes), and particle size of fiber and its effectiveness. Gut microbiologists are indebted to Hungate (1966) and Bryant (1978) for the development of adequate anaerobic techniques for culturing the more fastidious organisms. Rumen fluid remains the most satisfactory medium for culturing human gut microbes.

Digestion Studies with Primates

Digestion studies are available only in two primate species: howler monkeys (Milton et al., 1980) and chimpanzees (Milton and Demment, 1988). Digestion balances were conducted on howler monkeys on their natural diets, fruits and leaves from Ficus and Cecropia. Animals weighing 3–8 kg digested 75 percent cellulose, and 81 percent hemicellulose in fruit and 33 percent cellulose and 36 percent hemicellulose in leaves. There was no association between body size and digestive capacity. Yet fiber consumption (NDF) was 3–7 percent of body weight.

The chimpanzee balances were conducted with wheat bran as a fiber source so that results on digestion and passage could be compared with

Table 4. Digestibility of fiber components from AACC wheat bran in chimpanzees compared to humans and pigs

Species and diet	NDF Dietary content %	NDF Digestibility %	Cellulose Digestibility %	Hemicellulose Digestibility %
Chimpanzees				
Low fiber	15	71	68	77
High fiber	34	54	38	63
Human[a]				
High fiber	10–15	51	41	58
Pig[a]				
High fiber	17	65	24	74

[a] From Milton and Demment (1988).

trials done on humans and pigs (Milton and Demment, 1988). The data show that chimpanzees at low fiber intakes digest relatively more fiber than humans or pigs. Human values are similar to pigs, but the intake is much lower. Cellulose and hemicellulose digestibilities are significantly correlated with mean retention time in both chimpanzees (Milton et al., 1988) and in humans (Van Soest, 1977). The chimpanzee study also showed that larger animals tended to have higher digestion of fiber and longer retention times.

While the digestive patterns of chimpanzees and humans have similarities, the proportions of the gut devoted to fermentation is smaller in humans relative to body size than for other hominoids (Table 4). The hindgut volume in apes is about 52%, while for man this is about 17–20%. The fact that all of the non-human apes have relatively more of the digestive tract devoted to fermentation indicates that the situation in humans is evolutionarily derived and that human ancestors were decidedly herbivorous. Man apparently escaped the constraint of body size and digestive capacity through technological and social innovations that permitted improved net return from food gathering and a reduction in dietary bulk (Milton and Demment, 1988).

Fiber Requirements

That ruminants generally require adequate dietary fiber for normal rumen function is generally recognized. Ruminants may have fiber requirements on the order of 30% of the diet and some extreme nonruminant grazers are tolerant to diets containing 80% dietary fiber (Figure 4). However, positive effects of fiber in the diet also have been examined in several nonruminant species, e.g., pigs, guinea pigs and man. The optimum fiber for man has been estimated at 40g/day. Animal requirements are more often expressed as concentrations, reflecting the ratio of fiber to other dietary components. Forty grams of fiber may correspond to about 8–10% of daily dry matter intake, and compares well with data from pigs. The feeding of alfalfa to growing pigs affects gross feed efficiency and body composition. Up to a certain level (6–12% NDF in total diet) fiber does not alter use of digested energy and may even improve it (Kornegay, 1981). Feeding still more fiber generally elicits some loss in overall efficiency due to reduced food intake. However, one of the significant effects is the alteration in body composition. Fiber-fed pigs are leaner, with less fat, and have a larger gut fill and a heavier gut mucosa (Kass et al., 1980; Pond et al., 1988). The increased gut weight is probably the result of increased metabolism of butyrate and propionate.

The final question is whether increased intake of fiber and associated

VFA will induce caloric inefficiency and provide a basis for weight control in humans. Most animals attempt to eat to the level of their energy requirements, i.e., satiety. Thus dilution of the diet with inert bulk increases food intake to compensate for calories. However, dilution of the dietary energy by inert bulk usually discloses a level of bulk beyond which compensation is no longer possible (Baumgardt, 1970). In the aforementioned pig studies, fiber increased leanness, but did not decrease body weight because of compensatory increases in gut weight. An argument based on the model in Figure 4 is that moderate increase in fiber intake will (at least up to the optimal level) be compensated for by increased food intake, so that no reduction in net caloric intake will occur unless gut fill becomes limiting. This probably occurs past the optimum point and involves fiber intakes that most people will not accept. However, the argument from rumen metabolism is that acetate production is inefficient relative to ATP use so that heat increment is elevated, although caloric intake may not have changed. This is an aspect of ruminant studies that needs application and understanding in nonruminant and human nutrition.

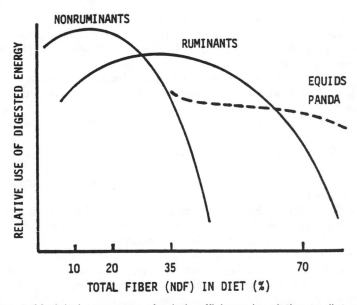

Figure 4. Modeled responses of caloric efficiency in relation to dietary fiber for various groups of animals (Van Soest, 1985). Ruminants fail on low quality very high fiber diets because of the cost of rumination and other digestive work required to eliminate lignified fiber from their complex gut. A few species, equids, elephants and pandas, can tolerate very high fibrous diets, but do not have much fermentation.

Conclusions

Rats and mice are very popular experimental animals for modeling human nutritional studies. However, for the purpose of dietary fiber research they have many disadvantages. They are small animals with inferior fermentation capacity. The main site of fermentation is in the cecum, whereas in man it is all in the colon. The rodents also consume their feces, which can confound results. Coprophagy may be prevented, but attempts to do so may lead to other complications (Gagnon, 1978). Pigs, chimps and baboons are much closer in feeding and "digestive" behavior to humans, but still have some differences. The apes have a larger portion of the digestive tract devoted to fermentation. All species differ in some way or another and there is no species that behaves exactly like humans.

References

Argenzio, R. A., J. E. Lowe, D. W. Pickard and C. E. Stevens. 1974. Digesta passage and water exchange in the equine large intestine. Amer. J. Physiol. 226:1035-1042.

Argenzio, R. A. and M. Southworth. 1974. Sites of organic acid production and absorption in gastrointestinal tract of the pig. Amer. J. Physiol. 228:454.

Argenzio, R. A. and C. E. Stevens. 1984. The large bowel—a supplementary rumen? Proc. Nutr. Soc. 43:13-23.

Bakker, R. 1986. The Dinosaur Heresies. Longman Scientific & Technical.

Banta, C. C., R. G. Warner and J. B. Robertson. 1975. Protein nutrition of the golden hamster. J. Nutr. 105:38-45.

Bauchop, T. and R. W. Martucci. 1968. Ruminant-like digestion of the Langur monkey. Science 161:698-699.

Bjornhag, G. 1972. Separation and delay of contents in the rabbit colon. Swedish J. Agr. Res. 2:125-136.

Bryant, M. P. 1978. Cellulose digesting bacteria from human feces. Amer. J. Clin. Nutr. Suppl. 31:S113-S115.

Cherbut, C. and Y. Ruckebusch. 1985. The effect of indigestible particles on digestive transit time and colonic motility in dogs and pigs. Br. J. Nutr. 53:549.

Clemens, E. T. and C. E. Stevens. 1980. A comparison of gastrointestinal transit time in ten species of mammal. J. Agric. Sci. Camb. 94:735-737.

Demment, M. and P. J. Van Soest. 1985. A nutritional explanation for body-size patterns of ruminant and nonruminant herbivores. The American Naturalist. 125:641-672.

Dierenfeld, E. S., H. F. Hintz, J. B. Robertson, P. J. Van Soest and O. T. Oftedal. 1982. Utilization of bamboo by the giant panda. J. Nutr. 112:636-641.

Ehle, F. R., J. L. Jeraci, J. B. Robertson and P. J. Van Soest. 1982. The influence of dietary fiber on digestibility, rate of passage and gastrointestinal fermentation in pigs. J. Anim. Sci. 55:1071-1081.

Ehle, F. R. and R. G. Warner. 1978. Nutritional implications of the hamster fore-stomach. J. Nutr. 108:1047.

Farlow, J. O. 1987. Speculations about the diet and digestive physiology of herbivorous dinosaurs. Paleobiology 13(1):60-72.

Foose, T. 1982. Trophic strategies of ruminant versus nonruminant ungulates. Ph.D. Thesis, Univ. Chicago, IL.

Gagnon, J. P. 1978. A harness for the prevention of coprophagy in the rat. MS Thesis, Cornell Univ., Ithaca, NY. pp.76.

Grajal, A., S. D. Strahl, R. Parra, M. G. Dominguez, A. Neher. 1989. Foregut fermentation in the hoatzin, a neotropical leaf-eating bird. Sci. 245:1236.

Grovum, W. L. and V. J. Williams. 1973. Rate of passage of digesta in sheep. IV. Passage of marker through the alimentary tract and the biological relevance of rate constants derived from the changes in concentration of marker in feces. Br. J. Nutr. 30:313-329.

Grovum, W. L. and V. J. Williams. 1977. Rate of passage of digesta in sheep. 6. The effect of level of food intake on mathematical predictions of the kinetics of digesta in the reticulorumen and intestines. Br. J. Nutr. 38:425-436.

Hackenberger, M. K. 1987. Diet digestibilities and ingesta transit times of captive Asian [Elephas maximus] and African [Loxodonta africana] elephants. MSc Thesis, Univ. of Guelph.

Heller, S. N., L. R. Hackler, J. M. Rivers, P. J. Van Soest, D. A. Roe, B. A Lewis and J. B. Robertson. 1980. Dietary fiber: the effect of particle size of wheat bran on colonic function in young adult men. Amer. J. Clin. Nutr. 33:1734-1744.

Hintz, H. F., C. J. Sedgewick and H. F. Schryver. 1976. Some observations on digestion of a pelleted diet by ruminants and non-ruminants. Internat. Zoo Yearb. 16:54-57.

Hoffmann, M., O. Steinhofel and R. Fuchs. 1987. Studies of the digestibility of crude nutrients in horses. 2. Comparative studies of the digestive capacities of thoroughbred horses, ponies and wethers. Arch. Tierernähr. 37:351.

Hofmann, R. R. 1989. Evolutionary steps of ecophysiological adaptation and diversification of ruminants: a comparative view of their digestive system. Oecologia 78:443-457.

Holmgren, V. C. 1972. The other panda. Animal Kingdom 75:6-10.

Hoover, W. H. and S. D. Clarke. 1972. Fiber digestion in the beaver. J. Nutr. 102:9-15.

Hume, I. D. 1982. Digestive Physiology and Nutrition of Marsupials. Monographs on Marsupial Biology. Cambridge Univ. Press.

Hungate, R. E. 1966. The Rumen and Its Microbes. Academic Press, NY.

Janis, C. M. 1976. The evolutionary strategy of the Equidae and the origins of rumen and cecal digestion. Evolution 30:757-774.

Janis, C. M. and D. Ehrhardt. 1988. Correlation of relative muzzle width and relative incisor width with dietary preference in ungulates. Zool. J. Linnean Soc. 92:267-284.

Janis, C. M. and M. Fortelius. 1988. On the means whereby mammals achieve increased functional durability of their dentitions, with special reference to limiting factors. Biol. Rev. 63:197-230.

Kass, M., P. J. Van Soest, W. G. Pond, B. L. Lewis, and L. E. McDonald. 1980. Utilization of dietary fiber from alfalfa by growing swine. I. Apparent digestibility of diet components in specific segments of the gastrointestinal tract. J. Anim. Sci. 50:175-197.

Keys, J. E., Jr. and P. J. Van Soest. 1970. Digestibility of forages by the meadow vole (*Microtus pennsylvanicus*). J. Dairy Sci. 53:1502-1508.

Keys, J. E., Jr., P. J. Van Soest and E. P. Young. 1970. Effect of increasing dietary cell wall content on the digestibility of hemicellulose and cellulose in swine and rats. J. Anim. Sci. 31:172.

Kornegay, E. T. 1981. Soybean hull digestibility by sows and feeding value for growing-finishing swine. J. Anim. Sci. 53:138-145.

Leng, R. A. 1970. Formation and production of volatile fatty acids in the rumen. In: Physiology of Digestion and Metabolism in the Ruminant. A.T. Phillipson, ed. Oriel Press, Newcastle upon Tyne, England. pp. 406-421.

Mason, V. C. 1984. Metabolism of nitrogenous compounds in the large gut. Proc. Nutr. Soc. 43:45-53.

McNeil, N. I., J. H. Cummings and W. P. T. James. 1978. Short chain fatty acid absorption by the human large intestine. Gut 19, 819-824.

Milton, K. and M. W. Demment. 1988. Digestion and passage kinetics of chimpanzees fed high and low fiber diets and comparison with human data. J. Nutr. 118:1082-1088.

Milton, K., P. J. Van Soest and J. B. Robertson. 1980. Digestive efficiencies of wild howler monkeys. Physiol. Zool. 53:402-409.

Moir, R. J. 1968. Ruminant digestion and evolution. In: Handbook of Physiology Section G: Alimentary Canal. Vol V. Bile Digestion, Ruminal Physiology. C. F. Code, ed. Am. Physiol. Soc., Washington, D.C. pp. 2673-2693.

Parra, R. 1978. Comparison of foregut and hindgut fermentation in herbivores. In: The Ecology of Arboreal Folivores. G. G. Montgomery, ed. Smithsonian Institution Press, Washington, D.C. p. 205.

Pond, W. G., H. G. Jung and V. H. Varel. 1988. Effect of dietary fiber on young adult genetically lean, obese and contemporary pigs: body weight, carcass measurements, organ weights and digesta content. J. Anim. Sci. 66:699-706.

Salyers, A. A., S. E. H. West, J. R. Vercellotti and T. D. Wilkins. 1977. Fermentation of mucins and plant polysaccharides by anaerobic bacteria from the human colon. Applied and Environ. Microb. 34:529-533.

Schaller, G. B., H. Jinchu, P. Wenshi, Z. Jine. 1985. The Giant Pandas of Wolong. Univ. of Chicago Press, Chicago.

Stevens, C. E. 1988. Comparative Physiology of the Vertebrate Digestive System. Cambridge Univ. Press, Cambridge and New York. pp. 300.

Udén, P. 1978. Comparable studies on rate of passage, particle size and rate of digestion in ruminants, equines, rabbits and man. Ph.D. Thesis, Cornell Univ., Ithaca, NY.

Uden, P., T. R. Rounsaville, G. R. Wiggans and P. J. Van Soest. 1982. The measurement of liquid and solid digesta retention in ruminants, equines and rabbits given timothy (*Phleum pratense*) hay. Br. J. Nutr. 48:329-339.

Uden, P. and P. J. Van Soest. 1982. Comparative digestion of timothy (*Phleum pratense*) fibre by ruminants, equines and rabbits. Br. J. Nutr. 47:267.

Van Dokkum, W., A. Wesstra and F. A. Schippers. 1982. Physiological effects of fibre-rich types of bread. 1. The effect of dietary fibre from bread on the mineral balance of young men. Br. J. Nutr. 47:451.

Van Soest, P. J. 1981. Some factors influencing the ecology of gut fermentation in man. In: Banbury Report 7: Gastrointestinal Cancer: Endogenous Factors. Cold Spring Harbor Laboratory, Cold Spring Harbor, NY. p. 61-69.

Van Soest, P. J. 1982. Nutritional Ecology of the Ruminant. 3rd Printing. Cornell University Press, Ithaca, NY.

Van Soest, P. J., P. Uden and K. F. Wrick. 1983. Critique and evaluation of markers for use in nutrition of humans and farm and laboratory animals. Nutr. Reports Interl. 27:17-27.

Varel, V. H., H. G. Jung and W. G. Pond. 1988. Effects of dietary fiber of young adult genetically lean, obese and contemporary pigs: rate of passage, digestibility and microbiological data. J. Anim. Sci. 66:707-712.

Vercellotti, J. R., A. A. Salyers, W. S. Bullard and T. D. Wilkins. Breakdown of mucin and plant polysaccharides in the human colon. Can. J. Biochem. 55:1190-1196.

Visek, W. J. and J. B. Robertson. 1973. Dried brewer's grains in dog diets. Proc. Cornell Nutr. Conf. pp. 40-49.

Warner, R. G. and W. P. Flatt. 1965. Anatomical developments of the ruminant stomach. In: Physiology of Digestion in the Ruminant. R. W. Dougherty, R. S. Allen, W. Burroughs, N. L. Jacobson and A. D. McGilliard, eds. Butterworths, Washington. pp. 24-38.

Wolin, M. J. 1975. Interactions between the bacterial species of the rumen. In: Digestion and Metabolism in the Ruminant. I. W. McDonald and A. C. I. Warner, eds. Univ. New England Publ. Unit, Newcastle upon Tyne, England. pp. 134-148.

Propionate as a Mediator of the Effects of Dietary Fiber

David L. Topping

CSIRO Division of Human Nutrition
Glenthorne Laboratory
O'Halloran Hill 5158,
Australia

Introduction

In obligate ruminant herbivores such as sheep and cattle the bacterial (and fungal breakdown of cellulosic and non-cellulosic non-starch polysaccharides [NSP]) supplies 60–70% of total energy through the generation of volatile fatty acids (VFA), principally acetate, propionate, and butyrate, which are absorbed and enter the hepatic circulation via the portal vein (1). The presence of the microflora at the beginning of the digestive process imposes certain constraints on ruminants as other dietary carbohydrates including starch and free glucose, are fermented more or less completely, which means that gluconeogenesis has to supply the needs of the animal for glucose. Endogenous glucose synthesis is driven to a large degree by the conversion of propionate which enters the citric acid cycle at succinate (2). There is evidence that propionate is limiting for some activities as its infusion into the rumen stimulates the growth of the mucosa. Conversely, fermentations that yield propionate at the expense of acetate depress milk fat production, presumably through lowering lipogenesis in adipose tissue or the mammary gland itself.

The importance of fiber fermentation in non-ruminant omnivores species is now generally recognized, as are the parallels with the rumen. The main end products of fermentation are the same major VFA, gases and an increased bacterial mass (3). As in ruminants, NSP are the principal fermentative substrates and, of the animals used commonly as models for human metabolism, only in the pig does it appear likely that appreciable fiber fermentation occurs in the upper gut, although this is still small relative to that occurring in the colon (4). The degree of NSP fermentation varies considerably, but in the cases of starch and of the many water-soluble polysaccharides eaten commonly in whole foods and also used widely in the food industry it appears to be reasonably complete. Of especial interest is the fact that these NSP have other attractive properties beside their technological attributes, notably cholesterol reduction and slowing of digestion (5).

NSP and Control of Plasma Cholesterol

Reduction of plasma cholesterol is recognized as an important step in the prevention of coronary heart disease, and dietary modification is an economic and effective means of attaining that end. Of the dietary maneuvers available, health authorities recommend reduction in total and saturated fat coupled with increased consumption of complex carbohydrates and fiber is a general recommendation. In controlled trials products such as oats and oat bran produce an independent reduction in plasma low density lipoprotein (LDL) cholesterol (6,7). The extent of the reduction varies depending on diet and quantity of food consumed but a 6–8% reduction at an intake of 80g of oat bran/day seems reasonable (7).

Propionate as a Mediator of Cholesterol Reduction by NSP

The mechanism whereby fiber lowers plasma cholesterol is a matter of debate, but viscosity in aqueous solution has been identified as an important characteristic. This property is thought to increase the viscosity of gut contents as to alter the digestion and/or absorption of fats and steroids (5). However, this proposition does not account for all of the attributes of NSP and an alternative has been proposed, namely that colonic NSP fermentation is responsible through a particular VFA-propionate (8). This is a very attractive hypothesis as propionate is a cheap and safe antifungal agent, used widely in the baking industry. The concept is based on several observations. Firstly, foods such as oat bran which lower cholesterol are fermented by the colonic microflora of experimental animal with a greater production of propionate that occurs with foods such as wheat bran that do not lower cholesterol (9). Secondly, propionate feeding lower plasma cholesterol in experimental animals including rats and pigs (10,11). Propionate inhibits cholesterol synthesis in isolated hepatocytes (9), an effect similar to that of certain drugs used to lower plasma cholesterol in humans with hypercholesterolemia (5).

Effect of Propionate in Vivo in Animal Models

The hypothesis that propionate is the mediator of ASP action is well supported. Firstly, the reduction in plasma cholesterol in rats fed a diet supplemented with propionate is as great as that obtained with foods such as oat bran. However, there are problems with the design of such model experiments. Propionate formed by large bowel fermentation is absorbed with quite a different time course to that of propionate ingested by mouth and in pigs with portal venous cannulae; dietary propionate gave a peak concentration 1–2 hours after feeding followed by a decline (11). After 4–6 hours, VFA concentrations rise and these raised levels are sustained for many hours, consistent with the onset and maintenance of large bowel fiber fermentation. In rats fed propionate-enriched diets, measurements of such a time course is impractical but determination of gut and portal venous VFA in the postabsorptive state shows that propionate concentrations are raised in the latter blood vessel. Propionate is raised also in the stomach but little appears in the small intestine (Table 1). In fact, in both rats and pigs most of the dietary propionate cannot be accounted for by portal transport and the question of its fate remains open. Given that propionate appears to be used by the rumen wall, it may be that the rodent and porcine stomach metabolize it also.

The peak concentrations of propionate we have measured after propionate feeding are in the region of 1 mmol/L. These compare favorably with those obtained in the portal venous plasma of rats fed dietary fibers preparations such as wheat bran aleurone (12). However, examination of plasma cholesterol in such animals shows that cecal propionate concentrations (which determine those in the portal vein) show no relationship to plasma cholesterol. A similar lack of relationship has also been found

Table 1. Concentrations of propionate in gut contents of rats fed a diet supplemented with 5% sodium propionate

Diet	Stomach	Duodenum	Ileum	Cecum
		(m/mol/L)		
Control	1	0	0	24
Propionate	116	1	1	24

in the pig (unpublished observations)—a species which considered to be a good model for human fiber and lipoprotein metabolism. The fact that, under some circumstances, large bowel propionate is elevated when plasma cholesterol is reduced in experimental animals has been taken to mean a causative relationship between propionate and sterol homeostasis. In fact, the opposite may be equally true. In a recent experiment with wheat milling fractions a strong negative correlation was found between cecal sterols (coprostanol and secondary bile acids) and plasma cholesterol in rats. In this experiment, a negative correlation was found between cecal propionate and plasma cholesterol (Table 2). However, an even stronger positive correlation was found between cecal butyrate and cholesterol. Moreover, as cecal secondary steroids increased, butyrate fell.

Much of the interest in propionate as mediator of fiber action comes from two complementary sets of observations—reduction of plasma cholesterol in animals and inhibition of cholesterol synthesis in vitro. It has been will documented that propionate inhibits hepatic cholesterol synthesis in isolated hepatocytes. Unfortunately, there are a number of aspects of this effect that are questionable. Firstly, isolated hepatocytes have relatively low rates of O_2 consumption (usually at high pO_2 values) and fatty acid and cholesterol synthesis relative to the liver in the intact animal. Comparison of those rates with livers perfused with whole blood at physiological flow rates shows that the perfused liver has much higher rates of O_2 uptake and of very low density lipoprotein production (13) than hepatocytes. In vivo the liver receives 30% of its supply via the hepatic artery at a pO_2 of 90–100 mm Hg and the rest through the portal vein at a lower pO_2. The latter vessel also supplies lactate, glu-

Table 2. Concentrations of plasma cholesterol and cecal butyrate and propionate in rats fed whole wheat (WW, wheat bran (WB), wheat pollard (WP) and white flour (WF)[1]

Diet	Plasma cholesterol	Cecal propionate	Cecal butyrate
		(m/mol/L)	
WW	3.11	20.0	32.6
WB	2.97	26.8	22.3
WP	2.81	26.7	28.4
WF	2.57	28.4	17.3
SE	0.17	3.0	4.3
r vs. cholesterol	—	−0.50 ($P < 0.01$)	+0.53 ($P < 0.01$)

[1] R. J. Illman, G. B. Storer, D. L. Topping (unpublished).

cose, VFA, and other substrates in response to diet and digestion. The concentrations of total VFA in the portal seldom exceed 2 mmol/L in the rat or pig and the highest concentration of propionate that we have found in animal studies is 1 mmol/L (12). At this concentration propionate does not affect cholesterol synthesis in perfused liver, although inhibition does occur at much higher concentrations (11). This situation may be analogous to that of acetate. The rat liver is in equilibrium with blood acetate and at a concentration below 0.2–0.3 mmol/L releases it but above that level, uptake occurs (13). There is a further set point that seldom is considered. At concentrations below 5 mmol/L acetate is directed largely towards fatty acid synthesis, but above that concentration, oxidation becomes activated (15). Put simply, the choice of substrate concentration dictates the observed metabolic effects.

Finally, we have to consider the choice of radioisotopic marker. Historically, radiolabelled acetate was used to measure de novo lipid synthesis. However, this tracer has a number of problems relating mostly to calculation of the true specific radioactivity of the precursor pool or acetyl-CoA. These difficulties have been overcome with $3H_2O$ and using that marker, cholesterol synthesis is found to be uninhibited by dietary propionate in the whole rat (11).

Conclusion

The hypothesis that propionate mediates some of the effects of dietary fiber on plasma cholesterol has stimulated much discussion and useful research. At present, it seems that the hypothesis is not supported by the evidence. However, much remains to be learned about the physiological effects of this metabolically important acid as well as its ultimate fate in humans and relevant model animal species. In furthering those investigations, the choice of experimental conditions seems to be critical.

References

1. E. F. Annison & D. G. Armstrong, Volatile fatty acid metabolism and energy supply in: "Physiology of Digestion and Metabolism in the Ruminant," A. T. Phillipson, ed., Oriel Press Newcastle upon Tyne (1970).
2. C. L. Davis & J. H. Clark, Ruminant digestion and metabolism, Dev. Ind. Microbiol. 22: 247 (1981).
3. S. E. Fleming and D. S. Acre, Volatile fatty acids: their production, Clin. Gastroenterol. 15: 787 (1986).
4. J. G. Fadel, R. K. Newman, C. W. Newman & H. Graham, Effects of baking hulless barley on the digestibility of dietary components as measured at the ileum and in the feces of pigs, J. Nutr. 119:722 (1989).

5. D. L. Topping, Soluble fibre polysaccharides: effects on plasma cholesterol and colonic fermentation, Nutr. Rev. 49:195 (1991).

6. R. W. Kirby, J. W. Anderson, B. Sieling, E. D. Rees, W.-J Chen, R. Miller & R. M. Kay, Oat bran intake selectively lowers serum cholesterol low-density lipoprotein concentrations of hypercholesterolemic men. Am. J. Clin. Nutr. 34:824 (1981).

7. M. Kestin, R. Moss, P. M. Clifton and P. J. Nestel, The comparative effects of three cereal brans on plasma lipids, blood pressure and glucose metabolism in mildly hypercholesterolemic men. Am. J. Clin. Nutr. 52: 661 (1990).

8. W.-J. Chen, J. W. Anderson and D. Jennings, Propionate may mediate the hypocholesterolaemic effects of certain soluble plant fibers in cholesterol-fed rats. Fed. Prod, Soc, Exp. Biol. Med. 75: 215 (1984).

9. R. J. Illman, D. L. Topping, K. Dowling, R. P. Trimble, G. R. Russell & Storer, Effects of solvent extraction on the hypocholesterolaemic action of oat bran in the rat. Brit. J. Nutr. 32:97 (1991).

10. R. J. Boila, M. D. Salomon, L. P. Milligan & F. X. Aherne, The effect of dietary propionic acid on cholesterol synthesis in swine. Nutr. Rep. Int. 23:1113 (1981).

11. R. J. Illman, D. L. Topping, G. H. McIntosh, R. P. Trimble, G. B. Storer, M. N. Taylor and B.-Q. Cheng, Hypocholesterolaemic effects of dietary propionate: studies in whole animals and perfused rat liver, Ann. Nutr. Metab. 32:97 (1988).

12. B.-Q. Cheng, R. P. Trimble, R. J. Illman, B. A. Stone & D. L. Topping, Comparative effects of dietary wheat bran and its morphological components (aleurone and pericarp-seed coat) on volatile fatty acid concentrations in the rat Br. J. Nutr. 57: 69 (1987).

13. D. L. Topping, G. B. Storer & R. P. Trimble, Effects of flow rate and insulin on triacylglycerol secretion by perfused rat liver, Am. J. Physiol. 255:E306 (1988).

14. B. M. Buckley and D. H. Williamson, Origins of blood acetate in the rat, Biochem. J. 166:539 (1977).

15. D. L. Topping, A. M. Snoswell, G. B. Storer, R. C. Fishlock & R. P. Trimble, Dependence on blood acetate concentration of the metabolic effects of ethanol in perfused rat liver, Biochem. Biophys. Acta 800:103 (1984).

In Vitro Methods That Anticipate the Colonic Influence of Dietary Fibre

W. Gordon Brydon

Gastrointestinal Laboratory
University Department of Medicine,
Western General Hospital,
Edinburgh EH4 2XU.

The fibre content of the diet is known to have a significant influence on stool weight.[1] Many studies have examined the effect which a variety of fibre sources have on faecal weight and constituents.[2,3] These have shown that in general fibre from cereals is more effective in increasing stool weight than either fruit or vegetable fibre sources or gel forming polysaccharides. These studies with human volunteers are demanding and time consuming. The chemical composition of the various complex carbohydrates (dietary fibres), gives little indication of the physiological potential of any particular fibre.[3]

In vitro methods which could identify fibre sources that can be used therapeutically to influence gastrointestinal function would be useful. The colon can be regarded as two organs—the right side, the caecum, a fermenter where a large mass of bacteria metabolise materials passing from the ileum, and the left side which is involved in stool formation and continence. This paper reviews in vitro methods which describe the influence of fibre on both these functions.

Early work in the water holding capacity (WHC) of fibre and its laxation properties was performed by Klecker[4] who demonstrated the swelling ability of water in a measuring cylinder, and Tainter and Buchanan[5] who demonstrated that the swelling power approximately predicted the laxative effects of these materials.

McConnel et al[6] described a method to measure water holding capacity in which the material was soaked in excess water for 24 hrs, and then centrifuged at 14000g for 1 hour, and the difference in weight between the dry fibre source and that of the centrifuged pellet gave a measure of the water held. Wheat bran, which is a concentrated fibre source, was shown to hold much more water than other fruits and vegetables, but when acetone dried powders were compared for WHC, bran was shown to hold much less water than, eg, carrots and cucumber.

Stephen and Cummings[7] examined the in vitro WHC properties of several dietary fibre preparations, measuring water uptake using the centrifugation technique and also a dialysis tecnique using PEG 4000 to create a suction pressure. This had originally been used by Blythe et al[8] in an attempt to mimic the pull of the colonic absorption forces. They compared their in vitro results with previous results when fibre was fed to human volunteers and found an inverse relationship between WHC and stool weight; eg, pectin with a WHC of 56 only increased stool weight by 19% whilst wheat bran had the lowest WHC, 4, but increased stool weight by 117%, providing evidence that fibre did not increase faecal weight simply by retaining water in the gut.

Subsequently, Stephen and Cummings[9] using a technique to fractionate faeces demonstated that bacteria provided the largest component of stool weight, and proposed that bacterial proliferation as a result of fibre fermentation contributed to the increase in stool weight. Fermentable fibres like cabbage extract, provide a readily useable substrate for microbial growth whilst cereal fibres are less readily fermented and retain water per se.

Robertson and Eastwood[10] showed that altering the conditions of fibre preparation or the WHC measurements may result in a very different WHC for a fibre source, eg, rapid gravity filtration of soaked fibre, gave lower values for WHC than centrifugation, and never dried potato fibre gave higher WHC values than air dried or roller dried. Differences in WHC within and between each fibre source, when measured by centrifugation, were attributed to structural differences which affected the amount of water that was trapped by the fibre. The same authors[11] further developed a dialysis model for in vitro measurements of WHC, using known suction pressures to measure how strongly water was held by the fibre, and this allowed a distinction to be made between water trapped and water bound, both of which are measured by centrifugation methods. WHC using this technique gave lower values than centrifugation methods, using potato, bran, and gum arabic as fibre sources (Table 1). Measurement of WHC using suction pressure has shown that bran has a poor ability to hold water compared with potato fibre which behaves like a gel, and gum arabic which is in solution. They used an osmoticum with MW 10000, since lower MW materials are slightly permeable and would cause inaccuracies in measured WHC. Using a suction pressure of 2 atmospheres best simulated normal colonic absorption forces.

McBurney et al[12] have examined the WHC of four sources of fibre using a suction/dialysis method with pectin and cellulose and extracts of lucerne and cabbage, both before and after in vitro fermentation. The potential WHC (PWHC)—a measure of the product of the residual fibre weight and the residual WHC, ranked the 4 fibres in the same order as in previous in vivo studies. They concluded that ethanol insoluble residues containing residual unfermented fibre and bacteria, should be used to calculate PWHC and used to predict the effects of fibre on faecal weight. Using the PWHC reverses the relationship seen by Stephen and Cummings, resulting in better prediction of stool weight. Also the neutral detergent residues yield the most accurate estimate of the digestibility of the fibre substrate but do not measure water soluble polysaccharides. Subsequent experiments by this group[13] using several inocula from different sources have shown that after 24 hour in vitro incubations, single inocula rank different substrates in the same order for fermentability as assessed by short chain fatty acids (SCFA), neutral detergent fibre, and gas production, but recommend the use of at least 3 donors to minimise differences and give a better prediction of in vivo effects. Armstrong et al[14] have used in vitro suction dialysis to measure the distribution of caecal and faecal water in the rat after supplementing a low fibre diet with bran and pectin. Dialysis of faeces and caecal contents against PEG 10000 for 72 hrs was used to remove free absorbable water. When supplementing a basal diet with 10% bran there was no increase in bound water, the increase in wet and dry weight being approximately the same. However supplementing with 10% pectin caused a significant increase in bound water. Caecal content wet and dry weight

Table 1. The water holding capacity (WHC: g water/g fibre) of selected fibres measured by centrifugation and suction pressure

	WHC					
			Suction Pressure			
	Centrifugation		1 atm		10 atm	
Fibre source	Mean	SE	Mean	SE	Mean	SE
Potato	23.8	4.0	3.3	0.5	1.7	0.3
Bran	3.7	1.7	1.4	0.2	1.0	0.4
Gum arabic	...	...	5.7	1.5	2.6	0.6

was increased by pectin but not bran; with bran caecal bound water increased but total water did not change. Pectin increased free water in both caecal contents and faeces.

Eastwood et al[3] summarised several in vivo experiments and indicated that it was not possible to predict the influence of dietary fibre on stool weight from the chemical structure of complex carbohydrates; also there was no simple relationship between changes in faecal output of cholesterol metabolites and serum cholesterol. In a subsequent experiment Adiotomre et al[15] have developed in vitro methods to assess the influence of fibre on biological function within the gastrointestinal tract and have compared these with in vivo results where possible.

Using a single human faecal inoculum at a final concentration of 4%, added to a reduced medium containing different fibre preparations, the gel forming and water soluble fibres in general produced the greatest concentration of SCFAs, pectin giving the highest concentration (Table 2).

When the amount of propionic acid produced by bacterial fermentation of each fibre was considered, guar produced the highest concentration which relates well to its potential to lower serum cholesterol, but gum arabic and tragacanth also produced high concentrations relative to the other fibres without having any effect in vivo.

To determine residual WHC, 5 ml of the the fermentation end products were added to dialysis bags, placed in 50 ml PEG 10000 and wet and dry weight calculated after 72 hrs. Carboxymethyl cellulose held the greatest amount of water after fermentation, followed by karaya and gellan. Karaya has a high predictive index but has no effect on stool weight in vivo. Although the 3 fibres which gave the greatest increase for in vivo stool weight also gave the greatest water held per residue, overall there was a poor relationship between in vitro and in vivo re-

Table 2. Evolution of short chain fatty acids after fibre fermentation

	Total	Acetate	Propionate	Butyrate
Pectin	82.2 (7.7)	58.5 (6.4)	12.2 (0.6)	7.0 (1.5)
Gum Arabic	74.0 (9.5)	50.5 (6.9)	14.5 (1.0)	6.1 (2.0)
Guar	71.4 (5.0)	41.2 (1.5)	19.4 (1.5)	5.7 (0.5)
Tragacanth	67.4 (5.5)	45.1 (4.0)	12.5 (0.7)	5.5 (1.5)
Kanthan	63.4 (4.3)	45.2 (3.9)	11.8 (0.7)	2.0 (0.7)
Gellan	37.2 (6.3)	23.0 (2.6)	7.3 (0.6)	2.6 (0.5)
Bran	34.3 (3.2)	17.8 (2.4)	3.9 (0.4)	6.6 (1.2)
CMC	25.8 (4.5)	14.4 (3.5)	4.4 (1.4)	2.5 (0.4)
Karaya	24.2 (4.9)	15.0 (5.1)	2.4 (0.3)	2.3 (0.6)
Control	15.5 (3.5)	6.5 (1.3)	2.4 (0.2)	1.6 (0.6)

SEM in parentheses.

sults, with little discrimination between fibres with a value <0.09 for total water held by residue (Table 2).

This model (Table 3) was set up not to produce absolute measurement of biological action, but to enable a hierarchy of potential biological activity to be predicted for unknown fibre sources and is currently being developed to improve in vivo predictability.

In vitro dialysis methods only measure water held by residual fibre and bacteria and take no account of the influence of smaller MW materials such as SCFA which may cause the retention of more water by faeces and so midght be expected to give lower than in vivo values.

McBurney et al[16] fermented aliquots of test foods, and freeze dried ileal effluent, or dietary fibre isolates from these foods, using a mixed human inoculum, in order to determine whether human ileostomy digestion studies could be avoided. SCFA production from ileal effluent correlated well with that from fibre isolates but not with production from whole foods, and they concluded that fibre isolates, rather than whole foods provide the nearest estimate of colonic SCFA production.

The same authors[17] showed that the profiles of production of SCFA were different for different fibre sources despite producing similar concentrations over a 24 hour period. Both tragacanth and pectin produced similar concentrations of SCFA over 24 hours and, whilst pectin was rapidly fermented (89% in 4 hours), tragacanth was more slowly fermented but over a sustained period.

Edwards and Eastwood[18] have demonstrated differences in the sites of fermentation of ispaghula and bran in the rat, with bran being fermented only in the caecum and giving increased butyrate production,

Table 3. The predictive indices for stool weight

	Fecal weight (humans)			In vitro experiments	
	Initial	Final	Percent Increase	WHC per g dry weight	Total water held by residue
CMC	140 (33)	242 (20)	73	11.9 (1.42)	0.79 (0.07)
Bran	120 (8)	183 (9)	63	1.9 (0.8)	0.14 (0.05)
Gellan	176 (50)	285 (56)	62	3.1 (0.6)	0.22 (0.05)
Tragacanth	125 (18)	188 (21)	50	2.1 (0.5)	0.09 (0.02)
Kanthan	187 (27)	242 (39)	30	2.2 (0.3)	0.09 (0.01)
Pectin	142 (17)	177 (15)	24	2.2 (1.1)	0.09 (0.04)
Guar	68 (6)	76 (16)	11	1.9 (0.8)	0.09 (0.04)
Gum Arabic	147 (18)	161 (199)	10	2.1 (1.0)	0.08 (0.04)
Karaya	134 (11)	139 (17)	3	4.7 (0.5)	0.38 (0.03)

SEM in parentheses.

while ispaghula was fermented throughout the colon and gave increased propionate. In vitro experiments correctly predicted the increase in individual SCFA production, without indicating the differences in duration of fermentation as in the in vivo experiment.

Stevens and Selvendran[19] have used an in vitro fermentation system to measure changes in composition and structure of wheat bran. Wheat bran cell wall preparation was incubated with human faecal bacteria for 24–72 hrs and structural changes were measured using methylation analysis. Of the carbohydrate content, about 39% was degraded in 24 hrs, and only a further 5% after 72 hrs. Arabinoxylans and mixed linkage B-D glucans from the aleurone layer were degraded preferentially.

Gray et al[20] have used an in vitro system to measure the time course of release of CO_2 from ^{14}C labelled spinach cell walls, and compared this with in vivo release. Only 15% of the label was evolved as $^{14}CO_2$ compared with 25% of the label when administered orally to rats. Part of the difference may have been due to liver metabolism of labelled SCFA to CO_2.

In conclusion, in vitro methods have been used to measure the rate and amount of colonic fermentation of DF using NDF difference measurements or the production of metabolites such as SCFAs and have also been used to also predict changes in stool weight, with suction/dialysis methods best simulating colonic absorption. Such methods have also been used to complement or replace ileostomy studies, and to measure changes in structure and composition of fibre.

References

1. M. A. Eastwood, W. G. Brydon, J. D. Baird, R. A. Elton, S. Helliwell, J. Smith, and J. L. Pritchard. Faecal weight and composition of serum lipids and diet amongst subjects aged 18–80 years not seeking health care. Am. J. Clin. Nutr. 46:628 (1984).
2. J. A. Cummings, D. A. T. Southgate, W. Branch, H. Houston, D. J. A. Jenkins, and W. P. T. James. Colonic response to dietary fibre from carrot, cabbage, apple, bran, and guar gum. Lancet 1:5 (1979).
3. M. A. Eastwood, W. G. Brydon and D. M. W. Anderson. The effect of the polysaccharide composition and structure of dietary fibresin caecal fermentation and faecal excretion. Am. J. Clin. Nut. 44:51 (1986).
4. E. Klecker. Eine methode zur Messungdes Quellungsvermogens pharmakologisch verwendeter Quellstoffe. Archiv fur experimentelle Pathologie und Pharmacologie. 161:596 (1931).
5. M. L. Tainter and O. H. Buchanan. Quantatative comparisons of colloidal laxatives. Annals of New York Academy of Science. 58:438 (1954).
6. A. A. McConnell, M. A. Eastwood, and W. D. Mitchell. Physical characteristics of vegetable foodstuffs that could influence bowel function. J. Sci. Fd.

Agric. 25:1457 (1974).

7. A. M. Stephen and J. H. Cummings. Water holding capacity of dietary fibre in vitro and its relationship to faecal output in man. Gut 20:722 (1979).

8. R. H. Blythe, J. J. Gulesich, and H. L. Tuthill. Evaluation of hydrophilic properties of bulk laxatives including the new agent sodium carboxymethylcellulose. J. Amer. Pharm. Assoc. 38:59 (1947).

9. M. Stephen and J. H. Cummings. Mechanism of action of dietary fibre in the human colon. Nature 284:283 (1980).

10. A. Robertson and M. A. Eastwood. An investigation of the experimental conditions which could affect water holding capacity of dietary fibre. J. Sci. Food Agric. 32:819 (1981).

11. J. A. Robertson and M. A. Eastwood. A method to measure the water holding properties of dietary fibre using suction pressure. Br. J. Nutr. 46:247 (1981).

12. M. I. McBurney, P. J. Horvath, J. L. Jeraci, and P. J. Van Soest. Effect of an in vitro fermentation using human fecal inoculum on the water holding capacity of dietary fibre. Br. J. Nutr. 53:17 (1985).

13. M. I. McBurney and L. U. Thompson. Effect of human faecal donor on in vitro fermentation variables. Scand. J. Gastroenterol. 24:359 (1989).

14. E. H. Armstrong, Brydon, W. G., and Eastwood, M. A. Fibre metabolism and colonic water. in Dietary Fibre, Eds D. Kritchevsky, C. Bonfield, and J. W. Anderson: Plenum Press, New York p. 179 (1990).

15. J. Adiotomre, M. A. Eastwood, C. A. Edwards, and W. G. Brydon. Dietary fiber: in vitro methods that anticipate nutrition and metabolic activity in humans. Amer. J. Clin. Nutr. 52:128 (1990).

16. M. I. McBurney, L. U. Thompson, D. J. Cuff, and D. J. A. Jenkins. Comparison of ileal effluents, dietary fibers, and whole foods in predicting the physiological importance of colonic fermentation. Amer. J. Gastroenterol. 83:536 (1988).

17. M. I. McBurney and L. U. Thompson. In vitro fermentabilities of purified fiber supplements. J. Food Sci. 54:347 (1989).

18. C. A. Edwards and M. A. Eastwood. Comparison of the effect of ispaghula and wheat bran on rat caecal and colonic fermentation. Gut (1992) in press.

19. B. J. Stevens and R. R. Selvendran. Changes in composition and structure of wheat bran resulting from the action of human faecal bacteria in vitro. Carbohyd. Res. 183:311 (1988).

20. D. F. Gray, M. A. Eastwood, and W. G. Brydon. Fermentation and subsequent disposition of ^{14}C plant cell wall material in the rat. in press.

Fiber and Aspects of Lipid and Cholesterol Metabolism

David Kritchevsky, Ph.D.

The Wistar Institute
3601 Spruce Street
Philadelphia PA 19104-4268

The literature relating dietary fiber to cholesterol or lipid metabolism is rich in studies of effects on serum or plasma cholesterol of animals and man but relatively poor in other aspects of fat metabolism. Cholesterol is a precursor of corticosteroids, sex hormones and bile acids. Only the last of these has been studied in reference to fiber. The conversion of cholesterol to bile acids requires initial hydroxylation at the 7 α position. Recent data suggest that the 7 α hydroxylation reaction and activity of HMG-CoA reductase (one of the key steps in cholesterol biosynthesis) are interrelated through phosphorylation-dephosphorylation reactions (Heuman et al., 1988; Vlahcevic et al., 1989; Shefer et al., 1991). Bjorkhem (1985) has reviewed biological factors which modify both HMG-CoA reductase and cholesterol 7 α hydroxylase activity (Table 1). As the interest in and understanding of dietary fiber have expanded in the past decade, it is time perhaps to broaden our horizons vis-a-vis fiber and lipid metabolism.

Among the earliest studies relating to the metabolic effects of fiber were those of Portman. Portman and Murphy (1958) found that changing rats from a commercial to a semi-purified diet doubled cholic acid half life, reduced the cholate pool by 54% and cut cholate and neutral steroid excretion by 79 and 42%, respectively. Portman (1960) also showed that lipid extraction of the commercial diet did not affect any parameters of cholate metabolism nor did addition of the lipid extracts to a semi-purified diet restore them. The non-lipid nature of the component of commercial ration which affected lipids was confirmed in stud-

353

ies which showed that solvent extracted commercial rabbit diet retained anti-atherogeneic properties, whereas addition of the extract to a semi-purified diet did not lower its atherogenicity (Kritchevsky and Tepper, 1965, 1968).

The bile acids are considered to be of importance in the two major diseases of Western man—heart disease (because of their relation to cholesterol metabolism) and cancer (because secondary bile acids may act as promoters in experimental carcinogenesis). While the ratio of primary to secondary bile acids in the feces has not been shown to be related epidemiologically to cancer, the concentration of fecal bile acids has been implicated in this disease (Crowther et al., 1976). Recently the ratio of lithocholic to deoxycholic acid has been suggested as an important etiological factor in colorectal cancer (Owen et al., 1984).

The foregoing made it logical to investigate the bile acid or bile salt-binding proclivities of various dietary fibers. Eastwood and Hamilton (1968) found that cholic acid was indeed bound to plant materials. Story and Kritchevsky (1976) examined the binding of cholic, chenodeoxy-cholic and deoxycholic acids to four fiber-rich materials or fibers (alfalfa, bran, cellulose and lignin). They found that each ligand exhibited a specific and unique affinity for every bile acid and bile salt. In general, cellulose was the weakest binder and lignin the strongest. Vahouny et al. (1980, 1981) showed that various fibers when incubated with tauro-cholate-phospholipid micelles bound cholesterol and phosphatidyl choline as well as the bile salt. Palmitic, oleic and linoleic acids also were bound to various fibers. Story and Lord (1987) showed that the binding facility of bran does not change when lipids or saponins have been extracted but falls sharply after removal of lignin. The binding of fiber to foods and mixed diets has been tested in few instances (Story and Kritchevsky, 1975; Tepper et al., 1984) and could bear exploitation.

The influence of fiber on cholesterol metabolism as reflected by steroid excretion has been studied to some extent. Story and Furumoto

Table 1. Factors which modify activities of both HMG CoA reductase and cholesterol 7α hydroxylase[*]

Increase	Decreases
Bile fistula	Adrenalectomy
Dark period (diurnal)	Fasting
Glucocorticoids	Thyroidectomy
Glucose re-feeding	
Lymph drainage	
Thyroid hormone	

[*] After Bjhorkhem, 1985.

(1990) examined the effects of wheat, corn or barley bran and of apple, carrot and potato fibers in rats fed a cholesterol-free or cholesterol-rich diet. Varying levels of steroid excretion and differences in fecal bile acid spectrum. For instance, changing from cellulose to potato fiber resulted in a 4- to 5-fold increase in muricholic acid excretion. The ratios of neutral fecal steroids (cholesterol, cholestanol, coprostanol and coprostanone) of rats change as a function of dietary fiber (Vahouny et al., 1987). The ratio of coprostanol to coprostanone, for instance, in rats fed alfalfa, pectin or psyllium is 2.83, 5.73 and 1.53, respectively. These findings suggest that it might be of interest to examine steroid excretion as a function of intestinal microflora in fiber-fed rats.

Fiber influences lipid absorption and excretion, as has been demonstrated frequently. The distribution of endogenous or exogenous cholesterol and metabolites was studied in rabbits; regardless of the cholesterol source, dietary fiber reduced appearance in blood and tissues and enhanced excretion as neutral and acidic steroid (Kritchevsky et al., 1975). These findings may be relevant to fiber effects in experimental atherosclerosis. When monkeys were fed cholesterol-free, semi-purified diets containing cellulose, alfalfa or wheat straw. Aortic sudanophilia (%) if cellulose is taken as 1.00 was 1.08 in monkeys fed alfalfa and 0.39 those fed wheat straw. Hepatic cholesterol 7α-hydroxylase activity (cellulose = 1.00) was 0.76 and 1.71 in monkeys fed alfalfa or wheat straw, respectively (Kritchevsky et al., 1981). The data show less severe sudanophilia in aortas of monkeys exhibiting the highest ratio of bile acid synthesis. This observation is another which might be followed up in other species. Neither pectin nor cellulose influence aortic sudanophilia in vervet monkeys fed a semi-purified diet ± 0.1% cholesterol (Kritchevsky et al., 1986) or a "Western" diet which contained 0.61 mg cholesterol/kcal (150 mg cholesterol/100 g diet) (Kritchevsky et al., 1988a).

The question of fiber effects on whole body cholesterol was addressed by Mueller et al. (1983). Rats were fed semi-purified diets containing cellulose, hemicellulose, pectin or lignin. The only difference in plasma lipids was lower triglyceride levels in rats fed pectin or lignin. Liver cholesterol levels were highest (541 ± 62 mg/g) in cellulose fed rats and similar in the other three groups (average 312 ± 14 for the three groups). Hepatic cholesterol 7 α hydroxylase levels were only elevated in rats fed cellulose (compared to controls) and HMG-CoA reductase activity was reduced in all rats except those fed pectin. Carcass lipids were determined and the cellulose-fed rats had the highest levels of carcass cholesterol and triglyceride. The heaviest epididymal and perirenal fat pads were found in the lignin-fed rats (Table 2). Rotenberg and Jakobson (1978) determined the lipid composition of liver and epididymal fat pads in pectin-fed rats but there are few data relating to effects of dietary fiber on carcass lipid or lipid in any organ save the liver.

Investigation in greater depth of fiber effects on lipids other than cholesterol might be warranted. Kritchevsky et al. (1988 b) examined the liver phospholipids of rats fed fibers. In general, lecithin levels were significantly elevated, sphingomyelin levels were significantly depressed and levels of phosphatidyl ethanolamine, lysolicithin and (Phosphatidyl inositol plus phosphatidyl serine) were unaffected (Table 3).

It would also be interesting to obtain more data on fiber effects in small rodents other than rats and mice. This is especially pertinent since

Table 2. Influence of fiber on carcass lipids in rats* (values given as g/100g carcass lipid)

Fiber	Cholesterol	Triglyceride	Phospholipid
Cellulose	1.9 ± 0.3 a	58.6 ± 5.7 ijkl	2.4 ± 0.9 s
Hemicellulose	1.2 ± 0.2 b	34.6 ± 2.0 imno	5.2 ± 1.1
Pectin	1.2 ± 0.2 c	24.3 ± 4.2 jmp	2.9 ± 0.9
Lignin	1.1 ± 0.2 ad	24.4 ± 3.9 knq	5.4 ± 0.9 s
Fiber-free	1.9 ± 0.2 bcd	284 ± 4.2 lr	2.6 ± 1.0
Stock	1.7 ± 0.4	57.4 ± 8.1 opqr	3.3 ± 0.8

* After Mueller *et al.*, 1983.
Rats (8/gp) fed 40% dextrose, 25% casein, 14% corn oil, 15% fiber, 5% salt mix, 1% vitamin mix for 22 days.
Values bearing the same letter are significantly different.

Table 3. Phospholipid distribution in livers of rats fed fiber supplements* (% ± SEM)

| Fiber (% fed) | PHOSPHOLIPID | | | | |
	PC	PE	Sph	LPC	PI + PS
None	43 ± 2	34 ± 0.4	9 ± 1	6 ± 0.4	8 ± 0.3
Particulate					
Alfalfa (10)	54 ± 1	30 ± 1	4 ± 0.3	6 ± 0.3	7 ± 0.4
Cellulose (10)	46 ± 1	34 ± 1	7 ± 0.5	6 ± 0.4	8 ± 0.2
Wheat bran (10)	47 ± 1	30 ± 1	7 ± 2	6 ± 0.2	9 ± 0.1
Soluble ionic					
Pectin (5)	53 ± 2	29 ± 1	6 ± 0.5	5 ± 0.4	7 ± 0.4
Soluble non-ionic					
Guar gum (5)	48 ± 0.4	30 ± 1	7 ± 1	7 ± 0.2	8 ± 0.4
Psyllium (10)	47 ± 2	32 ± 1	7 ± 1	7 ± 0.4	8 ± 0.3

*After Kritchevsky *et al.*, 1988[b].
‡PC, phosphatidycholine; PE, phosphatidyl ethanolamine; Sph, sphingomyelin; LPC, lysophosphatidyl choline; PI, phosphatidyl insitol; PS, phosphatidyl serine.

the gerbil, hamster and guinea pig are replacing the rat in studies of dietary influences on cholesterol metabolism. Wells and Ershoff (1962) studied the effects of adding 5% pectin to the diets of rabbits, hamsters, guinea pigs and rats who were also being fed 1% cholesterol. They compared three dietary groups in each species. One group was fed a basal cholesterol and fiber-free diet, one was fed a diet containing 1% added cholesterol and the third group was fed 1% cholesterol and 5% citrus pectin. Adding cholesterol to the diet of rats led to a 53% increase in plasma cholesterol and a 13.5-fold increase in liver cholesterol. When the diet contained 1% cholesterol and 5% pectin the plasma cholesterol increase was 9%, the liver cholesterol increased 4.7-fold. Addition of 1% cholesterol to the diets of rabbits, hamsters and guinea pigs by 750, 275, and 650%, respectively. Liver cholesterol level increases were 6.2-fold, 28.8-fold and 12-fold in rabbits, hamsters and guinea pigs, respectively. Addition of 5% pectin to the diet further increased plasma and liver cholesterol levels in the rabbits and had no effects in hamsters or guinea pigs.

The foregoing has been a brief review of the salient studies involving mainly dietary fiber and aspects of lipid metabolism other than plasma or liver lipids. Much work remains before we can delineate accurately the overall effect(s) of dietary fiber on lipid metabolism.

References

Bjorkhem, I., 1985, Mechanism of bile acid synthesis in mammalian liver, in: "Sterols and Bile Acids," H. Danielsson and J. Sjovall, eds., Elsevier, Amsterdam.

Crowther, J. S., Drasar, B. S., Hill, M. J., MacLennan, R., Magnin, D., Peach, S., and Teah-Chan, C. H., 1976, Fecal steroids and bacteria and large bowel cancer in Hong Kong by socioeconomic groups. Br. J. Cancer 34:191.

Eastwood, M. A. and Hamilton, D., 1968, Studies on the adsorption of bile salts to nonabsorbed components of diet. Biochim. Biophys. Acta 152:165.

Heuman, D. M., Vlahcevic, L. R., Barley, M. L., and Hylemon, P. B., 1988, Regulation of bile acid synthesis II. Effect of bile acid feeding on enzymes regulating hepatic cholesterol and bile acid synthesis in the rat. Hepatology 8:892.

Kritchevsky, D., Davidson, L. M., Goodman, G. T., Tepper, S. A., and Mendelsohn, D., 1986, Influence of dietary fiber on lipids and aortic composition of vervet monkeys. Lipids 21:338.

Kritchevsky, D., Davidson, L. M., Krendel, D. A., Vander Watt, J. J., Russell, D., Friedland, S., and Mendelsohn D., 1981, Influence of dietary fiber on aortic sudanophilia in vervet monkeys. Ann. Nutr. Metab. 25:125.

Kritchevsky, D., Davidson, L. M., Scott, D. A., Vander Watt, J. J., and Mendelsohn, D., 1988a, Effects of dietary fiber in vervet monkeys fed "Western" diets. Lipids 23:164.

Kritchevsky, D. and Tepper, S. A., 1965, Factors affecting atherosclerosis in rabbits fed cholesterol-free diets. Life Sci. 4:1467.

Kritchevsky, D. and Tepper, S. A., 1968, Experimental atherosclerosis in rabbits fed cholesterol-free diets: Influence of chow components. J. Atheroscler. Res. 8:357.

Kritchevsky, D., Tepper, S. A., Kim, H. K., Moses, D. E., and Story, J. A., 1975, Experimental atherosclerosis in rabbits fed cholesterol-free diets 4. Investigation into the source of cholesterolemia. Exp. Mol. Pathol. 22:11.

Kritchevsky, D., Tepper, S. A., Satchithanandam, S., Cassidy, M. M., and Vahouny, G. V., 1988b, Dietary fiber supplements: effects on serum and liver lipids and on liver phospholipid composition in rats. Lipids 23:318.

Mueller, M. A., Cleary, M. P., and Kritchevsky, D., 1983, Influence of dietary fiber on lipid metabolism in meal-fed rats. J. Nutr. 113:2229.

Owen, R. W., Dodo, M., Thompson, M. H., and Hill, M. J., 1984, The faecal ratio of lithocholic to deoxycholic acid may be an important aetological factor in colorectal cancer. Biochem. Soc. Trans. 12:861.

Portman, O. W. and Murphy, P., 1958, Excretion of bile acids and hydroxysterols by rats. Arch. Biochem. Biophys. 76:367.

Portman, O. W., 1960, Nutritional influences on the metabolism of bile acids. Am. J. Clin. Nutr. 8:462.

Rotenberg, S. and Jakobson, P. E., 1978, The effect of dietary pectin on lipid composition of blood, skeletal muscle and internal organs of rats. J. Nutr. 108:1384.

Shefer, S., Nguyen, L. B., Salen, G., Ness, G. C., Tint, G. S., and Batta, A. K., 1991, Regulation of cholesterol 7a hydroxylase by hepatic 7a hydroxylated bile acid flux and newly synthesized cholesterol supply. J. Biol. Chem. 266:2693.

Story, J. A. and Furumoto, 1990, Dietary fiber and bile acid metabolism, in: "Dietary Fiber: Chemistry, Physiology and Health Effects," D. Kritchevsky, C. Bonfield and J. W. Anderson, eds., Plenum, New York.

Story, J. A. and Kritchevsky, D., 1976, Comparison of binding of various bile acids and bile salts in vitro by several types of fiber. J. Nutr. 106:1292.

Story, J. A. and Kritchevsky, D. 1975, Binding of sodium taurocholate to various foodstuffs. Nutr. Rep. Int. 11:161.

Story, J. A., and Lord, S. L., 1987, Bile salts, in vitro studies with fibre components. Scand. J. Gastroenterol. 22: Suppl. 129:174.

Tepper, S. A., Goodman, G. T., and Kritchevsky, D., 1984, Diet nutrition intake and metabolism in populations at high and low risk for colon cancer. Binding of bile salts to dietary residues. Am. J. Clin. Nutr. 40:947.

Vahouny, G. V., Khalafi, R., Satchithanandam, S., Watkins, D. W., Story, J. A., Cassidy, M. M., and Kritchevsky, D., 1987, Dietary fiber supplementation and fecal bile acids, neutral steroids and divalent cations in rats. J. Nutr. 117:2009.

Vahouny, G. V., Tombes, R., Cassidy, M. M., Kritchevsky, D., and Gallo, L. L., 1980, Dietary Fiber V. Binding of bile salts, phospholipids and cholesterol from mixed micelles by bile acid sequestrants and dietary fiber. Lipids 15:1012.

Vahouny, G. V., Tombes, R., Cassidy, M. M., Kritchevsky, D., and Gallo, L. L., 1981, Dietary Fibers VI. Binding of fatty acids and monoolein from mixed micelles containing bile salts and lecithin. Proc. Soc. Exp. Biol. Med. 166:12.

Vlahcevic, L. R., Heuman, D. H., and Hylemon, P. B., 1989, Physiology and patho-physiology of enterohepatic circulation, in: "Hepatology, 2nd Edition," D. Zakim and T. Boyer, eds., W. B. Saunders, Philadelphia.

Wells, A. F., and Ershoff, B. H., 1962, Comparative effects of pectin NF administration on the cholesterol-fed rabbit, guinea pig, hamster and rat. Proc. Soc. Exp. Biol. Med. 111:147.

In Vitro and In Vivo Models for Predicting the Effect of Dietary Fiber and Starchy Foods on Carbohydrate Metabolism

Thomas M.S. Wolever, M.D., Ph.D.
Department of Nutritional Sciences,
Clinical Nutrition and Risk Factor Modification Center,
St. Michael's Hospital, University of Toronto,
Toronto, Ontario, Canada M5S 1A8

Introduction

The identification of simple in vitro and in vivo tests to predict the physiologic effects and long-term health benefits of dietary fiber and carbohydrate foods would have widespread implications for the scientific and lay communities in both the public and private sectors. Such knowledge would further understanding of the mechanism(s) by which carbohydrate foods produce health benefits; help improve dietary recommendations; facilitate the design and development of foods or food processing techniques with health benefits; allow regulatory agencies to develop legislation regarding appropriate health claims for high fiber foods; and help the food industry assess carbohydrate foods in order to validate health claims.

Dietary fiber and high fiber foods are believed to affect carbohydrate metabolism by two major mechanisms: reducing the rate of absorption of carbohydrate from the gastrointestinal tract; and increasing colonic fermentation.

A number of lines of evidence suggest that slowing the rate of absorption of nutrients influences systemic metabolism. The ability of purified dietary fibers to slow the diffusion of glucose out of dialysis sacs in vitro is directly related to their blood glucose and insulin lowering ability (Jenkins et al., 1986). The rates of digestion of foods in vitro are related to their blood glucose (O'Dea et al., 1981; Jenkins et al., 1982; Brand JC et al., 1985; Thorburn AW et al., 1987; Bornet et al., 1987) and insulin responses (Bornet et al., 1987; Wolever et al., 1988). Sipping glucose solution or liquid formula diet slowly over 3 hours compared to taking the same amount as a bolus, as a model of slow absorption, mimics the reduced blood glucose and insulin responses seen with viscous fibers and slowly digested foods (Jenkins et al., 1990; Wolever, 1990a). Thus, the acute blood glucose response can be used as an index of slow absorption.

By definition, dietary fiber is not broken down by human digestive enzymes and enters the colon. In addition, 5–20% of dietary starch escapes digestion in the small intestine and enters the colon (Stephen et al., 1983; Englyst and Cummings, 1985; Englyst and Cummings, 1986; Wolever et al., 1986; Levitt et al., 1987). Carbohydrate entering the colon is fermented with the production of the short chain fatty acids acetic, propionic and butyric acids which are absorbed from the colon and may mediate some of the long-term effects of high fiber diets (Royall et al., 1990).

This paper will review the utility of some in vitro models in predicting the effects of dietary fiber and different carbohydrate foods on blood glucose responses and colonic fermentation. In addition, the use of the glycemic index as an in vivo model of carbohydrate metabolism will be reviewed to see if it predicts the long-term effects of high carbohydrate diets on carbohydrate and lipid metabolism in diabetes.

In Vitro Models

Dietary Fiber Analysis

The dietary fiber content of foods appears to be a fairly good predictor of the digestibility of starch in foods, but a relatively weak predictor of their blood glucose responses.

Between 5 and 20% of dietary starch escapes digestion in the small intestine and enters the colon, where it is fermented (Stephen et al., 1983; Englyst and Cummings, 1985; Englyst and Cummings, 1986; Wolever et al., 1986; Levitt et al., 1987). Variation in starch digestibility is probably due to many factors, but there are insufficient data to allow the role of dietary fiber to be assessed with certainty. In addition, it is not known if the values for starch digestibility derived using different methods can be compared directly. We measured the amount of available carbohydrate in ileostomy effluent using a standard method for 20 different foods (Jenkins et al., 1987a). Although only one subject with an ileostomy tested all the foods, we found a very close positive correlation between the amount of available carbohydrate in ileostomy effluent and total dietary fiber in the test foods measured using the AOAC gravimetric technique (Prosky et al., 1984) (r=0.885). Using Englyst's published dietary fiber values (Englyst et al., 1988, 1989), we found a similar positive correlation between available carbohydrate in ileal effluent and total non-starch polysaccharides (NSP) (Figure 1). Most dietary fiber fractions correlated highly with available carbohydrate in ileal effluent, but total insoluble NSP was the best predictor (Figure 1, Table 1). The relationship between total fiber intake and carbohydrate digestibility has recently been confirmed in a larger number of subjects with an ileostomy (Steinhart et al., 1992).

The dietary fiber contents of foods are not closely related to their blood glucose responses (Table 2). The relationship obtained depends upon the number and type of foods studied. The first glycemic index (GI) paper found no correlation between total dietary fiber and GI for over 60 foods (Jenkins et al., 1981). It was thought at the time that this was because total fiber analysis did not distinguish between soluble and

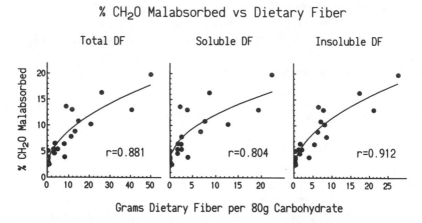

Figure 1. Relationship between dietary fiber content of foods (g/80g available carbohydrate portion) and % carbohydrate malabsorbed (MAL). Carbohydrate digestibility determined by recovery in ileal effluent (Jenkins et al., 1987a). Regressions equations: total fiber (TDF), %MAL = 1.66+2.28* TDF^0.5; soluble fiber (SDF), %MAL = 3.00+2.85*SDF^0.5; insoluble fiber (IDF), %MAL = 1.26+3.21*IDF^0.5.

insoluble fibers and that only the former would reduce blood glucose. Therefore, it was surprising that there was no relationship between Anderson's soluble fiber values (Anderson and Bridges, 1988) and GI for the 25 foods for which both values were available (Wolever, 1990b). Even more unexpected was the fact that cellulose was closely related to GI, since purified cellulose has no effect on blood glucose responses in vivo. It was subsequently reported that soluble fiber was significantly related to the blood glucose responses of foods (Nishimune et al., 1991); however, only 16 foods were studied and oats were not included. Englyst has published fiber values for over 50 foods for which GI values are known (Englyst et al., 1988, 1989), and the relationship between

Table 1. Percent of available carbohydrate (CHO) in ileal effluent, weight (W) and Soluble (SDF) insoluble (IDF) and total (TDF) fiber content of 20 foods

	% CHO in ileal effluent	Composition (g/80g CHO)			
		WT	**SDF**	**IDF**	**TDF**
Cereal products					
Barley	13.0	115	3.9	7.8	11.7
Bulgur	6.4	115	2.5	5.4	7.9
Instant rice	5.1	98	0.0	0.4	0.4
Long grain white rice	3.9	104	0.0	0.4	0.4
Parboiled white rice	3.6	102	0.0	0.4	0.4
Pumpernickel bread 1	8.8	174	6.8	6.3	13.1
Pumpernickel bread 2	10.8	197	7.7	7.1	14.8
Spaghetti	4.6	115	1.7	1.6	3.3
White bread	5.4	188	1.7	1.3	3.0
White Macaroni	6.5	115	1.8	1.7	3.6
Wholemeal bread	7.8	216	2.6	8.6	11.2
Wholemeal rye bread	3.9	183	4.0	4.1	8.1
Breakfast cereals					
Corn chex	2.5	95	0.4	0.5	0.9
Oat bran	10.2	168	12.8	8.1	20.8
Rice chex	2.9	96	0.1	0.4	0.5
Legumes					
Canned chick peas	16.3	544	8.7	17.4	26.1
Canned kidney beans	13.0	607	19.4	21.2	40.7
Canned pinto beans	19.8	605	22.4	27.8	50.2
Red lentils	13.6	180	2.3	6.5	8.8
Vegetables					
Instant mashed potato	5.4	97	2.6	2.1	4.8

Carbohydrate digestibility from (Jenkins et al., 1987a). Dietary fiber calculated from (Englyst et al., 1988, 1989).

Table 2. Glycemic index (GI) values, weight and soluble (SDF), insoluble (IDF) and total (TDF) dietary fiber content (g/50g available carbohydrate) of 53 foods

	GI	Weight	SDF	IDF	TDF
Cereal products					
Barley	36	59.8	2.0	4.1	6.1
Brown rice	81	62.3	0.0	1.2	1.2
Buckwheat	78	70.0	0.7	0.8	1.5
Cornmeal	99	65.1	0.2	0.9	1.1
Millet	103	68.0	0.1	1.22	1.3
Pumpernickel bread	68	109.9	4.3	4.0	8.2
Rye bread	89	102.0	3.8	3.7	7.4
Rye grain	47	65.9	2.6	4.9	7.5
Ryvita	95	70.8	2.8	5.5	8.3
Wheat grain	63	76.0	1.6	5.9	7.4
White Bread	100	100.6	1.0	0.7	1.7
White Macaroni	64	59.5	1.0	0.9	1.8
White rice	81	60.0	0.0	0.2	0.2
White spaghetti	67	59.5	0.9	0.8	1.7
Whole wheat bread	100	119.6	1.4	4.8	6.2
Whole wheat spagetti	61	68.0	1.4	4.4	5.7
Breakfast cereals					
All bran	74	116.3	4.8	23.7	28.5
Bran flakes	110	76.1	2.3	6.3	8.6
Cornflakes	121	58.8	0.2	0.3	0.5
Muesli	96	75.5	1.3	3.4	4.7
Oat bran	80	105.0	8.8	5.6	14.4
Oatmeal	89	68.7	3.1	2.2	5.3
Puffed rice	132	56.8	0.1	0.2	0.3
Shredded wheat	97	73.6	1.5	5.7	7.2
Weetabix	109	71.1	2.2	4.7	6.9
Cookies					
Digestives	82	75.8	0.8	0.8	1.7
Rich tea	80	66.0	0.7	0.4	1.1
Shortbread	88	76.3	0.6	0.5	1.1
Water biscuits	100	66.0	1.2	0.9	2.0
Legumes					
Baked beans	70	485.4	10.2	6.8	17.0
Butter beans	46	100.4	6.3	9.7	16.1
Chick peas	47	100.0	3.3	7.4	10.7
Dried peas	50	100.0	1.6	3.9	5.5
Frozen peas	65	694.4	11.1	25.0	36.1
Haricot beans	54	109.9	8.7	10.0	18.7
Kidney beans	43	111.1	7.7	9.8	17.4
Peanuts	15	581.4	11.0	25.0	36.0
Red lentils	38	94.0	1.2	3.4	4.6
Soya beans	20	212.8	14.5	18.9	33.4
Vegetables					
Beetroot	93	833.3	10.0	10.8	20.8
Canned corn	80	211.0	0.2	2.7	3.0
Carrots	94	925.9	13.0	9.3	2.2
New Potato	80	273.2	1.6	1.4	2.7
Parsnip	139	442.5	10.2	7.5	17.7
Potato chips	77	101.4	2.7	2.2	5.0
Sweet potato	70	232.6	2.6	3.0	5.6
Yam	74	154.3	0.8	1.2	2.0
Fruit					
Apples	52	420.2	2.9	4.2	7.1
Banana	84	260.4	1.8	1.0	2.9
Orange juice	71	531.9	0.5	0.0	0.5
Oranges	59	588.2	8.2	4.1	12.4
Raisins	93	77.6	0.9	0.8	1.6

these confirms the earlier observations using Anderson's values. Total and soluble NSP were weakly related to GI, but insoluble NSP was a better predictor (Figure 2). For both Anderson's and Eglyst's values, uronic acids in insoluble fiber was the strongest predictor of GI (Figure 2), accounting for 49% of the variability in GI.

Fiber Viscosity

Fiber viscosity has not been measured in most studies. Nevertheless, the fibers can be classified as viscous or non-viscous, and this appears to

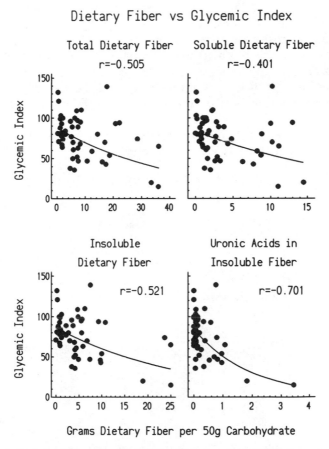

Figure 2. Relationship between dietary fiber content of foods and glycemic index (GI) for 52 foods. Regression equations: total fiber (TDF), GI = 87xe^(-0.023 x TDF); soluble fiber (SDF), GI = 83xe^ (-0.043 x SDF); insoluble fiber (IDF), GI = 86xe^ (-0.036 x IDF); uronic acids in IDF (UA), GI = 84xe^ (-0.51 x UA).

be a fairly accurate way to predict whether purified fiber will reduce acute blood glucose responses (Figure 3) (Wolever and Jenkins, 1992) and in longer term studies improve blood glucose and lipid control in diabetic patients (Figure 4).

In the two studies where viscosity was measured, viscosity was shown to be related to the ability of various purified fibers to flatten blood glucose and insulin responses in human subjects (Jenkins et al., 1978; Edwards et al., 1987). Unfortunately, the data cannot be pooled because the viscosity measurements are not comparable, being measured at different fiber concentrations using different techniques and different viscosity units. In future studies in the area a number of factors should be considered. At least some viscous fibers form solutions which are pseudoplastic in nature, that is, the viscosity is a function of the shear rate. Viscosity measurements might most physiologically be carried out at a low shear rate as found in the intestine. The effect of pH changes designed to mimic passage through the stomach and duodenum should be considered since it has been shown that some fibers maintain their viscosity under these conditions, while others do not (Edwards et al., 1987).

There has been no attempt made, to my knowledge, to relate the viscosity of carbohydrate foods to physiologic responses in human sub-

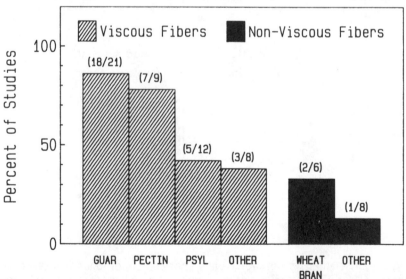

Figure 3. Percent of studies reporting a significant reduction in acute blood glucose response after various purified viscous and non-viscous fiber (Wolever and Jenkins, 1992).

jects. Both fiber and starch may contribute to viscosity, but the viscosity due to starch would be reduced rapidly during the digestion process. This would complicate the interpretation of viscosity measurements of whole foods. However, continuous viscosity monitoring during the course of in vitro digestion might yield useful information.

In Vitro Fiber Fermentation

Different fibers are fermented to varying extents; however, the fermentability of fiber in foods may differ from that of purified fiber. For example virtually no purified cellulose is broken down after 24h in vitro fermentation (Jeraci and Van Soest, 1986; McBurney and Thompson, 1989), whereas about 50% of the cellulose in the diet disappears upon passage through the human GI tract (Cummings et al., 1986). In addition other factors such as transit time (Van Soest, 1982) and the nature of the bacterial population in the colon (Weaver et al., 1989) will influence the extent of fiber fermentation and the exact products released.

We studied breath hydrogen and methane levels of healthy subjects for 12h after they took 20g of guar, pectin, psyllium, soy polysaccharide, or cellulose (Wolever and Robb, 1992) and compared the results to

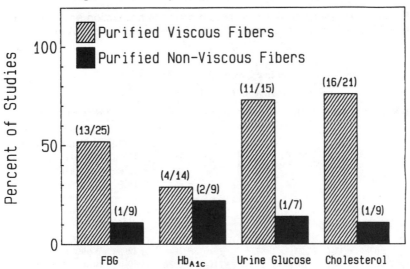

Figure 4. Percent of studies reporting significant reductions in fasting blood glucose (FBG), glycosylated hemoglobin (HbA1c), insulin dose and serum cholesterol after treatment of diabetes with viscous or non-viscous purified fiber (Wolever and Jenkins, 1992).

in vitro fermentation of the same fibers (McBurney and Thompson, 1989). Despite a 10-fold range of rates of digestion of the fibers in vitro, none of the fibers increased breath hydrogen levels. However, there were small changes in breath methane which related significantly to the in vitro fermentability of the fibers (Figure 5). Breath gases and blood acetate responses have been assessed after adding pectin, guar and psyllium to polysaccharide-free diets.

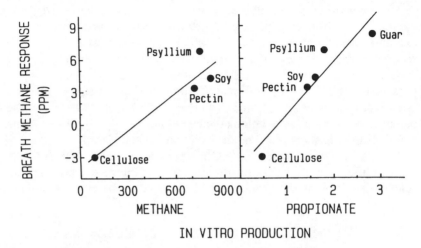

Figure 5. Relationship between breath methane production and in vitro fermentability of five purified dietary fibers (Wolever and Robb, 1992).

Table 3. Long-term effects of low glycemic index (GI) diets

| WK | SUB | Change on Low GI Diet | | | | | | Reference |
		GI	PPBG	GlyPr	In/CP	CHOL	TG	
2	6H	−39%	−37%*	−37%*	−2%n	−11%+	−13%n	Jenkins et al. 1987a
2	8N	−26%		−3%n	−3%n	−3%n	0%n	Jenkins et al. 1988
2	15N	−31%	−29%*	−3%+	−3%+	−7%+	−12%n	Wolever et al. 1992c
3	8I	−23%		−22%*	−22%*	0%n	−16%+	Fontvieille et al. 1988
4	12T	−16%				−9%*	−16%*	Jenkins et al. 1985
4	24T	−13%				−9%*	−19%*	Jenkins et al. 1987b
4	6C	−13%				−3%n	−1%n	Jenkins et al. 1987b
4	24D	−12%	−13%n	9%n	0%n			Calle-Pascual 1988
6	7I	−15%		−27%+	−14%+	−9%*	−3%n	Collier et al. 1988
6	6N	−33%		−8%n		−7%*	−22%n	Wolever et al. 1992
12	16N	−14%	−14%+	−11%+	−11%+	0%n	+6%n	Brand et al. 1991

WK = length of diet periods in weeks; SUB = subjects, H = healthy, N = NIDDM, I = IDDM, D = diabetic (both IDDM and NIDDM); T = hypertriglyceridemic, C = hypercholesterolemic (type 2a); GI = diet glycemic index; PPBG = post-prandial blood glucose response area; GlyPr = glycosylated albumin or hemoglobin; In/CP = insulin dose (in IDDM subjects) or urine c-peptide output; CHOL = serum cholesterol; TG = serum triglycerides; n = non-significant; + = p < 0.05; * = p < 0.01.

Table 4. Effects in diabetic patients of increasing fiber intake from whole foods with no change in available carbohydrate

| GI | % Change on high fiber diet | | | | | Reference |
	FBG	PPBG	UGO	CHOL	TG	
L	−34%*	−37%**	−82%+	−14%*	−12%*	Rivellese *et al.* 1980
L	−6%ns	−24%++		−20%**	ns	Riccardi *et al.* 1984
L	−24%++	−18%++				Garcia *et al.* 1982
L	−38%**	−30%***	−76%**			Kinmouth *et al.* 1982
L		−20%*	−19%ns	0%ns		Manhire *et al.* 1981
L		+1%ns		−5%ns	−26%ns	Venhous *et al.* 1988
L	−9%ns	−5%fns		−13%*		Stephens *et al.* 1985
H	−6%*	−13%**	−37%*	+2%ns	+11%ns	Karlström *et al.* 1984
H	+10%ns	ns	−10%ns	+5%ns	+8%ns	Hollenbeck *et al.* 1986
H	−14%	−15%				Nygren *et al.* 1984
H	−6%**	+6%ns		−4%+	+10%ns	Hagander *et al.* 1988
H	−7%f			−6%ns	−7%ns	Silvis *et al.* 1990

GI = fiber increased with low (L) or high (H) glycemic index (H) foods; FBG = fasting blood glucose; PPBG = postprandial blood glucose; UGO = urinary glucose output; CHOL = serum cholesterol; TG = serum triglyceride; *$p < 0.05$; +$p < 0.025$; **$p < 0.01$; ++$p < 0.005$; ***$p < 0.001$.
f change in HbA1c (ns).

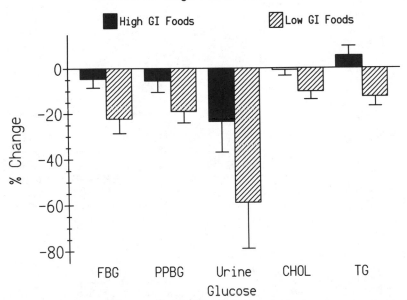

Figure 6. Mean ± SEM % changes in fasting (FBG) and postprandial (PPBG) blood glucose levels, urine glucose output, and serum cholesterol (CHOL) and triglycerides (TG) after increasing dietary fiber intake with high or low glycemic index (GI) foods (data from Table 4).

In one study, pectin increased breath hydrogen and serum acetate, but methane was not measured (Pomare et al., 1985). Guar had no effect on breath hydrogen, but increased breath methane and serum acetate, whereas psyllium had no effect on hydrogen, methane or acetate (Wolever et al., 1992a). These studies suggest that the fermentation of fibers which are readily fermented in vitro can be detected in vivo. However, breath hydrogen may not be the best marker of fermentation, and increased concentrations of breath gases and serum acetate may not be seen for slowly fermented fibers such as psyllium.

In Vivo Model

Gycemic Index

The glycemic index is a classification of foods according to their blood glucose responses. The definition and methods used to determine the

Table 5. Effects of high carbohydrate, high fiber diets

GI	% Change on high fiber carbohydrate diet					
	FBG	HbAlc	U/I/B	CHOL	TG	Reference
L	−13%ns		U-56%***	−19%***	+23%ns	Rivillese et al. 1980
L	−7%ns		B-15%+	−16%+	ns	Riccardi et al. 1984
L	0%ns		B-20%*	−18%*	−6%ns	Parillo et al. 1988
L	−26%++		I-56%+	−24%***	−15%ns	Kiehm et al. 1976
L	−7%ns		I-58%***	−29%***	−2%ns	Anderson et al. 1989
L	−5%*			−22%***	+21%ns	Fukagawa et al. 1990
L	+5%ns		U-11%ns	−10%ns	ns	Abbott et al. 1989
L	−15%***	−10%+	U-94%*	−14%**	−14%ns	Simpson et al. 1981
L	−38%ns	−2%ns	U-80%*	−15%*	−18%ns	Simpson et al. 1981
L	−23%*	−19%*		−15%*		Stevens et al. 1985
L	−5%	−12%**	U-64%ns	−4%ns	+11%ns	Bruttomesso et al. 1989
L	−25%***		I-90%***	−5ns	−43%++	Anderson et al. 1978
L	−18%*			−13%*	−15%*	Barnard et al. 1983
H	−11%ns		B ns			Lindsay et al. 1984
H	−18%**		U-33%ns	−10%***	+10%ns	Simpson et al. 1988
H	−1%ns		U-14%ns	−22%*	+20%**	Hollenbeck et al. 1985a
H	−12%**	−11%**	R+26%+	−14%***	−6%ns	Simpson et al. 1979a
H	−36%**	+1%ns	I −6%**	−10%***	−9%ns	Simpson et al. 1979b
H	−1%ns	+2%ns	I 0%ns	−22%*	+61%**	Hollenbeck et al. 1985b
H		−15%***		−2%ns	−17%*	Dodson et al. 1984
H		+19%**				McCulloch et al. 1985
H		−30%	I-65%*			Ney et al. 1982
H	+17%**	+6%ns	B +7%			Scott et al. 1988

GI = fiber increased with low (L) or high (H) glycemic index foods; FBG = fasting blood glucose; HbAlc = glycosylated hemoglobin; U = urine glucose; I = insulin dose; R = glucose disposal rate during insulin clamp; B = mean blood glucose; CHOL = serum cholesterol; TG = serum triglyceride; *p < 0.05; +p < 0.025; **p < 0.01; ++p < 0.005; ***p < 0.001.
Duplicate citation is for different patient groups (IDDM, NIDDM)

glycemic index of foods have been reviewed elsewhere (Wolever et al., 1991). There have been a number of studies showing that reducing the glycemic impact of the diet, with no change in total carbohydrate or dietary fiber intakes, improves overall blood glucose and lipid control in patients with diabetes (Table 3). This suggests that this may be a useful model for predicting the long-term effects of high fiber diets.

Twelve studies have been reviewed where dietary fiber intake was increased using normal foods with no change in overall carbohydrate intake (Table 4). There were consistent reductions of blood glucose and lipids in the 7 studies where dietary fiber was increased using low glycemic index foods such as legumes and pasta. Smaller and less consistent changes were seen when fiber was increased using cereal products with a high glycemic index such as wholemeal bread (Figure 6). Similarly, the effects of increasing carbohydrate and fiber intakes on blood glucose and lipid control were more desirable in the 13 studies where carbohydrate and fiber intakes were increased using low glycemic index foods, than in the 10 studies where high glycemic index foods were used (Table 5; Figure 7).

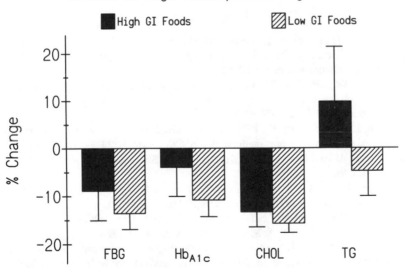

Figure 7. Mean ± SEM % changes in fasting blood glucose (FBG), HbA1c, and serum cholesterol (CHOL) and triglycerides (TG) after increasing carbohydrate and fiber intakes with high or low glycemic index (GI) foods (data from Table 5).

Conclusion

Dietary fiber analysis, rate of digestion, viscosity, and fermentability have been used as in vitro models of fiber, and measurement of the blood glucose response is a simple in vivo test. In general, these models are useful for identifying purified fibers and high fiber foods with beneficial effects on carbohydrate metabolism. Foods which are slowly digested in vitro and viscous purified fibers reduce acute blood glucose responses and improve blood glucose and lipid control in diabetic patients. The dietary fiber content of foods predicts the overall digestibility of their available carbohydrate, with high fiber foods resulting in increased amounts of available carbohydrate entering the colon. In addition, high fiber foods tend to have low blood glucose responses. However, the relationship between fiber and glycemic index is not very strong due to the many other food factors which influence glycemic responses. Unexpectedly, the insoluble fiber content of foods is a better predictor of their glycemic indices than soluble fiber. Fermentable purified fibers increase breath methane and serum acetate levels in vivo, but do not increase breath hydrogen levels. The ability to reduce acute blood glucose responses indicates that a starchy food or purified fiber is likely to improve diabetic blood glucose control, reduce insulin requirements, and reduce blood lipid levels.

References

Abbott, W. G. H., Boyce, V. L., Grundy, S. M., and Howard, B. V., 1989, Effects of replacing saturated fat with complex carbohydrate in diets of subjects with NIDDM. Diabetes Care 12:102-107.

Anderson, J. W. and Ward, K., 1978, Long-term effects of high carbohydrate, high fiber diets on glucose and lipid metabolism: a preliminary report in patients with diabetes. Diabetes Care 1:77-82.

Anderson, J. W. and Ward, K., 1979, High carbohydrate, high fiber diets for insulin treated men with diabetes mellitus. Am. J. Clin. Nutr. 32:2312-2321.

Anderson, J. W. and Bridges, S. R., 1988, Dietary fiber content of selected foods. Am. J. Clin. Nutr. 47:440-447.

Barnard, R. J., Massey, M. R., Cherny, S., O'Brien, L. T., and Pritikin, N., 1983, Long-term use of a high-complex-carbohydrate, high-fiber, low-fat diet and exercise in the treatment of NIDDM patients. Diabetes Care 6:268-273.

Bornet, F. R. J., Fontvieille, A. M., Rizkalla, S., Colonna, P., Blayo, A., Mercier, C., and Slama, G., 1987, Insulin and glycemic responses in healthy humans to native starches processed in different ways: correlation with in vitro alpha-amylase hydrolysis. Am. J. Clin. Nutr. 45:588-595.

Brand, J. C., Colagiuri, S., Crossman, S., Allen, A., Roberts, D. C. K., and Truswell, A. S., 1991, Low glycemic index foods improve long term glycemic control in non-insulin-dependent diabetes mellitus. Diabetes Care 14:95-101.

Brand, J. C., Nicholson, P. L., Throburn, A. W., and Truswell, A. S., 1985, Food processing and the glycemic index. Am. J. Clin. Nutr. 42:1192-1196.

Bruttomesso, D., Briani, G., Bilardo, G., Vitale, E., Lavagnini, T., Marescotti, C., Duner, E., Giorato, D., and Tiengo, A., 1989, The medium-term effect of natural or extractive dietary fibers on plasma amino acids and lipids in type 1 diabetes. Diab. Res. Clin. Prac. 6:149-155.

Calle-Pascual, A.L., Gomez, V., Leon, E., and Bordiu, E., 1988, Foods with a low glycemic index do not improve glycemic control of both type 1 and type 2 diabetic patients after one month of therapy. Diabete Metab. (Paris) 14:629-633.

Collier, G. R., Giudici, S., Kalmusky, J., Wolever, T. M. S., Helman, G., Wesson, V., Ehrlich, G. R., and Jenkins, D. J. A., 1988, Low glycaemic index starchy foods improve glucose control and lower serum cholesterol in diabetic children. Diab. Nutr. Metab. 1:11-19.

Cummings, J. H., Englyst, H. N., and Wiggins, H. S., 1986, The role of carbohydrates in lower gut function. Nutr. Rev. 44:50-54.

Dodson, P. M., Pacy, P. J., Bal, P., Kubicki, A. J., Fletcher, R. F., and Taylor, K. G., 1984, A controlled trial of a high fibre, low fat and low sodium diet for mild hypertension in Type 2 (non-insulin-dependent) diabetic patients. Diabetologia 27:522-526.

Edwards, C. A., Blackburn, N. A., Craigen, L., Davison, P., Tomlin, J., Sugden, K., Johnson, I. T., and Read, N. W., 1987, Viscosity of food gums determined in vitro related to their hypoglycemic actions. Am. J. Clin. Nutr. 46:72-77.

Englyst, H. N. and Cummings, J. H., 1985, Digestion of the polysaccharides of some cereal foods in the human small intestine. Am. J. Clin. Nutr. 42:778-787.

Englyst, H. N. and Cummings, J. H., 1986, Digestion of the carbohydrates of banana (Musa Paradisiaca sapientum) in the human small intestine. Am. J. Clin. Nutr. 44:42-50.

Englyst, H. N., Bingham, S. A., Runswick, S. A., Collinson, E., and Cummings, J. H., 1988, Dietary fibre (non-starch polysaccharides) in fruit, vegetables and nuts. J. Hum. Nutr. Dietet. 1:247-286.

Englyst, H. N., Bingham, S. A,. Runswick, S. A., Collinson, E., and Cummings, J. H., 1989, Dietary fibre (non-starch polysaccharides) in cereal products. J. Hum. Nutr. Dietet. 2:253-271.

Fontvieille, A. M., Acosta, M., Rizkalla, S. W., Bornet, F., David, P., Letanoux, M., Tchobroutsky, G., and Slama, G., 1988, A moderate switch from high to low glycaemic-index foods for 3 weeks improves the metabolic control of Type I (IIDM) diabetic subjects. Diab. Nutr. Metab. 1:139-143.

Fukagawa, N. K., Anderson, J. W., Hageman, G., Young, V. R., and Minaker, K. L., 1990, High-carbohydrate, high-fiber diets increase peripheral insulin sensitivity in healthy young and old adults. Am. J. Clin. Nutr. 52:524-528.

Garcia, R., Garza, S., De La Garza, S, Espinosa-Campos, J., and Ovalle-Berumen, F., 1982, Dieta alta in fibras preparada con alimentos regionales como complemento in il control de la diabetes. Rev. Invest. Clin. (Mex) 34:105-111.

Hagander, B., Asp, N.-G., Efendic, S., Nilsson-Ehle, P., and Scherstén, B., 1988, Dietary fiber decreased fasting blood glucose levels and plasma LDL concentration in noninsulin-dependent diabetes mellitus patients. Am. J. Clin. Nutr. 47:852-858.

Hollenbeck, C. B., Connor, W. E., Riddle, M. C., Alaupovic, P., and Leklem, J. E., 1985a, The effects of a high-carbohydrate low-fat cholesterol-restricted diet on plasma lipid, lipoprotein, and apoprotein concentrations in insulin-dependent (Type I) diabetes mellitus. Metabolism 34:559-566.

Hollenbeck, C. B., Riddle, M. C., Connor, W. E., and Leklem, J. E., 1985b, The effects of subject-selected high carbohydrate, low fat diets on glycemic control in insulin dependent diabetes mellitus. Am. J. Clin. Nutr. 41:293-298.

Hollenbeck, C. B., Coulston, A. M., and Reaven, G. M., 1986, To what extent does increased dietary fiber improve glucose and lipid metabolism in patients with non-insulin-dependent diabetes mellitus (NIDDM)? Am. J. Clin. Nutr. 43:16-24.

Jenkins, D. J. A., Wolever, T. M. S., Leeds, A. R., Gassull, M. A., Dilawari, J. B., Goff, G. V., Metz, G. L., and Alberti, K. G. M. M., 1978, Dietary fibres, fibre analogues and glucose tolerance: importance of viscosity. Brit. Med. J. 1:1392-1394.

Jenkins, D. J. A., Wolever, T. M. S., Taylor, R. H., Barker, H. M., Fielden, H., Baldwin, J. M., Bowling, A. C., Newman, H. C., Jenkins, A. L., and Goff, D. V., 1981, Glycemic index of foods: a physiological basis for carbohydrate exchange. Am. J. Clin. Nutr. 34:362-366.

Jenkins, D. J. A., Ghafari, H., Wolever, T. M. S., Taylor, R. H., Barker, H. M., Fielden, H., Jenkins, A. L., and Bowling, A. C., 1982, Relationship between the rate of digestion of foods and post-prandial glycaemia. Diabetologia 22:450-455.

Jenkins, D. J. A., Wolever, T. M. S., Kalmusky, J., Giudici, S., Giordano, C., Wong, G. S., Bird, J. H., Patten, R., Hall, M., Buckley, G. C., and Little, J. A., 1985, Low glycemic index foods in the management of hyperlipidemia. Am. J. Clin. Nutr. 42:604-617.

Jenkins, D. J. A., Jenkins, M. A., Wolever, T. M. S., Taylor, R. H., and Ghafari, H., 1986, Slow release carbohydrate: mechanism of action of viscous fibers. J. Clin. Nutr. Gastroenterol. 1:237-241.

Jenkins, D. J. A., Cuff, D., Wolever, T. M. S., Knowland, D., Thompson, L. U., Cohen, Z., and Prokipchuk, E., 1987a, Digestibility of carbohydrate foods in an ileostomate: relationship to dietary fiber, in vitro digestibility, and glycemic response. Am. J. Gastroenterol. 82:709-717.

Jenkins, D. J. A., Wolever, T. M. S., Kalmusky, J., Giudici, S., Giordano, C., Patten, R., Wong, G. S., Bird, J. N., Hall, M., Buckley, G., Csima, A., and Little, J. A., 1987b, Low-glycemic index diet in hyperlipidemia: use of traditional starchy foods. Am. J. Clin. Nutr. 46:66-71.

Jenkins, D. J. A., Wolever, T. M. S., Collier, G. R., Ocana, A., Rao, A. V., Buckley, G., Lam, Y., Mayer, A., and Thompson, L. U., 1987c, The metabolic effects of a low glycemic index diet. Am. J. Clin. Nutr. 46:968-975.

Jenkins, D. J. A., Wolever, T. M. S., Buckley, G., Lam, Y., Giudici, S, Kalmusky, J., Jenkins, A. L., Patten, R. L., Bird, J., Wong, G. S., and Josse, R. G., 1988, Low glycemic-index starchy foods in the diabetic diet. Am. J. Clin. Nutr. 48:248-254.

Jenkins, D. J. A., Wolever, T. M. S., Ocana, A. M., Vuksan, V., Cunnane, S. C., Jenkins, M., Wong, G. S., Singer, W., Bloom, S. R., Blendis, L. M., and Josse,

R. G., 1990, Metabolic effects of reducing rate of glucose ingestion by single bolus versus continuous sipping. Diabetes 39:775-781.

Jeraci, J. L. and Van Soest, P. J., 1986, Interaction between human gut bacteria and fibrous substrates, in: Handbook of Dietary Fiber and Nutrition, (G. Spiller, ed.), CRC Press Inc., Boca Raton, Florida, pp. 299-303.

Karlström, B., Vessby, B., Asp, N.-G., Boberg, M., Gustafsson, I.B., Lithell, H., and Werner, I., 1984, Effects of an increased content of cereal fibre in the diet of Type 2 (non-insulin-dependent) diabetic patients. Diabetologia 26:272-277.

Kiehm, T. G.; Anderson, J. W., and Ward, K., 1976, Beneficial effects of a high carbohydrate high fiber diet in hyperglycemic men. Am. J. Clin. Nutr. 29:895-899.

Kinmouth, A.-L., Angus, R. M., Jenkins, P. A., Smith, M. A., and Baum, D., 1982, Whole foods and increased dietary fibre improve blood glucose control in diabetic children. Arch. Dis. Child. 57:187-194.

Levitt, M. D., Hirsh, P., Fetzer, C. A., Sheahan, M., and Levine, A. S., 1987, H_2 excretion after ingestion of complex carbohydrates. Gastroenterology 92:383-389.

Lindsay, A. N., Hardy, S., Jarrett, L., and Rallinson, M. L., 1984, High-carbohydrate, high-fiber diet in children with type I diabetes mellitus. Diabetes Care 7:63-67.

Manhire, A., Henry, C. L., Hartog, M., and Heaton, K. W., 1981, Unrefined carbohydrate and dietary fibre in treatment of diabetes mellitus. J. Hum. Nutr. 35:99-101.

McBurney, M. I. and Thompson, L. U., 1989, In vitro fermentabilities of purified fiber supplements. J. Food. Sci. 54:347-350.

McCulloch, D. K., Mitchell, R. D., Ampler, J., and Tattersall, R.B., 1985, A prospective comparison of 'conventional' and high carbohydrate/high fibre/low fat diets in adults with established Type 1 (insulin dependent) diabetes. Diabetologia 28:208-212.

Ney, D., Hollingsworth, D. R., and Cousins, L., 1982, Decreased insulin requirement and improved control of diabetes in pregnant women given a high-carbohydrate, high-fiber, low-fat diet. Diabetes Care 5:529-533.

Nishimune, T., Yakushiji, T., Sumimoto, T., Taguchi, S., Konishi, Y., Nakahara, S., Ichikawa, T., and Kunita, N., 1991, Glycemic response and fiber content of some foods. Am. J. Clin. Nutr. 54:414-419.

Nygren, C., Hallmans, G., and Lithner, F., 1984, Effects of high-bran bread on blood glucose control in insulin-dependent diabetic patients. Diabete Metab (Paris) 10:39-43.

O'Dea, K., Snow, P., and Nestel, P., 1981, Rate of starch hydrolysis in vitro as a predictor of metabolic responses to complex carbohydrate in vivo. Am. J. Clin. Nutr. 34:1991-1993.

Parillo, M., Riccardi, G., Pancioni, D., Iovine, C., Contaldo, F., Isernia, C., DeMarco, F., Perrotti, N., and Rivellese, A., 1988, Metabolic consequences of feeding a high-carbohydrate, high-fiber diet to diabetic patients with chronic kidney failure. Am. J. Clin. Nutr. 48:255-259.

Pomare, E. W., Branch, W. J., and Cummings, J. H., 1985, Carbohydrate fermentation in the human colon and its relation to acetate concentrations in venous blood. J. Clin. Invest. 75:1448-1454.

Prosky, S., Asp, N.-G., Furda, I., DeVries, J. W., Schweizer, T. F., and Harland, B. F., 1984, Determination of total dietary fiber in foods, food products, and total diets: interlaboratory study. J. Assoc. Off. Anal. Chem. 67:1044-1052.

Riccardi, G., Rivellese, A., Pacioni, D., Genovese, S., Mastranzo, P., and Mancini, M., 1984, Separate influence of dietary carbohydrate and fibre on the metabolic control in diabetes. Diabetologia 26:116-121.

Rivellese, A., Riccardi, G., Giacco, A., Pancioni, D., Genovese, S., Mattioli, P. L., and Mancini, M., 1980, Effect of dietary fibre on glucose control and serum lipoproteins in diabetic patients. Lancet 2:447-450.

Royall, D., Wolever, T. M. S., and Jeejeebhoy, K. N., 1990, Clinical significance of colonic fermentation. Am. J. Gastroenterol. 85:1307-1312.

Scott, A. R., Attenborough, Y., Peacock, I., Fletcher, E., Jeffcoate, W. J., and Tattersall, R. B., 1988, Comparison of high fibre diets, basal insulin supplements, and flexible insulin treatment for non-insulin dependent (type II) diabetics poorly controlled with sulphonylureas. Brit. Med. J. 297:707-710.

Silvis, N., Vorster, H. H., Mollentze, W. F., de Jager, J., and Huisman, H. W., 1990, Metabolic and haemostatic consequences of dietary fibre and n-3 fatty acids in black type 2 (NIDDM) diabetic subjects: a placebo controlled study. Int. Clin. Nutr. Rev. 10:362-380.

Simpson, H. R. C., Simpson, R. W., Lousley, S., Carter, R. D., Geekie, M., Hockaday, T. D. R., and Mann, J. I., 1981, A high carbohydrate leguminous fibre diet improves all aspects of diabetic control. Lancet 1:1-5.

Simpson, R. W., Mann, J. I., Eaton, J., Moore, R. A., Carter, R, and Hockaday, T. D. R., 1979a, Improved glucose control in maturity onset diabetes treated with high carbohydrate-modified fat diet. Brit. Med. J. 1:1752-1756.

Simpson, R. W., Mann, J. I., Eaton, J., Carter, R, and Hockaday, T. D. R., 1979b, High carbohydrate diets in insulin-dependent diabetes. Brit. Med. J. 2:523-525.

Simpson, R. W., McDonald, J., Wahlqvist, M. L., Balasz, N., Sissons, M., and Atley, L., 1988, Temporal study of metabolic change when poorly controlled non-insulin-dependent diabetics change from low to high carbohydrate and fiber diet. Am. J. Clin. Nutr. 48:104-109.

Stephen, A. M., Haddad, A. C., and Phillips, S. F., 1983, Passage of carbohydrate into the colon: direct measurements in humans. Gastroenterology 85:589-595.

Stevens, J., Burgess, M. B., Kaiser, D. L., and Sheppa, C. M., 1985, Outpatient management of diabetes mellitus with patient education to increase dietary carbohydrate and fiber. Diabetes Care 8:359-366.

Steinhart, A. H., Jenkins, D. J. A., Mitchell, S., Cuff, D., and Prokipchuk, E.J., 1992, Effect of dietary fiber on total carbohydrate losses in ileostomy effluent. Am. J. Gastroenterol. 87:48-54.

Thorburn, A. W., Brand, J. C., and Truswell, A. S., 1987, Slowly digested and absorbed carbohydrate in traditional bushfoods: a protective factor against diabetes? Am. J. Clin. Nutr. 45:98-106.

Van Soest, P. J., 1982, Nutritional Ecology of the Ruminant, O & B Books, Corvallis, Oregon.

Venhous, A. and Chantelau, E., 1988, Self-selected unrefined and refined carbohydrate diets do not affect metabolic control in pump-treated diabetic patients. Diabetologia 31:153-157.

Weaver, G. A., Krause, J. A., Miller, T. L., and Wolin, M. J., 1989, Constancy of glucose and starch fermentations by two different human faecal microbial communities. Gut 30:19-25.

Wolever, T. M. S., 1990a, Metabolic effects of continuous feeding. Metabolism 39:947-951.

Wolever, T. M. S., 1990b, Relationship between dietary fiber content and composition in foods and the glycemic index. Am. J. Clin. Nutr. 51:72-75.

Wolever, T. M. S., 1990c, The glycemic index, in: Aspects of Some Vitamins, Minerals and Enzymes in Health and Disease. World Rev. Nutr. Diet. (G.H. Bourne, ed.), S. Karger, Basel, vol. 62, pp.120-185.

Wolever, T. M. S. and Robb, P. A., 1992, Effect of guar, pectin, psyllium, soy polysaccharide and cellulose on breath hydrogen and methane in healthy subjects. Am. J. Gastroenterol. 87:305-310.

Wolever, T. M. S., and Jenkins, D. J. A., 1992, Effect of fiber and foods on carbohydrate metabolism, in: Handbook of Dietary Fiber in Human Nutrition (G. Spiller, ed.), CRC Press Inc., Boca Raton, Florida, in press.

Wolever, T. M. S., Cohen, Z., Thompson, L. U., Thorne, M. J., Jenkins, M. J. A., Prokipchuk, E. J., and Jenkins, D. J. A., 1986, Ileal loss of available carbohydrate in man: comparison of a breath hydrogen method with direct measurement using a human ileostomy model. Am. J. Gastroenterol. 81:115-122.

Wolever, T. M. S., Jenkins, D. J. A., Collier, G. R., Lee, R., Wong, G. S., and Josse, R. G., 1988, Metabolic response to test meals containing different carbohydrate foods: 1. Relationship between rate of digestion and plasma insulin response. Nutr. Res. 8:573-581.

Wolever, T. M. S., Jenkins, D. J. A., Jenkins, A. L., and Josse, R. G., 1991, The glycemic index: methodology and clinical implications. Am. J. Clin. Nutr. 54.

Wolever, T. M. S., ter Wal, P., Spadafora, P., and Robb, P. A., 1992a, Guar, but not psyllium, increases breath methane and serum acetate concentrations in human subjects. Am. J. Clin. Nutr. 55:719-722.

Wolever, T. M. S., Jenkins D. J. A., Vuksan, V., Jenkins, A. L., Wong, G. S., and Josse, R. G., 1992b, Beneficial effect of low-glycemic index diet in overweight NIDDM subjects. Diabetes Care in press.

Wolever, T. M. S., Jenkins, D. J. A., Vuksan, V., Jenkins, A. L., Buckley, G. C., Wong, G. S., and Josse, R. G., 1992c, Beneficial effect of a low-glycaemic index diet in type 2 diabetes. Diabetic Med. in press.

Animal Models of Obesity: Diet, Inactivity, and Genetics

Linda J. Magrum,[1] Barbara A. Horwitz,[2] and
Judith S. Stern[1,3]
[1]Department of Nutrition
[2]Section of Animal Physiology
[3]Division Clinical Nutrition & Metabolism
University of California Davis, CA 95616

Introduction

Obesity is a significant public health problem in developed nations, largely because of its association with chronic diseases such as cardiovascular disease, diabetes, hypertension, and some forms of cancer (National Research Council [NRC], 1989). In comparison to the early part of the 20th century, obesity has reached epidemic-like proportions. The incidence of obesity increases with increased level of affluence (Dulloo and Miller, 1987). As many as 20% of children and 30% of adults in the United States are considered to be obese, and the numbers appear to be increasing (NRC, 1989). This increase has been attributed, in part, to increased intake of dietary fat and decreased physical activity. Figure 1 illustrates the per capita increase in dietary fat intake in the United States from 1910 to 1980.

It is not clear, however, if the change in incidence of obesity from the early 1900s to the present day reflects our increased intake of dietary fat or changes in other nutrients. During this same period, intake of dietary fiber decreased (NRC, 1989). Given this observation, it is hard to distinguish the effects of decreased dietary fiber from those of increased dietary fat. While epidemiological studies have suggested that fiber intake may be related to body weight, clinical studies are not definitive (Table

1) (Stevens, 1988). The case linking dietary fat and obesity in humans has not yet been proven (NRC, 1989), although the evidence strongly suggests cause and effect. A diet high in fat may result in increased energy intake and energetic efficiency. Data from the laboratory of Lissner and colleagues (1987), for example, reveal that as percent dietary fat increased from 15–20% to 45–50%, energy intake during a 14-day period also increased (Figure 2). Furthermore, the work of Danforth and his colleagues (1985) dramatically illustrates that when adults purposefully overeat in order to gain weight, a comparable amount of weight is

Table 1. Effects of dietary fiber on body weight in humans (From Stevens 1988)

Fiber type	Authors	Reduced body wt
Methyl cellulose	Yudkin 1959	Yes
	Michelsen *et al.* 1979	Yes
	Duncan *et al.* 1960	No
	Evans & Miller 1975	No
Psyllium	Frati-Munari *et al.* 1983	Yes
	Stevens *et al.* 1987	No
Food	Russ & Atkinson, 1985	No
	Baron *et al.* 1986	No

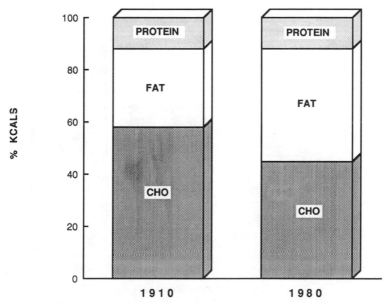

Figure 1. Changes in U. S. diet from 1910 to 1980.

gained in fewer days of overeating a high fat diet than a mixed diet (Figure 3). The use of animal models, and in particular, rodent models of obesity, allows researchers to examine the etiology of obesity in more detail. All obesities are defined by increased white adipose tissue mass, although molecular, cellular, metabolic, and behavioral characteristics may differ. This chapter will discuss several animal models of obesity in more detail, including animals that become obese because of alterations in diet composition, changes in physical activity or genetic predisposition. These models have been chosen in part because of their potential usefulness in studying the effects of dietary fiber on development and maintenance of obesity.

Diet-Induced Obesity

Diet-induced obesity in experimental animals may be produced experimentally by a variety of techniques including increasing energy intake, increasing energetic efficiency by changing the pattern of eating from nibbling to meal feeding, and by altering the composition of the diet from low fat to high fat. Overfeeding to the point of obesity can be achieved by either tube feeding part of the daily energy intake while allowing voluntary intake to continue (Rothwell and Stock, 1984a) or by forcing experimental animals which are normally nibblers to consume

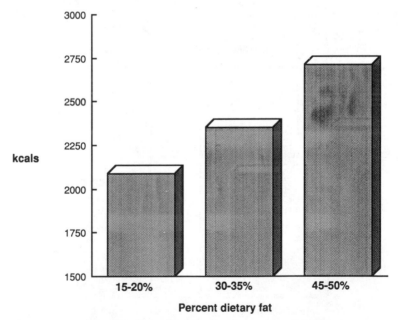

Figure 2. Energy intake during 14-day treatment (from Lissner et al., 1987).

their calories in discrete meals (Fabry, 1967). Rats also become obese when they are allowed to eat either diets high in fat, diets high in fat and sugar, or diets that provide a variety of palatable foods, the so-called cafeteria diet (Sclafani and Springer, 1976). When laboratory rodents are given a diet containing 30% or more of the calories as fat (standard laboratory chow diet contains only 10% of energy as fat), most initially increase their energy intake, become more efficient in energy utilization, and become obese. Over a six week period, daily energy intake of rats fed a high fat diet is typically comparable to that of rats fed a low fat diet; however, body weight gain is often higher on the high fat diet (Figure 4; Applegate et al., 1984).

The effect of a high fat diet depends, in part, on the type of fat in the diet, with diets high in saturated fatty acids promoting greater fat gain than diets high in polyunsaturated fatty acids (PUFAs) (Mercer and Trayhurn, 1987); the type of PUFAs, with corn or soy oil promoting greater fat gain than black current oil (Thurmond et al., 1992); the gender of the animal, with females generally being more susceptible than males (Sinha et al., 1977; Schemmel et al., 1970); and the age at which the diet is fed, with younger animals being less susceptible than older

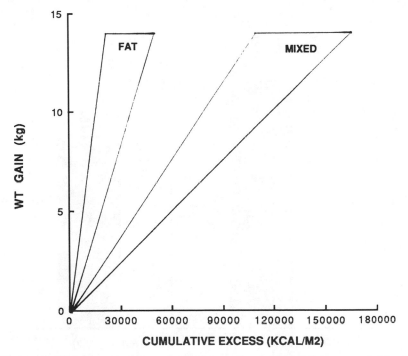

Figure 3. Weight gained by overfeeding a mixed diet for 7 mos. vs. fat for 3 mos. (from Danforth, 1985).

ones (Bray et al., 1989).

The genetic background of the animal also plays a role. Classical work of Fenton and Chase (1951), for example, demonstrated that only susceptible mice become obese on a high fat diet. Similarly, rat strains vary in their susceptiblity to diet-induced obesity. The Osborne-Mendel rat demonstrates a much greater weight gain on a high fat diet than does the S5B/Pl strain (Bray et al., 1989). When rats are returned to a standard low fat chow diet after becoming obese on a high fat diet, they reduce food intake, lose weight, and adipocytes return to normal size (Faust et al., 1976, 1978). If, however, the number of adipocytes has increased, total body fat remains elevated even though food intake may return to normal (Faust et al., 1976, 1978). This increase in fat cell number as measured by incorporation of ^{3}H-thymidine into adipocyte DNA occurs within a week of rats being placed on a high fat diet and is seen in rats as old as 18 months of age (Ellis et al., 1990).

There are also different responses to a high fat diet within a given strain. Approximately 25% of female Sprague-Dawley rats become morbidly obese when fed a diet containing over 80% of energy from fat (Figure 5; Landerholm and Stern, 1992). Prior to consuming the high fat

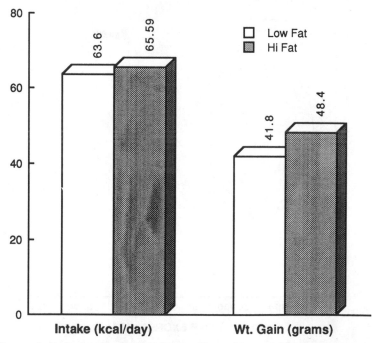

Figure 4. Daily intake (kcals) and total weight gain (g). Rats were fed low and high fat diets for 6 wks. (from Applegate et al., 1984).

diet, obesity-prone rats released less glycerol from adipose tissue in response to catecholamine stimulation. They were also more efficient than obesity resistant rats when fed the high fat diet (Landerholm and Stern, 1992). The addition of sucrose, fructose, glucose or polysaccharides to the diet in liquid form increases energy intake in laboratory rodents from 10 to 20% and results in a gradual increase in body weight and fat accumulation (Kanarek and Hirsch, 1977; Kanarek and Orthen-Gambill, 1982). Feeding saccharides in powdered as opposed to liquid form produces some, but not as high a degree of hyperphagia and adiposity (Ramirez, 1987b). In reviewing numerous studies on the substitution in rat diets of sugar for starch, Sclafani (1987a) found that there was little change in body fat or weight gain even if the amount of diet consumed decreased. This suggests that the high sugar diets may have increased food efficiency. Sucrose-induced obesity follows the same pattern as fat-induced obesity in relation to genetic strain, gender, and age differences. Osborne-Mendel rats are highly susceptible to sucrose-induced obesity while rats of the S5B/Pl strain show an actual decrease in weight when given sucrose solutions (Schemmel et al., 1982b). Female rats more consistently become obese when given sucrose than do male rats

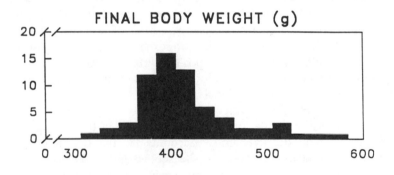

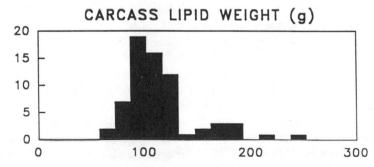

Figure 5. Distribution of final weight and carcass composition (from Landerholm and Stern, 1992).

(Hirsch et al., 1982), and young rats tend not to gain excessive weight when given sucrose solutions, even though intake may increase (Hirsch et al., 1982; Kanarek and Marks-Kaufman, 1979).

Rats and mice provided a variety of palatable foods in addition to laboratory chow increase their energy intake by as much as 60% and gain from 50 to 200% more than control animals provided only with chow (Sclafani and Springer, 1976; Gale and Sclafani, 1977). Weight gained in response to the cafeteria diet follows the trends seen in other diet-induced obesities, with female rats becoming more obese than male rats and older rats becoming more obese than younger rats (Sclafani and Gorman, 1977). Increased adiposity reflects an increase in both size and number of fat cells (Mandenoff et al., 1982). As seen with animals on high fat diets, when cafeteria-fed rats are fed only chow, food intake falls and weight is reduced; however, weight generally remains above that of control animals (Armitage et al., 1983). A problem with the use of this type of diet is that it is extremely hard to precisely replicate the diet in terms of macronutrient and micronutrient composition (Moore, 1987). Palatability, the hedonistic response to foods due to taste, smell, texture and temperature (Young and Green, 1953), also contributes to diet-induced obesity (Sclafani and Springer, 1976). After becoming obese on either a high fat (Maller, 1964) or a cafeteria diet (Sclafani and Springer, 1976), rats show increased rejection of less palatable foods compared to controls. In a model proposed by Bray and coworkers (1989), palatability may provide a positive afferent feedback signal acting on the central nervous system (CNS) to increase food intake or to suppress negative feedback signals. Through the use of sham feeding experiments where food is ingested but removed from the system by means of a gastric fistula, diet-induced increases in thermogenesis are found to be biphasic. Palatability accounts for the first phase while postabsorptive factors account for the second phase (Diamond et al., 1985; LeBlanc et al., 1984). LeBlanc and coworkers (1984) have suggested that these sensory-stimulated increases in thermogenesis are mediated by the sympathetic nervous system.

There is additional evidence that altered autonomic nervous system function occurs in diet-induced obesity. Schwartz and coworkers (1983) reported that animals eating a high fat diet had higher turnover of norepinephrine (NE) in brown adipose tissue (BAT), indicating increased sympathetic activity. In the obesity resistant S5B/Pl rat, NE turnover in BAT was increased 3-fold after 2 weeks on a high fat diet, while the increase in NE turnover in BAT from obesity prone Osborne-Mendel rat was smaller (Yoshida et al., 1987). Sprague Dawley rats also respond to a high fat diet with alterations in sympathetic activity if the diet is provided for more that one week (Bray et al., 1989). There is increased thermogenesis in BAT when animals are initially fed a high fat diet and decreased thermogenesis in BAT of animals chronically fed a high fat diet.

The medial hypothalamus is the most likely site for integration of signals regarding fat content of the diet (Bray et al., 1989). A useful animal model to study the role of the hypothalamus is a rat that has specific hypothalamic lesions. Rats with injury to the ventromedial nucleus (VMN) (Corbit and Stellar, 1964) or the paraventricular nucleus (PVN) (Bartness et al., 1985) are particularly responsive to high fat diets, while rats with injury to the dorsomedial nucleus of the hypothalamus are particularly responsive to highly palatable cafeteria diets. Using obesity resistant S5B/Pl rats, Oku and coworkers (1984b) showed that bilateral parasagittal hypothalamic knife cuts produced hyperphagia and obesity when rats were provided with a 30% but not a 10% fat diet. These lesions, which produce an obesity similar to that produced by PVN lesions, also disturbed the diurnal feeding pattern, resulting in increased consumption during the light period.

Among the signals which act on the hypothalamus to regulate feeding is the neurotransmitter serotonin (5HT or 5-hydroxytryptophan). Increased levels of 5HT are associated with reduced feeding; decreased levels of 5HT are associated with increased food intake (Bray et al., 1989). The metabolism of tryptophan, the precursor of serotonin, is altered in the diet-sensitive Osborne-Mendel rat (Weekley et al., 1982). Levels of 5HT in the VMN are lower in the Osborne-Mendel rat than in the S5B/Pl rat. When placed on a high fat diet, Osborne-Mendel rats showed increased 5HT in the VMN while S5B/Pl rats showed a decrease (Bray et al., 1989). In contrast, a major metabolite of serotonin, 5-hydroxyindoleacetic acid (5-HIAA), did not differ between strains, but did increase in both when rats were fed a high fat diet. The use of specific pharmacologic agents which alter 5HT metabolism also differentiates obesity-prone from obesity-resistant animals. Osborne-Mendel rats are more sensitive to fenfluramine, a 5HT reuptake inhibitor, than are S5B/Pl rats (Fisler and Bray, 1986; Bray et al., 1989). This implies that Osborne Mendel rats are more sensitive to serotonergic stimulation. Administration of fenfluramine prevents obesity caused by high fat feeding in Osborne Mendel rats largely by reducing food intake (Underberger et al., 1987). Similarly, it causes reduced food intake and weight loss in cafeteria-fed rats (Blundell, 1986). Fenfluramine stimulates the sympathetic nervous system and BAT thermogenesis, as indicated by increased mitochondrial GDP binding and BAT temperature (Rothwell and Stock, 1987b; Lupien and Bray, 1985). The adrenergic neurotransmitters, NE and dopamine, also play roles in diet-induced obesity. Measurements of NE and DOPAC, a metabolite of dopamine, in the

VMN of Osborne-Mendel and S5B/Pl rats show a pattern similar to that of 5HT, being higher in the S5B/Pl rat, but increasing only in the Osborne-Mendel rat when a high fat diet was fed. Similar to the apparent increased sensitivity of Osborne-Mendel rats to serotonergic stimulation is their apparent increased sensitivity to a-adrenergic stimulation (Leibowitz, 1970). Hyperinsulinemia is not a prominent feature of diet-induced obesity; however, some abnormalities in insulin secretion and sensitivity have been reported. Animals that are most susceptible to diet-induced obesity have modestly elevated plasma insulin levels (Levin et al., 1985). Rats consuming diets high in sucrose content have higher than normal insulin levels due to the increased glucose load (Sundin and Nachad, 1983). While a high fat diet does not consistently alter insulin levels, whole body glucose utilization is decreased in all animals studied (Bray et al., 1989).

Adrenal steroids play a fundamental role in the expression of obesity. Adrenalectomy counters the development of obesity in most animal models including, to some degree, diet-induced obesity. Castonguay and Stern (1983) found that adrenalectomy reduces the fat intake of lean Zucker rats given macronutrient choices. Adrenalectomy prevents the development of obesity in cafeteria-fed rats due to a depression of both food intake and energetic efficiency (Rothwell et al., 1984). Following adrenalectomy there is an increase in energy expenditure, and increased thermogenesis in BAT of both stock diet-fed and cafeteria-fed rats (Rothwell et al., 1984; Rothwell and Stock, 1986). The role of adrenal steroids in the expresssion of obesity may relate to abnormalities in the synthesis and metabolism of corticotropin releasing factor (CRF). Infusion of CRF into the third ventricle led to suppression of food intake to a greater extent in Osborne-Mendel than in S5B/Pl rats on a low fat diet. This suppression was partly overcome in Osborne-Mendel rats when a high fat diet was given (Bray et al., 1989).

As is true in other animal models of obesity, dietary obesity is characterized by abnormalities of fat metabolism. A number of studies have reported that rats eating a high fat diet show decreased insulin-stimulated lipogenesis as well as activity of the enzymes involved in this process. These include enzymes which generate NADPH, glucose-6-phosphate dehydrogenase and malic enzyme (Lavau et al., 1979), and fatty acid synthetase (Robeson et al., 1981). In addition, β-oxidation of fatty acids is increased, resulting in increased ketone formation (Triscari et al., 1985).

Products of fat metabolism, glycerol, fatty acids such as 3-hydroxy-butyrate, and ketones play a role in food intake and may account for some of the differences seen between rat strains in relation to diet-induced obesity. The resistant S5B/Pl rat has a higher blood ketone concentration (Yoshida et al., 1987) and a higher rate of transport of 3-hydroxybutyrate across the blood-brain barrier (Bray et al., 1989). Injection of 3-hydroxybutyrate into either the PVN or VMN of Sprague-Dawley rats caused a significant and dose-dependant increase in the firing rate of the sympathetic nerves to BAT (Sakaguchi et al., 1988). While it is clear that not all experimental animals are equally susceptible to diet-induced obesity, this model is one that is highly relevant to the human condition. Over the past 80 years, the addition of foods high in fat and the concomitant decrease in foods rich in complex carbohydrate and fiber, as well as a decrease in physical activity are thought to play major roles in the epidemic of obesity seen in developed nations.

Physical Inactivity

While obese individuals are not always less active than normal weight individuals, inactivity is often associated with obesity. In a classical study of adult-onset obese individuals, Greene (1939) traced the onset of obesity to forced inactivity in 68% of his patients. Inactivity in experimental animals can be more precisely documented and may also promote obesity in normally lean rats (Ingle, 1949) as observed by Greene (1939) in his patients that became inactive. A more complete understanding of the effects of exercise on humans is limited, in part, because of problems with the control and measurement of energy intake and expenditure and the inaccuracies of in-vivo body composition methodologies (Stern et al., 1987). By using experimental animals, we can more easily control such factors as age, sex, and genetic background. However, results may be influenced by the strain and sex of rats, diet composition, and the duration, type, intensity, and frequency of exercise. While forced running or swimming programs produce slower weight gain and lower final body weights in exercised males in comparison to controls, exercised females typically gain weight at comparable rates to controls (Stern et al., 1987).

Exercise tempers fat gain when rats are fed a high fat diet (Applegate et al., 1984). Genetically obese rodents are usually less active than their lean littermates and the degree and the onset of inactivity varies. The onset of inactivity in *obob* mice, as judged by a brief 5 minute motor test, is at one to two weeks of age (Mayer 1953). The onset of inactivity, as judged by daily revolutions in an activity wheel, in the morbidly obese Zucker (*fafa*) rat is coincident with weaning (Stern and Johnson, 1977). When obese Zucker rats are calorically restricted and comparably active to lean rats resulting in a body weight that is less than that in inactive ad-libitum-fed lean rats, the obese rats are still considerably fatter than the lean rats (Stern et al., 1987).

Regular physical activity results in a number of alterations including diminished body fat, decreased intake of fat (Miller, Dimond, and Stern, manuscript in preparation), increased oxidative capacity of muscles, and changes in a number of circulating hormones such as insulin, epinephrine, and glucocorticoids (for review see Stern et al., 1987). Exercise also prevents the increase in fat intake associated with "yo-yo" dieting (Gerardo-Gettens et al., 1990). Such adaptations to exercise appear to be transient and are reversed following discontinuation of exercise. In Osborne-Mendel rats, exercise termination resulted in increased plasma insulin (by 48 hrs after termination), increased food intake (by 60 hrs after termination), and enhanced adipose tissue lipoprotein lipase activity (by 84 hrs after termination) (Applegate and Stern, 1987). These alterations may result in permanent increases in adipose tissue mass in formerly active animals compared with their sedentary controls. This phenomenon was observed in formerly active lean and obese Zucker rats 4 months after exercise termination (Stern and Johnson, 1977). There is excellent evidence that routine physical activity is key to weight maintenance in humans (Kayman et al., 1990) and cessation of activity leads to weight gain.

Genetic Models of Obesity

Genetically obese animals are categorized as to whether the trait is expressed through single gene dominant, single gene recessive, or polygenic inheritance (for review see Johnson et al., 1991). Models in which obesity is transmitted through a single gene recessive defect, such as hyperglycemic obese (*obob*) and diabetic obese (*dbdb*) mice and Zucker fatty (*fafa*) and Wistar Diabetic Fatty (*fafa*) rats are frequently studied genetic models of obesity. Their attractiveness may be due in part to the opportunity they provide to isolate a single protein responsible for triggering the obese condition (Dulloo and Miller, 1987).

When obesity is fully developed, the many different genetic models share similar alterations in metabolic pathways. Metabolic abnormalities in autosomal recessive rodent models, Zucker (*fafa*) and Wistar Diabetic Fatty (WDF) (*fafa*) rats, *obob* and *dbdb* mice, have been reviewed by Johnson and her colleagues (1991). Common characteristics include hyperphagia, glucose intolerance, blunted BAT thermogenesis, increased white adipose tissue mass, hyperplastic and hypertrophic white adipose tissue, pancreatic islet hypertrophy, and impairment of the sympathetic nervous system. Adrenalectomy tends to reverse the aforementioned changes.

Energy imbalance resulting in obesity in genetically obese rodents is characterized by both increased food intake and by marked elevation in the efficiency of food utilization reflecting decreased energy expenditure (Dulloo and Miller, 1987; Bray et al., 1989). All genetically obese rodents show some degree of hyperphagia during the development of obesity (Bray and York, 1971, 1979). The obese condition is not dependent on increased food intake since it occurs even when the animals are pair-fed (Cox and Powley, 1977, Cleary et al., 1980) or yoke-fed (Coleman, 1978) with lean controls. In addition, increased adiposity precedes hyperphagia, the former having been observed in the first week of life (Romsos, 1981). A reduction in physical activity is also not critical in the early development of obesity in the Zucker *fa/fa* rat (Stern and Johnson, 1977, Stern 1984). The high energy efficiency in genetically obese rodents may be brought about by reduced energy expenditure for thermoregulatory thermogenesis (Trayhurn and James, 1978, Berce et al., 1986). Reduced metabolic rate has been observed in these animal models as early as the first week of life (Romsos, 1981). Low oxygen consumption and low body temperature have been described in the first few days of life of *obob* mice and Zucker *fafa* rats (Bray and York, 1979, Moore, et al., 1985; Berce, et al., 1986). Brown adipose tissue (BAT) has long been recognized as a major site of heat production in hibernators and neonates, and more recently for its role in the thermogenic response to cold and overfeeding in adult laboratory rodents (Dulloo and Miller, 1987). BAT is responsible for more than 50% of the increased metabolic rate during NE infusion in both cold-acclimated and cafeteria-overfed rats (Dulloo and Miller, 1987). There are conflicting reports concerning impairment of BAT thermogenesis in genetically obese rodents in response to cold, with some, such as *obob* mice, showing severe impairments in their thermogenic response to cold (Saito and Bray, 1984), while others show a normal response to cold acclimation (Bray et al., 1989). On the other hand, genetically obese rodents are uniformly characterized by an impairment in diet-related BAT thermogenesis. This is characterized by the failure to show the normal increase in oxygen consumption after feeding (Bray et al., 1989) and has been associated with reduced stimulation of BAT by the sympathetic nervous system (Bray, 1991).

The hypothesis that the primary defect in obesity lies within the CNS gained widespread acceptance during the 1950's on the basis of experiments which showed that damage to the VMH led to hyperphagia and obesity (Hetherington and Ranson, 1940) and damage to the lateral hypothalamus (LH) resulted in anorexia and weight loss (Anand and Brobeck, 1951). The similarities between obesity induced by these lesions and genetic obesity in animal models have given rise to a great deal of research on these areas of the brain. Guillaume-Gentil and co-workers (1990) propose that a CNS defect in *obob* and *dbdb* mice and *fafa* rats leads to hyperphagia, hyperinsulinemia, alterations in sympathetic and parasympathetic outflow, and altered regulation of the hypothalamohypophysial-adrenal axis. These alterations may be associated with abnormalities in hypothalamic nuclei involved in the control of glycemia, insulinemia and circadian corticosterone secretion (Bestetti et al., 1990). The work of Plotsky and coworkers (1992) suggests that reduced hypothalamic release of corticotropin releasing factor (CRF) by obese Zucker rats may be central to the etiology of obesity in these animals. The development of many of the abnormalities seen in Zucker obese rats is dependent on the presence of glucocorticoids (Freedman et al., 1986; Castonguay and Stern, 1983, Castonguay et al., 1984), the secretion of which is regulated by a neuroendocrine cascade initiated by hypothalamic release of CRF. It is hypothesized that reduced hypothalamic CRF tone seen in obesity may be due to dysregulation of the hypothalamic-pituitary-adrenal axis at a site involving the CRF system that mediates glucocorticoid feedback regulation (Plotsky et al., 1992). Investigation of a possible CNS defect as a primary lesion in obesity has also been approached in autosomal recessive animal models from the perspective of neuropeptides, and opioid peptide concentrations, binding

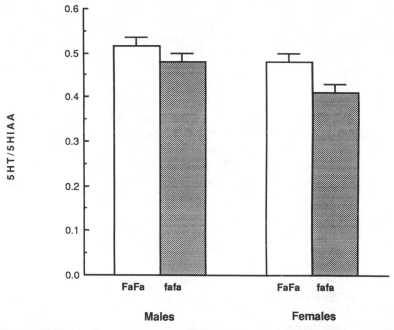

Figure 6. Ratio of concentrations of 5HT/5HIAA in the VMN from 11-wk-old obese (fafa) and lean (FaFa) Zucker rats (male obese vs. lean $p < .01$, female vs. lean $p < .001$).

and turnover in the brain. With respect to the former, Zucker obese rats (11–13 wks of age) have lower VMN serotonergic activity than their lean counterparts. This is true of both males and females (Figure 6; data from Routh et al. 1992 and Routh et al., unpublished data, 1993). Zucker obese rats have higher hypothalamic levels than their lean littermates of Neuropeptide Y (NPY), a potent stimulator of food intake in rats (Morley et al., 1985). In addition, Schwartz and coworkers (1991) reported that insulin inhibits the expression of the gene encoding NPY in the hypothalamus of lean but not obese Zucker rats.

A number of other neuropeptides have been examined in genetically obese animals. A clear relationship between food intake and tissue opioid peptide concentrations in genetically obese rodents has not yet been established; however, consistent reports of increased sensitivity to opiate receptor antagonists provide to a more reliable indicator of the involvement of opioid peptides in obesity (Bray et al., 1989). Increased responsiveness to opioid peptides may contribute to hyperphagia, hyper-insulinemia, and sterility typically seen in a number of genetic obesities (Bray et al., 1989).

Although *ob* and *db* map to different chromosomes (Table 2), they cause similar if not identical diabetes-obesity syndromes when maintained on the same inbred background. Coleman has suggested that these mice may differ in their ability to either produce or respond to a satiety signal (Coleman, 1973; Coleman and Hummel, 1969). Cholecystokinin (CCK), an intestinal peptide hormone that acts as a satiety signal, is a potential site of the genetic defect in *obob* mice. Although initial reports of decreased CCK concentration in the brains of *obob* mice (Strauss and Yallow, 1979) were not confirmed by later work (Oku et al., 1984b; Schneider et al., 1979; Finkelstein and Steggles, 1981); McLaughlin and workers (1985), studying more highly defined regions of the hypothalamus, reported increased CCK in the ventromedial, anterior and dorsal hypothalami of Zucker obese rats; while opiate control of CCK release was normal. Differences in CCK receptor binding have also been identified in *obob* mice and obese Zucker rats. Increased CCK

Table 2. The proposed chromosomal locations of the defect in several autosomal recessive rodent models of obesity (From: Johnson *et al.*, 1991).

Animal model	Mutant alleles	Chromosomes
Hyperglycemic obese mouse	*ob*	6
Diabetic mouse	*db*	4
Yellow obese mouse	Ay *et al.* at Agouti locus	2
Zucker obese rat	*fa*	5
Wistar diabetic fatty rat	*fa*	5

binding has been reported in the cortex of both genotypes and additionally in the hippocampus and midbrain of obese Zucker rats, while binding in the hypothalamus was normal in both genotypes (McLaughlin et al., 1985). Contrary to the hypothesis that the primary defect in genetic obesity lies within the CNS is the view that the primary lesion(s) responsible for the development of obesity are located in the peripheral tissues. Candidates for a peripheral mechanism responsible for the onset of obesity include a number of hormones, glucose transporters, enzymes involved in the metabolism of fat, guanine nucleotide regulatory proteins (G proteins), and abnormalities of the pancreas.

Among the hormones that play a key role in the development of obesity are the adrenal glucocorticoids, known to be essential for the development of genetically inherited forms of obesity in animal models. Adrenalectomy prevents or suppresses the development of obesity in *obob, dbdb,* and *AYa,* mice and in Zucker and WDF *fafa* rats (Johnson et al., 1991; Bray et al., 1989). As summarized by Bray et al. (1989) there are three likely mechanisms by which adrenalectomy influences the development of obesity, these being normalization of food intake, restoration of normal sympathetic activity and thus normal BAT thermogenesis, and the suppression of insulin secretion. The cumulative effect of these changes is to restore energy balance to levels seen in lean littermates. In addition to the obvious effect of suppressing the weight gain and fat deposition seen in obesity, adrenalectomy tends to reverse many other abnormalities associated with the manifestation of obesity in these animal models. These include abnormal diurnal pattern of feeding, preference for fat macronutrient diets, insulin insensitivity, attenuated BAT thermogenesis, decreased basal glucose transport, low brain weight, adipocyte hyperplasia, and infertility in male rats. Genetically obese rodents to which replacement glucocorticoids are given after adrenalectomy have been shown to have increased sensitivity to the exogenous hormone compared to lean controls. Increased responsiveness in the obese animals has been reported in relation to food intake, serum insulin, lipogenesis and its related enzyme activities, BAT function, weight gain, and fat deposition (Saito and Bray, 1984).

Another hormone which may play a key role in the development of genetic obesity is calcitonin (CT), an enzyme synthesized in the thyroid and involved in the regulation of calcium metabolism. Obese Zucker rats have higher circulating levels of CT, as well as higher thyroid content at 10-weeks of age than do lean controls (Flynn et al., 1983, Margules et al., 1979). Changes in CT mRNA were followed in lean and obese Zucker rats by Segond and coworkers (1986) who found that mRNA in obese rats was 50% lower than lean rats at 30 days of age, but higher than that of lean rats in 12-week old animals. Developmental changes in thyroid CT mRNA in the obese Zucker rat were found to parallel those of plasma insulin (Zucker and Antoniades, 1972). Rat CT and insulin genes are known to be located on the same chromosome (Todd et al., 1985) and thus it has been proposed that alterations in the DNA around these two loci may be responsible for altering the expression of both these genes (Segond et al., 1986). That the hormone insulin may play a primary role in the development and expression of obesity is suggested by the fact that all genetically obese animal are characterized by hyperinsulinemia (Bray and York, 1979). It has been proposed that hyperinsulinemia may result from increased stimulation of the pancreas by the parasympathetic nervous system as well as increased sensitivity of the pancreas to that stimulation (Rohner-Jeanrenaud et al., 1983b). Genetically obese rodents also exhibit some degree of hyperglycemia, peripheral insulin resistance, pancreatic islet hypertrophy and often hyperplasia, and altered insulin receptor function, including defects in insulin binding and in the phosphorylation of the insulin receptor β subunit (Johnson et al., 1991). Insulin plays a role in the stimulation of lipid deposition, the regulation of food intake, sympathetic nerve activity, and body weight (Bray and York, 1979). Five week-old *dbdb* mice have a four-fold elevation in plasma insulin and in pancreatic proinsulin mRNA that decreases as the animals age and become increasingly glucose intolerant (Orland et al., 1985). In contrast, WDF *fafa* rats at 5 and 14 weeks of age show no differences in pancreatic preproinsulin mRNA levels or in insulin content when compared to lean animals (Koh et al., 1990). A comparison of the levels of preproinsulin mRNA in Zucker and WDF *fafa* rats indicates that insulin genes are subject to differing regulation in these two animal models of obesity, resulting in the development of frank diabetes in WDF *fafa* but not in the Zucker *fafa* rats (Koh et al., 1990). Pancreatic preproinsulin mRNA and plasma insulin increase to a greater extent with age in obese than in lean Zucker rats, suggesting that increased fat deposition is associated with enhanced insulin gene expression in these animals. Although insulin appears to play a role in the expression of the obese phenotype, hyperinsulinemia itself is not a necessary condition for the development of obesity in the Zucker obese rat (Chan and Stern, 1982).

The effects of insulin on the CNS have been examined in a number of experimental animals. Cerebroventricular injection of insulin into baboons and rats reduces food intake and body weight in a dose dependent manner (Brief and Davis, 1984; Porte and Woods, 1981). Injection of insulin into the VMH of rats reduces firing rate of the sympathetic nerves innervating BAT (Sakaguchi and Bray, 1987), while injection into the LH leads to increased firing rate of these sympathetic nerves (Sakaguchi and Bray, 1989). Although the level of insulin in the cerebrospinal fluid (CSF) is thought to reflect that in the blood, the Zucker *fafa* rat has a lower CSF insulin level than that predicted by the degree of peripheral hyperinsulinemia (Stein et al., 1983, 1985). In spite of increased levels of insulin in the blood and CSF of obese rats, there is evidence that the insulin concentration of various brain regions may be lower than that in lean controls, suggesting a possible abnormality in the transport of insulin into the CNS (Figlewicz et al., 1985, 1986).

Insulin release from the pancreas is associated with glucose transport into the pancreas through the action of the glucose transporter, GLUT-2 (Thorens et al., 1988). Impaired glucose-stimulated insulin secretion in a line of inbred Zucker rats which develop severe hyperglycemia as well as obesity has been found to be associated with lower levels of GLUT-2 and GLUT-2 mRNA than occur in lean controls (Johnson et al., 1991).

Insulin resistance of peripheral tissues is characteristic of most animal models of genetic obesity. This abnormality is thought to be the result of defects in the insulin-mediated transport of glucose (James et al. 1985, Kahn and Cushman, 1985). Given that most studies done to this point find few if any differences in the amount of GLUT-4, the most prevalent glucose transporter in muscle and adipose tissue, or of its mRNA in lean and obese animals, it is believed that the defect in glucose transport is likely to lie in signal transduction, functional activity of the transporter, or translocation of the transporter (Johnson et al., 1991). Altered activity of enzymes responsible for lipogenesis, glycolysis, and gluconeogenesis in liver and adipose tissue of genetically obese animals provides a potential peripheral mechanism for the onset of obesity (Johnson et al., 1991). Several lipogenic enzymes are increased in the adipose tissue of 7-day-old Zucker *fafa* rats prior to the onset of hyperinsulinemia (Gruen and Greenwood, 1981). This evidence supports the hypothesis that abnormalities in adipose tissue lie closer to the primary genetic lesion responsible for obesity than do the changes in insulin synthesis and secretion (Bazin et al., 1982). Greenwood (1985) proposed that the primary lesion in genetic obesity is the adipose tissue enzyme lipoprotein lipase (LPL) which acts as an adipocyte "gatekeeper" in that it is responsible for the breakdown of circulating triglyceride to free fatty acids and triglyceride just prior to their crossing the adipocyte plasma membrane. In addition to being one of the enzymes that is increased in the obese Zucker rat at an early stage of development, LPL turnover has been shown to be higher in obese than in lean Zucker rats (Johnson et al., 1991). Moreover, adrenalectomy tends to normalize LPL activity in obese Zucker rats and glucocorticoid administration causes activity to return to the level of sham-adrenalectomized animals (Freedman et al., 1986). Insulin enhances LPL synthesis (Fried et al., 1990), while insulin and glucocorticoids together decrease rates of LPL degradation in isolated human adipocytes (Johnson et al., 1991).

Another adipose tissue enzyme that may play a role in the development of obesity is glyceraldehyde-3-phosphate dehydrogenase (GAPDH). It has been proposed that this enzyme may act as a regulator of glycolysis in adipose tissue, thus influencing the supply of substrate for lipogenesis (Johnson et al., 1991). GAPDH activity in adipose tissue of obese Zucker rats was found to be slightly higher in 7-day-old animals, threefold higher in 16-day old animals, and tenfold higher in 30-day old weanlings than it was in lean controls (Dugail et al., 1988).

There is evidence that the etiology of obesity may involve G-proteins, part of the guanine nucleotide regulatory mechanism, which function in the activation of adenyl cyclase and hence the synthesis of cAMP. Studies of metabolic systems involving G-proteins in adipose tissue, liver, and pancreas of genetically obese animals have revealed a number of abnormalities (Johnson et al., 1991). These proteins function in adipose tissue by coupling adrenergic receptors to adenylate cyclase, thus resulting in increased synthesis of cAMP and activation of lipolysis. Abnormalities in this system identified in the *obob* mouse could account for the abnormal response of the adipose tissue to lipolytic hormones (Johnson et al., 1991). In the pancreatic islets of obese mice, the ATP-sensitive K^+-activated and the Ca^{2+}-activated ion channels display abnormalities that can be related to altered synthesis of a G-protein or another component of a second messenger system (Begin-Heick, 1990). Another adipose tissue factor that has been suggested as a possible primary lesion in the development of obesity is adipsin, a serine protease with complement D factor activity (Johnson et al., 1991). Adipsin synthesis has been linked to specific stages in the differentiation of adipocytes (Spiegelman et al., 1989). Adipsin mRNA and circulating protein are greatly reduced in adult *obob, dbdb,* and MSG-treated obese mice and Zucker obese rats (Johnson et al., 1991). One study reported that adipsin levels were 30% lower in 2-week-old *dbdb* mice than in lean controls (Lowell et al., 1990), while another found levels to be similar between lean and obese mice at this age, but 65% lower in obese mice by 30 days of age (Dugail et al., 1990). Spiegelman and coworkers demonstrated that adipsin expression is regulated by adrenal glucocorticoids (Spiegelman et al., 1989) as are a number of other metabolic processes that differ between lean and obese animal models.

Increased body fat in animals with genetic obesity is due in all cases to increased fat cell size; however, in homozygous recessive animal models of obesity, there is an accompanying increase in fat cell number as well (Bray et al., 1989). Examples of hyperplasia also occur in polygenically inherited obesities, such as the NZO mouse, when the animals are fed a highly palatable diet (Herberg et al., 1974).

Research with genetic models of obesity has now focused on trying to identify the precise chromosomal location of the defect. *Obob* and *dbdb* mice carry autosomal recessive mutations that map to different chromosomes (Table 2). Clearly, the mutation for Zucker obese *fafa* and WDF obese *fafa* rats is the same. Truett and coworkers (1991) have evidence that *fa* and *db* are sentenic and are located on different chromosomes in the mouse and in the rat. Although no widespread human homozygous recessive genetic defect for obesity is known, as early as 1965, Dr. Jean Mayer (1965) wrote that there was strong circumstantial evidence for an underlying genetic cause for obesity. This concept is supported by the observations that obesity is known to run in families, that identical twins have similar body weights even when brought up separately (MacDonald and Stunkard, 1990), and by direct evidence for the inheritability of skinfold thickness (Dulloo and Miller, 1987). According to Bouchard (1991), the heritability of percent body fat is about 25%.

Normal weight children of obese parents have a lower metabolic rate than do the children of non-obese parents (Griffiths and Payne, 1976). Although there is little evidence that the obese have a reduced basal metabolic rate (BMR), the greater weight of the obese is accompanied by an increase in lean body mass as well, this being highly correlated with the BMR (Halliday et al., 1979; Dulloo and Miller, 1987). Upon substantial weight loss, formerly obese people have a lower BMR and a reduced energy requirement for maintenance than do lean controls (Leibel and Hirsch, 1984).

A predisposition to obesity may be more closely related to a reduction in the heat production following a meal than to BMR, this being supported by a study in which obese subjects demonstrated a thermogenic response to food that was one third of normal (Dulloo and Miller, 1987). Additional evidence in support of this hypothesis is provided by reports of subnormal thermogenic responses to food in obese (Jequier, 1983), post-obese, (Bessard et al., 1983), and in subjects maintaining weight on a relatively low food intake (Morgan et al., 1982). The potentiation of diet-induced thermogenesis observed in lean subjects (Miller et al., 1967) is reported to be reduced in the obese (Segal and Gutin, 1983). There is support for the concept that individuals with a genetic predisposition to obesity are metabolically more efficient than the lean and that such a thermogenic defect can make a significant contribution to weight gain in the absence of controlled food intake (Dulloo and Miller, 1987). Readers are referred to several excellent reviews in this area (Bouchard and Perusse, 1988; Bouchard, 1991; Price, 1987).

Future Directions in Obesity Research

It is generally accepted that obesity in humans is associated with both genetic and environmental factors (Dulloo and Miller, 1987; Bouchard, 1991). The obese phenotype in humans is sensitive to environmental and behavioral factors including dietary patterns, abundance and variety of foods available, physical activity, psychological factors, and social factors, thus making it difficult to assess the genetic aspects of this disorder, although there are human populations with known pedigree that are being intensively studied. For this reason, animal models of obesity have been extremely useful in determining the likely genetic and metabolic abnormalities in human obesity (Leibel et al., 1990; Fuller and Yen, 1987).

There is no doubt that much work is needed to continue to elucidate the metabolic and biochemical differences between lean and obese individuals in animal models of obesity and to carry these investigations to the cellular and molecular level. Efforts are also needed to understand the interrelationship between obesity and numerous other disease states associated with it such as diabetes, heart disease, and hypertension, through the use of animal models that demonstrate combined disorders. In this area as well, future research will provide information about the cellular and molecular mechanisms involved in the etiologies of these disorders. At the forefront of obesity research in the future will be the effort to elucidate the genetic basis of obesity through the techniques of molecular biology. These techniques include the mapping and cloning of the genes associated with the metabolic processes involved in obesity and elucidating the factors that regulate the expression of these genes. The sum of information provided about obesity through the use of animal models will provide direction for the study of human obesity and eventually, as the human genome is mapped, the molecular basis of the genetic component of human obesity will no doubt become clear.

Literature Cited

Anand, B., and Brobeck, J. R., 1951, Hypothalamic control of food intake in rats and cats, Yale J. Biol. Med. 24:123.

Applegate, E. A., and Stern, J. S., 1987, Exercise termination effects on food intake, plasma insulin, and adipose lipoprotein lipase activity in the Osborne-Mendel rat, Metabolism 36:709.

Applegate, E. A., Upton, D. E., and Stern, J. S., 1984, Exercise and detraining: Effect on food intake, adiposity and lipgenesis in Osborne-Mendel rats made obese by a high fat diet. J. Nutr. 114:447.

Armitage, G., Hervey, G. R., Rolls, B. J., Rowe, E. A., and Tobin, G., 1983, The effects of supplementation of the diet with highly palatable foods upon energy balance in the rats, J. Physiol. 342:299.

Bartness, T. J., Bittman, E. L. and Wade, N. G., 1985, Paraventricular nucleus lesions exaggerate dietary obesity but block photoperiod-induced weight gains and suspension of estrous cyclicity in Syrian hamsters, Brain Res. Bull. 14:427.

Bazin, R., and Lavan, M., 1982, Development of hepatic and adipose tissue lipogenic enzymes and insulinemia during suckling and weaning on to a high fat diet in Zucker rats, J. Lipid Res. 23:839.

Begin-Heick, N., 1990, Quantification of the alpha and beta subunits of the transducing elements (Gs and Gi) of adenylate cyclase in adipocyte membranes from lean and obese (*ob/ob*) mice, Biochem. J. 268:83.

Berce, P. J., Moore B. J., Horwitz, B. A., Stern, J. S., 1986, Metabolism at thermoneutrality and in the cold is reduced in the neonatal preobee Zucker fatt (fafa) raat, J. Nutr. 116:2478.

Bessard,T., Schultz, Y., and Jequier, E., 1983, Energy expenditure and postprandial thermogenesis in obese women before and after weight loss. Am. J. Clin. Nutr. 38:680.

Bestetti, G. E., Abramo, F., Guillaume-Gentil, C., Rohner-Jeanrenaud, F., Jeanrenaud, B., and Rossi, G. L., 1990, Changes in the hypothalamo-pituitary-adrenal axis of genetically obese fa/fa rats: a structural, immunocytochemical, and morphometrical study, Endocrinology 126:1880.

Blundell, J. E., 1986, Serotonin manipulations and the structure of feeding behavior, Appetite 7:39.

Bouchard, C., 1991, Current understanding of the etiology of obesity: genetic and nongenetic factors, Am. J. Clin. Nutr. 53:1561.S.

Bouchard, C., and Perusse, L., 1988, Heredity and body fat, Ann. Rev. Nutr., 8:259.

Bray, G. A., 1991, Obesity, a disorder of nutrient partitioning: the MONA LISA hypothesis, J. Nutr.121:1146.

Bray, G. A. and York, D. A., 1971, Genetically transmitted obesity in rodents, Physiol. Rev. 51:598.

Bray, G. A. and York, D. A., 1979, Hypothalamic and genetic obesity in experimental animals: an autonomic and endocrine hypothesis, Physiol. Rev. 59:719.

Bray, G. A., York, D. A. and Fisler, J. S., 1989, Experimental obesity: a homeostatic failure due to defective nutrient stimulation of the sympathetic nervous system, Vit. and Hor. 45:1.

Brief, D. J., and Davis, J. D., 1984, Reduction in food intake and body weight by chronic intraventricular insulin infusion, Brain Res. Bull. 12:571.

Castonguay, T. W., Dallman, M., and Stern, J. S., 1984, Corticosterone prevents body weight loss and diminished fat appetite following adrenalectomy, Nutr. and Behav. 2:115-125.

Castonguay, T. W., and Stern, J. S., 1983, The effect of adrenalectomy on dietary component selection by the genetically obese Zucker rat, Nutr. Rep.Int. 28:725.

Chan, C. P. and Stern, J. S., 1982, Adipose lipoprotein lipase in insulin-treated diabetic lean and obese Zucker rats, Am. J. Physiol. 242:E445.

Cleary, M. P., Vaselli, J. R., and Greenwood, M. R. C., 1980, Development of obesity in the Zucker obese (fa/fa) rat in absence of hyperphagia, Am. J. Physiol. 238:E292.

Coleman, D. L., 1973, Effects of parabiosis of obese with diabetes and normal mice,

Diabetologia 9:294.

Coleman, D. L., 1978, Obese and diabetes: two mutant genes causing diabetes-obesity syndromes in mice, Diabetologia 14:141.

Coleman, D. L., and Hummel, K. P.,1969, Effects of parabiosis of normal with genetically diabetic mice, Am. J. Physiol. 217:1298.

Corbit, J. D., and Stellar, E., 1964, Palatability, food intake and obesity in normal and hyperphagic rats, J. Comp. Physiol. 58:63.

Cox, J. E. and Powley, T. L., 1981, Prior vagotomy blocks VMH obesity in pair-fed rats, Am. J. Physiol. 240: E573.

Danforth, Jr., E., 1985, Diet and Obesity, Amer. J. Clin. Nutr.41:1132.

Diamond, P., Brondel, L., and LeBlanc, J., 1985, Palalability and postprandial thermogenesis in dogs, Am. J. Physiol. 248:E75.

Dugail, I., Quignard-Boulange, A., Brigant, L., Etienne, J. Noe, L. and Lavau, M., 1988, Increased lipoprotein lipase content in the adipose tissue of suckling and weaning obese Zucker rats, Biochem. J. 249:45.

Dugail, I., Quignard-Boulange, A., Le Liepvre, X., and Lavau, M., 1990, Impairment of adipsin expression is secondary to the onset of obesity in db/db mice. J. Biol. Chem. 265:1831.

Dulloo, A. G. and Miller, D. S., 1987, Obesity: a disorder of the sympathetic nervous system, Wld. Rev. Nutr. Diet. 50:1.

Ellis, J. R., McDonald, R. B., and Stern, J. S., 1990, A diet high in fat stimulates adipocyte proliferation in older (22 months) rats, Exper. Gerontology 25:141.

Fabry, P., 1967, Metabolic consequences of the pattern of food intake, in Code, Handbook of Physiology, sect. 6, vol. 1, pp 31.

Faust, I. M., Johnson, P. R., and Hirsch, J., 1976, Noncompensation of adipose mass in partially lipectomized mice and rats. Am. J. Physiol. 231:538.

Faust, I. M., Johnson, P. R., Stern, J. S., and Hirsch, J., 1978, Diet-induced adipocyte number increase in adult rats: a new model of obesity. Am. J. Physiol. 235:E279.

Fenton, P. F., and Chase, H. B., 1951, Effect of diet on obesity of yellow mice in inbred lines, Proc. Soc. Exp. Biol. Med. 77:420.

Figlewicz, D. P., Ikeda, H., Stein, L. J. Baskin, D. G., Paguette, T., Greenwood, M. R. C., Woods, S. C. and Porte, D., 1985, Brain and liver insulin binding is decreased in Zucker rats carrying the fa gene, Endocrinology 117:1537.

Figlewicz, D. P., Ikeda, H., and Stein, L. J., 1986, Brain insulin binding is decreased in Wistar Kyoto rats carrying the fa gene, Peptides 7:61.

Finkelstein, J. A. and Steggles, A.-W., 1981, Levels of gastrin-cholecystokinin like immunoreactivity in the brains of genetically obese and non-obese rats, Peptides 219.

Fisler, J. S., and Bray, G. A., 1986, Effect of fenfluramine on food intake and body weight of S5B/Pl and Osborne-Mendel rats, Am. J. Clin. Nutr. 43:54A.

Flynn, J. J., Margules, D. L., Peng, T. C., and Cooper, C. W., 1983, Serum calcitonin, calcium and thyroxine in young and old fatty Zucker rats (fafa), Physiol. Behav. 31:79.

Freedman, M. R., Horowitz, B. A., and Stern, J. S. 1986, Effect of adrenalectomy and glucocorticoid replacement on development of obesity, Am. J. Physiol. 250:R595.

Fried, S. K., Turkenkopf, I. J., Goldberg, I. J., Doolittle, M. H., Kirchgessner, T. G., Schotz, M. G., Johnson, P. R., and Greenwood, M. R. C., 1991, Mechanisms of increased lipoprotein lipase in fat cells of obese Zucker rats, Am. J. Physiol. 261:E653.

Fuller, R. W., and Yen, T. T., 1987, The place of animal models and animal experimentation in the study of food intake regulation and obesity in humans, Annals NY Acad. Sci. 499:167.

Gale, S. K., and Sclafani, A., 1977, Comparison of ovarian and hypothalamic obesity syndromes in the female rat: effects of diet palatability on food intake and body weight, J. Comp. Physiol. 91:381.

Greene, J. A. 1939, Clinical study of the etiology of obesity, Ann. Intern. Med. 12:1797.

Gerrardo-Gettens, T., Miller, G. D., Horwitz, B. A., McDonald, R. B., Brownell, K. D., Greenwood, M. R. C., Roden, J., and Stern, J. S., 1991, Exercise decreases fat selection in females during weight cycling, Am. J. Physiol., 260:518.

Greenwood, M. R. C., 1985, Normal and abnormal growth and maintenance of adipose tissue, In: Recent Advances In Obesity Research: IV, J. Hirsch, and T. Van Itallie, eds, John Libbey, London, p. 20.

Griffiths, M. and Payne, P. R., 1976, Energy expenditure in small children of obese and non-obese parents, Nature 260:698.

Gruen, R. K., and Greenwood, M. R. C., 1981, Adipose tissue lipoprotein lipase and glycerol release in fasted Zucker (fa/fa) rats, Am. J. Physiol. 241:E76.

Guillaume-Gentil, C., Rohner-Jeanrenaud, F., Abramo, F., Bestetti, G. E., Rossi, G. L., and Jeanrenaud, B., 1990, Abnormal regulation of the hypothalamo-pituitary-adrenal axis in the genetically obese *fa/fa* rat, Endocrinology 126:1873.

Halliday, D., Hesp., R., Stalley, S. F., Warwick, P., Atlman, D. G. and Garrow, J. S., 1979, Resting metabolic rate, weight, surface area and body composition of obese women, Int. J. Obes. 3:1.

Herberg, L., Doeppen, W., Major, E., and Gries, F. A., 1974, Dietary induced hypertrophic-hyperplastic obesity in mice, J. Lipid Res. 6:580.

Hetherington, A. W., and Ranson, S. W., 1940, Hypthalamic lesions and adiposity in the rat, Anat. Rec. 78:149.

Hirsch, J., Dubose, C., and Jacobs, H. L., 1982, Overeating, dietary selection patterns and sucrose intake in growing rats, Physiol. Behav. 28:819.

Ingle, D. J., 1949, A simple means of producing obesity in the rat. Proc. Soc. Exp. Biol. Med. 72:604.

James, D. E., Burleigh, K. M., and Kraegen, E. W., 1985, Time dependence of insulin action in muscle and adipose tissue in the rat in vivo: an increasing response in adipose tissue with time, Diabetes 34:1049.

Jequier, E., 1983, Does a thermogenic defect play a role in the pathogenesis of human obesity? Clin. Physiol. 3:1.

Johnson, P. R., Greenwood, M. R. C., Horowitz, B. A. and Stern, J. S., 1991, Animal models of obesity: genetic aspects, Annu. Rev. Nutr., 11:325.

Kahn, B. B., and Cushman, S. W., 1985, Subcellular translocation of glucose transporters: role in insulin action and its perturbation in altered metabolic states, Diabetes Metab. Rev. 1:203.

Kanarek, R. B. and Hirsch, E., 1977, Dietary-induced overeating in experimental animals, Fed. Proc., Fed. Am. Soc. exp. Biol. 36:154.

Kanarek, R. B. and Marks-Kaufman, R., 1979, Developmental aspects of sucrose-induced obesity in rats, Physiol. Behav. 23:881.

Kanarek, R. B. and Orthen-Gambill, N., 1982, Differential effects of sucrose, fructose and glucose on carbohydrate-induced obesity in rats. J. Nutr. 112:1546.

Kayman S., Bruvold, W., and Stern, J. S., 1990, Maintenance and relapse after weight loss in women: behavioral aspects, Am. J. Clin. Nutr., 52:800.

Koh, G., Seino, Y., Usami., M., Matsuo, T., and Ikeda, H., 1990, Importance of impaired insulin-gene expression in occurrence of diabetes in obese rats, Diabetes 39:1050.

Landerholm, T. E., and Stern, J. S., 1992, Adipose tissue lipolysis in vitro: a predictor of diet-induced obesity in female rats, Amer J. Physiol. 263: in press.

Lavau, M., Fried, S. K., Susini, C., and Freychet, Pl, 1979, Mechanism of insulin resistance in adipocytes of rats fed a high fat diet, J. Lipid Res. 20:8.

LeBlanc, J., Cabanac, M., and Samson, P., 1984, Reduced postprandial heat production with gavage as compared with meal feeding in human subjects, Am. J. Physio. 246:E95.

Leibel, R. L., Bahary, N., and Friedman, J. M., 1990, Genetic variation and nutrition in obesity: approaches to the molecular genetics of obesity, Wld. Rev. Nutr. Diet. 63:90.

Leibel, R. L., and Hirsch, J., 1984, Diminished energy requirements in reduced obese patients, Metabolism 33:164.

Leibowitz, S. F., 1970, Reciprocal hunger-regulating circuits involving alpha and beta-adrenergic receptors located, respectively, in the ventromedial and lateral hypothalamus, Proc. Natl. Acad. Sci. U.S.A. 67:1063.

Levin, B. E., Finnegan, M. B., Triscari, J., and Sullivan, A. C., 1985, Brown adipose and metabolic features of chronic diet-induced obesity, Am. J. Physiol. 248:R717.

Lissner, L., Levitsky, D. A., Strupp, B. J., Kalkwarf, H. J., and Roe, D. A., 1987, Dietary fat and the regulation of energy intake in human subjects, Amer. J. Clin. Nutr. 46:886.

Lowell, B. B., Napolitano, A., Usher, P., Dulloo, A. G. and Rosen, B. S.,1990, Reduced adipsin expression in murine obesity: effects of age and treatment with the sympathomimetic-thermogenic drug mixture ephedrine and caffeine, Endocrinology 126:1514.

Lupien, J. R., and Bray, G. A., 1985, Influence of fenfluramine on GDP-binding to brown adipose tissue mitochondria, Pharmacol., Biochem. Behav. 23:509.

MacDonald, A., and Stunkard, A. J., 1990, Body mass indexes of British separated twins, New Eng. J. Med., 322:1530.

Maller, O., 1964, The effect of hypothalamic and dietary obesity on taste preferences in rats, Life Sci. 3:1281.

Mandenoff, A., Lenoir, T., and Apfelbaum, M., 1982, Tardy occurrence of adipocyte hyperplasia in cafeteria-fed rats, Am. J. Physiol. 242:R349.

Margules, D. L., Flyn, J. J., Walker, J. and Cooper, C. W., 1979, Elevation of calcitonin immunoreactivity in the pituitary and thyroid glands of genetically obese rats (fafa), Brain Res. Bull. 4:589.

Mayer, J., 1953, Decreased activity and energy balance in the hereditary obesity-diabetes syndrome of mice, Science 117:504.

Mayer, J., 1965, Genetic factors in human obesity, Ann. N.Y. Acad. Sci. 131: 412.

Mercer, S. W., and Trayhurn, P., 1987, Effect of high fat diets on energy balance and thermogenesis in brown adipose tissue of lean and genetically obese ob/ob mice, J. Nutr. 2117:2147.

McLaughlin, C. L., Baile, C. A., Dellaferra, M. A. and Kasser, T. G., 1985, Meal-stimulated increased concentration of CCK in the hypothalami of Zucker obese and lean rats, Physiol. Behav. 35:215.

Miller, D. S., Mumford, P. M., and Stock, M. J., 1967, Gluttony. II. Thermogenesis in overeating man, Am. J. Clin. Nutr. 20:1223.

Moore, B. J., 1987, The cafeteria diet—an inappropriate tool for the study of thermogenesis, J. Nutr. 118:1594.

Moore, B. J., Armbruster, S. J., Horwitz, B. A., and Stern, J. S., 1985, Energy expenditure is reduced in preobese 2-day Zucker *fafa* rats. Am. J. Physiol. 249:R262.

Morgan, J. B., York, D. A., Wasilewska, A., and Portman, J., 1982, The study of the thermogenic responses to a meal and to a sympathomimetic drug (ephedrine) in relation to energy balance in man, Br. J. Nutr. 47:21.

Morley, J. E., Levine, A. S., Gosnell, B. A., and Krahn, D. D., 1985, Peptides as central regulators of feeding, Brain Res. Bull., 14:511.

National Research Council, 1989, Obesity and eating disorders, in : Diet and Health, National Academy Press, Washington, D. C.

Oku, J., Bray, G. A., Fisler, J. S.,and Schemmel, R., 1984a, Ventromedial hypothalamic knife cut lesions in rats resistant to dietary obesity, Am. J. Physiol. 246:R943.

Oku, J., Inoue, S., Glick, Z., Bray, G. A. and Walsh, J. H., 1984b, Cholecystokinin, bombesin, and neurotensin in brain tissue from obese animals, Int. J. Obes. 8:171.

Orland, M. J., Chyn, R., and Permutt, M. A., 1985, Modulation of proinsulin mRNA after partial pancreatectomy in rats, J. Clin. Invest. 84:305.

Plotsky, P. M., Thrivikraman, K. V., and Watts, A. T., 1992, Hypothalamic-pituitary-adrenal axis function in the Zucker obese rat, Endocrinology 130:1931.

Porte Jr., D., and Woods, S. C., 1981, Regulation of food intake and body weight by insulin, Diabetologia 20:274.

Price, R. A., 1987, Genetics of human obesity, Ann. Behav., Med., 9:9.

Ramirez, I., 1987b, Feeding a liquid diet increases energy intake, weight gain and body fat in rats, J. Nutr. 117:2127.

Robeson, B. L., Eisen, E. J., and Leatherwood, M. J., 1981, Adipose cellularity, serum glucose, insulin and cholesterol in polygenic obese mice fed high fat or high carbohydrate diets, Growth 45:198.

Rohner-Jeanrenaud, F. Hochstrasser, A.-C., and Jeanrenaud, B., 1983b, Hyper-insulinemia of preobese and obese *fa/fa* rats is partly vagus nerve mediated, Am. J. Physiol. 244:E317.

Romsos, D. R., 1981, Efficiency of energy retension in genetically obese animals and in dietary-induced thermogenesis, Fed. Proc. 40: 2524.

Rothwell, N. J. and Stock, M. J., 1984a, Brown adipose tissue, Recent Adv. Physiol. 10:349.

Rothwell, N. J. and Stock, M. J., 1986, Energy balance and brown fat activity in adrenalectomized male, female, and castrated male rats, Metab. Clin. Exp. 36:128.

Rothwell, N. J. and Stock, M. J., 1987b, Effect of diet and fenfluramine on thermogenesis in the rat: possible involvement of serotonergic mechanisms, Int. J. Obes. 11:319.

Rothwell, N. J. and Stock, M. J., and York, D. A., 1984, Effects of adrenalectomy on energy balance, diet-induced thermogenesis, and brown adipose trissue in cafeteria-fed rats, Comp. Biochem. Physiol. A 78:565.

Routh, V. H., Stern, J. S., and Horwitz, B. A., 1992, Adrenalectomy (ADX) does not reverse the altered ventromedial hypothalamic serotonergic actiavity of the obese Zucker rat, FASEB J. 6:A1784.

Routh, V. H., Gietzen, G. W., Stern, J. S., and Horwitz, 1993, Ventromedial (VMN) serotonergic activity is lower in male and female obese (fa/fa) versus lean (FaFa) Zucker rats. FASEB J., in press.

Saito, M., and Bray, G. A., 1984, Adrenalectomy and food restriction in the genetically obese (ob/ob) mouse, Am. J. Physiol. 248:E20.

Sakaguchi, T., and Bray, G. A., 1987, Intrahypothalamic injection of insulin decreases firing rate of sympathetic nerves, Proc. Natl. Acad. Sci. USA 84:2012.

Sakaguch, T., Takahashi, M., and Bray, G. A., 1988, The lateral hypothalamus and sympathetic firing rate, Am. J. Physiol., 255:R507.

Sakaguchi, T., and Bray, G. A., 1989, Effect of norepinephrine, serotonin, and tryptophan on the firing rate of sympathetic nerves, Brain Res., 492:271.

Schemmel, R., Mickelson, O., and Gill, J. L.,1970, Dietary obesity in rats: body weight and body fat accretion in seven strains of rats, J. Nutr. 100:1040.

Schemmel, R. A., Teague, R. J., and Bray, G. A., 1982b, Obesity in Osborne-Mendel and S5B/Pl rats: effects of sucrose solutions, castration, and treatment with estradiol or insulin, Am. J. Physiol. 243:R347.

Schneider, B., Monahan, J., and Hirsch, J., 1979, Brain cholecystokinin and nutritional status in rats and mice. J. Clin. Invest. 64:1348.

Schwartz, J. H., Young, J. B., and Landsberg, L., 1983, Effect of dietary fat on sympathetic nervous system activity in the rat, J. Clin. Invest. 72:361.

Schwartz, M. W., Marks, J. L., Sipols, A. J., Baskin, D. G., Woods, S. C., Kahn, S. E., and Porte Jr., D., 1991, Central insulin administration reduces Neuropeptide Y mRNA expression in the arcuate nucleus of food-deprived lean (Fa/Fa) but not obese (fa/fa) Zucker rats, Endocrinology 128:2645.

Sclafani, A., 1987a, Carbohydrate taste, appetite, and obesity: an overview, Neurosci. Biobehav. Rev. 11:131.

Sclafani, A., and Gorman, A. N., 1977, Effects of age, sex, and prior body weight on the development of dietary obesity in adult rats, Physiol. Behav. 18:1021.

Sclafani, A., and Springer, D., 1976, Dietary obesity in adult rats: similarities to hypothalamic and human obesity syndromes, Physiol. Behav.17:461.

Segal, K. R., and Gutin, B., 1983, Thermic effects of food and exercise in lean and obese women, Metabolism 32:581.

Segond, N., Tahri, E. H., Besnard, P., Legendre, P., Jullienne, A., and Garel, J. M.,

1986, Calcitonin mRNA activity in genetically obese rats, Biomed. Pharmocother. 40:207.

Sinha, Y. N., Thomas, J. W., Salocks, C. B., Wickes, M. A., and Vanderlaan, W. P., 1977, Prolactin and growth hormone secretion in diet-induced obesity in mice, Horm. Metab. Res. 9:277.

Spiegelman, B. M., Lowell, B., Napolitano, A., Dubuc, P., and Barton, D., 1989, Adrenal glucocorticoids regulate adipsin gene expression in genetically obese mice, J. Biol. Chem. 264:1811.

Stein, L. J., Dorsa, D. M., Baskin, D. G., Figelwicz, D. P., Ikeda, H., Frankman, S. P., Greenwood, M. R. C., Porte Jr., D., and Woods, W. C., 1983, Immunoreactive insulin levels are elevated in the cerebrospinal fluid of genetically obese Zucker rats, Endocrinology 113:2299.

Stein, L. J., Figelwicz, D. P., Dorsa, D. M., Baskin, D. G., Reed, D., Braget, D., Midkiff, M., Porte Jr., D., and Woods, W. C., 1985, Effect of insulin infusion on cerebrospinal fluid in heterozygous lean and obese Zucker rats, Int. J. Obes. 9:A145.

Stern, J. S., 1984, Is obesity a disease of inactivity?, In.: Eating Disorders, Stunkard, A. J. and Stellar, E., eds, pp. 131-9, Raven Press, New York.

Stern, J. S. and Johnson, P. R., 1977, Spontaneous activity and adipose cellularity in the genetically obese Zucker rat (fafa). Metabolism. 26:371.

Stern, J. S., Titchenal, C. A., and Johnson, P. R., 1987, Obesity: does exercise make a difference? In: Recent Advances in Obesity Research, John Libby, London, pp. 337-349.

Stevens, J., 1988, Does dietary fiber affect food intake and body weight?, J. Am. Diet. Assoc. 88:939.

Stern, J. S., and Keesey, R. E., 1981, The effect of ventromedial lesions on adipose cell number in the rat, Nutr. Rep. Int. 23:295.

Straus, E., and Yallow, R. S., 1979, Cholecystokinin in the brain of obese and non-obese mice. Science 203:68.

Sudin, W., and Nachad, M., 1983, Tropic response of rat brown fat by glucose feeding: involvement of sympathetic nervous system, Am. J. Physiol. 244:C142.

Thorens, B., Sarker, H. K., Kaback, H. R., and Lodish, H. F., 1988, Cloning and functional expression in bacteria of a novel glucose transporter present in liver, intestine, kidney, and beta pancreatic islet cells, Cell 55:281.

Thurmond, D. C., Tang, A. B., Nakamura, M. T., Stern, J. S., and Phinney, S. D., 1993, Time-dependent effects of progressive gamma-linolenate feeding on hyperphagia, weight gain and erythrocyte fatty acid composition during growth of Zucker obese rats. Obesity Res. 1(Supplement 1), 1993.

Todd, S., Yoshida, M. C., Fang, X. E., McDonald, L., and Jacobs, J., 1985, Genes for insulin I and II, parathryoid hormone and calcitonin are on rat chromosome I, Biochem. Biophys. Res. Commun. 131:1175.

Trayhurn, P., and James, W. P. T., 1978, Thermoregulation and non-shivering thermogenesis in the genetically obese (ob/ob) mouse, Pfluegers Arch. 373:189.

Triscari, J., Nause-Karol, C., Levin, B. E., and Sullivan, A. C., 1985, Changes in lipid metabolism in diet-induced obesity, Metab., Clin. Exp. 34:580.

Truett, G., Bahary, N., Friedman, J. M. and Leibel, R. L. 1991, Rat obesity gene fatty (*fa*) maps to chromosome 5: evidence for homology with the mouse gene diabetes (*db*), Proc. Nat. Acad. Sci. USA, 88:7806.

Underberger, S. J., Fisler, J. S., York, D. A., and Bray, G. A., 1987, Fenfluramine prevents dietary obesity in Osborne-Mendel rats, Clin. Res. 35:166A.

Weekley, L. B., Maher, R. W., and Kimbrough,T. D., 1982, Alterations of tryptophan metabolism in a rat strain (Osborne-Mendel) predisposed to obesity, Comp. Biochem. Physiol. A 72A:747.

Yoshida, T., Fisler, J. S., Fukushima, M., Bray, G. A., and Schemmel, R. A., 1987, Effects on diet, lighting, and food intake on norepinephrine turnover in dietary obesity, Am. J. Physiol. 252:R402.

Young, P. T., and Green, J. T., 1953, Quantity of food injested as a measure of relative acceptability, J. Comp. Physiol. Psychol. 46:288.

Zucker, L. M. and Antoniades, H.N., 1972, Insulin and obesity in the Zucker genetically obese rat "fatty", Endocrinology 90:1320.

Animal Models
of Colon Cancer

David M. Klurfeld

Wayne State University
Department of Nutrition and Food Science
3009 Science Hall
Detroit, MI 48202

Introduction

Animal models that reproduce all features of human colon cancer are an ideal that is yet to be realized. No existing model replicates the disease as an entity, but available models do approximate many of the characteristics of colonic carcinogenesis and metastasis. There are two "spontaneous" models of colon cancer if spontaneous is defined as obviating the requirement of administering a chemical carcinogen. However, most studies of experimental colonic carcinogenesis have been conducted using chemicals to induce tumors in several rodent species. These include the rat, mouse, hamster, and guinea pig. The spontaneous models include one strain each of rat and monkey.

Spontaneous Colon Cancer

Spontaneous colon tumors in nonhuman species are fairly rare. Adenomas and adenocarcinomas in dogs and cats account for less than one per cent of neoplasms reported (Squire et al, 1978). Spontaneous intestinal tumors have been reported from monkeys, mice, rats, hamsters, and the blue fox, but many of the tumors are of nonepithelial origin. A Wistar/Furth rat colony maintained at Osaka University was found to develop a 30% incidence of colon cancer (Miyamoto and Takizawa, 1975). It was subsequently reported that the majority of rats in this colony had acute colitis early in life and that Campylobacteria were isolated from most primary tumors and metastases (van den Berghe et al, 1985). Kitamura and Fujita (1986) wrote that "the incidence [of colon cancer in Wistar/Furth rats] fluctuates from time to time... the incidence decreased significantly when a part of the Wistar/Furth colony was moved to cleaner conditions." A strain of monkey that develops colon cancer spontaneously is maintained in a colony at Oak Ridge, Tennessee, and is *Saguinus oedipus oedipus* or the cotton-top tamarin (Clapp et al, 1985), a small new world primate that has fastidious eating habits and is recorded on the U.S. Department of Agriculture's endangered species list. It also appears that colonic carcinogenesis in this species is colitis-associated. Other primate centers in the U. S. had observed colon tumors in the same species of monkey but when sanitation in the colonies was improved, colitis was much less common and colon tumors were no longer found. Other species of monkey maintained under similar conditions that also acquired colitis did not, however, go on to develop colon tumors. It is well established that colitis is a promoter of colonic tumor growth in humans and in mice (Barthold, 1981).

Chemically Induced Colon Cancer

At present, one must presume that human colon cancer is, at least in part, due to exposure to initiating agents in unknown amounts and at unknown times during life. Therefore, the hypothesis that chemically induced cancers can teach us about the behavior and biology of human cancer is not only viable but of value. The first consistent production of intestinal cancer in animals as a result of administration of carcinogens was reported using dibenzanthracene or methylcholanthrene feeding to mice which resulted in tumors of the ileum (Lorenz and Stuart, 1941). But it was not until the discovery by Druckrey (1967) that dimethylhydrazine was a fairly specific colon carcinogen that extensive studies were conducted on pathogenesis and nutritional intervention in rats and mice. Since then a number of colonic carcinogens have been identified that fit into seven categories: 1) aflatoxins; 2) alkylnitrosamides and nitrosoureas such as methylnitrosourea, ethylnitrosourea, and methylnitronitroso-guanidine; 3) aromatic amines such as dimethylaminobenzidene and nitrosobisoxo-propylamine and numerous mutagens; 4) cholanthrenes; 5) cycasin and its derivatives such as azoxymethane, dimethylhydrazine, and methylazoxymethanol acetate; 6) irradiation from sources such as x-rays, strontium, and cerium; and 7) irritants such as dextran sulfate and undegraded carrageenan. It is not clear if compounds in the last group act as complete carcinogens or are simply strong tumor promoters.

Dimethylhydrazine-induced Carcinogenesis

By far, the most commonly used carcinogens are dimethylhydrazine (DMH) and its metabolites. It is of some interest that symmetrical DMH (1,2-dimethylhydrazine) which is usually used as the water soluble dihydrochloride salt is highly carcinogenic to rodents, but unsymmetrical DMH (1,1-dimethylhydrazine) is not carcinogenic in similar doses and time interval studied. DMH must be activated metabolically to an ultimate carcinogen and most of this activity occurs in the liver. The compound and most metabolites undergo substantial enterohepatic circulation, but studies have demonstrated clearly that the active carcinogen reaches the dividing cells at the base of the crypts via the bloodstream. DMH is converted to azomethane (most of which is exhaled) which is in turn metabolized to azoxymethane (AOM). Cycasin is also metabolized to AOM. This is converted to methylazoxymethanol (MAM) whose metabolism liberates formalin and a methyldiazonium ion. The methyldiazonium ion is transformed to a methylcarbonium ion which appears to be the ultimate carcinogen responsible for methylation of DNA and other macromolecules. Administration of DMH and related compounds results in alkylation of DNA primarily in the colon, liver, and kidney. Doses of 30 mg/kg of the dihydrochloride salt for five weeks result in a colon tumor incidence of approximately 70–100% in rats fed a purified diet *ad libitum*. In the small intestine, adenocarcinoma incidence varies from 20–50% and most of these tumors are found just distal to the common bile duct. Tumors of the ear are of two types: squamous cell carcinoma of the ear canal or of Zymbal's gland, a specialized sebaceous gland below the ear and tumor incidence varies from 5 to 20%. Incidence of small bowel and ear tumors seem to vary highly with each lot of DMH. Both kidney and liver tumors are generally observed in fewer than 1% of the animals; the only exception to this is when high levels of bile acids are added to the diet and this promotes both colon and liver tumorigenesis so that hepatocarcinomas appear in about a quarter of the rats. This presumably results from greatly increased hepatic flux of bile acids which also act as a tumor promoter in hepatocytes.

Pathology of Chemically-induced Tumors. In the broad sense, colon tumors induced in rats appear morphologically, histologically, and behaviorally to resemble adenocarcinoma of the colon in humans. But appreciation of the differences between the induced lesions in rodents and the spontaneous tumors in humans is essential. One pitfall in discussing the experimental tumors is that there is no universally accepted classification scheme. A strategy of categorization of chemically induced colonic tumors found in rats proposed by Pozharisski (1973) appears to be the most comprehensive treatment of the subject. At the gross level, most of the tumors that arise in the rat as a result of DMH treatment are exophytic pedunculated polyps. These are composed of relatively well-differentiated glandular elements that contain fewer goblet cells than normal colonic epithelium. These tumors generally have a narrow pedicle attaching them to the mucosa (Figure 1). The tumors are in contiguity with the intestinal lumen and are exposed to the intestinal contents. With the paradigm used in the author's laboratory (5 DMH treatments followed by about 6 months of feeding), the majority of polypoid tumors found are classified as adenomas. Only about 25% of the polypoid tumors are classified as adenocarcinomas and most of these are 4 mm or greater in size. A few fungiform carcinomas are usually found and one must wonder if different factors are active in promoting the growth of this type of tumor compared to the more commonly observed.

After the well-differentiated polypoid tumor, the next most commonly detected tumor is a poorly differentiated mucin-producing tumor that is usually observed within the lymphoid follicles of the proximal 2 cm of the colon (Figure 2). Although there are large pools of extracellular mucin, epithelial cells with a signet ring appearance are often found indicating excessive intracellular mucin storage. This tumor is usually not exposed to the lumenal contents and does not appear to respond to dietary manipulation. This particular tumor is the most

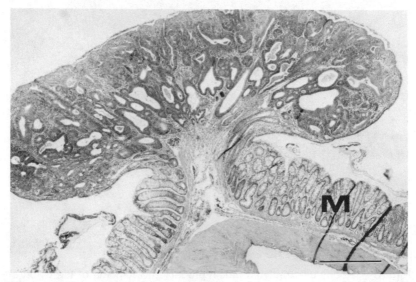

Figure 1. Adenomatous polyp exhibiting an absence of goblet cells and a wide diversity of glandular size and shape; a narrow pedicle attaches the tumor to the mucosa (M). Bar = 500 μm.

malignant of those induced by DMH and has a high propensity for metastasis to regional lymph nodes and visceral organs. One must question the usefulness of including these mucinous tumors in the total tumor response. There seems to be some disagreement as to the topographical distribution of DMH induced colonic tumors, with some authors finding relatively uniform distribution throughout the colon and others reporting a predilection for the distal colon. It is clear that tumors of the cecum and rectum are relatively uncommon, compared to those found in the colon itself. Complicating analysis of the location of tumors in the rodent colon is the use of terms for location in human colon which are not appropriate for the animal model. One significant difference between the DMH induced model and human colon cancer is that while the latter presents with a single tumor, the former generally displays multiple tumors which often have different morphologic and histologic characteristics.

Genetic Alterations in Experimental Colon Cancer

There are both similarities and differences in the genetic material of human colon cancer tissue compared with that from tumors of rats. While half of human colon carcinomas are aneuploid and another

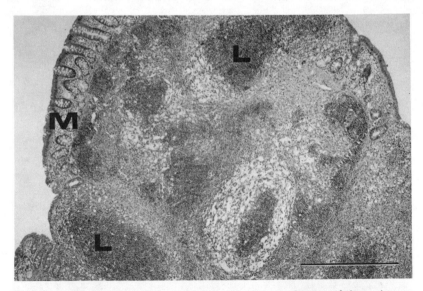

Figure 2. Poorly differentiated mucin-producing carcinoma of the colon associated with lymphoid aggregates (L) of the proximal colon that lies entirely beneath an intact mucosa (M). There are accumulations of pools of extracellular mucin and intracellular mucin within signet ring cells. Bar = 500 μm.

quarter are "near diploid," virtually all DMH induced tumors present diploid DNA with only a single tumor expressing a "near diploid" pattern (Fischbach et al, 1991). However, a variety of other genetic changes have been reported for chemically induced colonic carcinomas. Several groups have examined the expression of various oncogenes in carcinogen induced tumors and found enhanced levels of those genes. A marked increase in the abundance of c-*myc* was seen in all AOM induced colon tumors, including adenomas and carcinomas (Guillem et al, 1988). This same group (Tulchin et al, 1988) localized the expression of the c-*myc* protein using immunohistochemistry. They found elevated expression of this protein in normal tissue within the nuclei of cells in the base of the crypts where proliferation was taking place, in all levels of adenomatous polyps and intensely in a carcinoma *in situ*. H-*ras* oncogene expression was found in 64% of colon carcinomas induced with DMH (Yasui et al, 1987) but in none of the tumors classified as adenomas; all metastases showed strong reactivity for the oncoprotein. In the colon carcinomas, H-*ras* reactivity was stronger in deeply invasive tumors than in superficial tumors; there was no significant difference in oncogene expression between well- and poorly-differentiated tumors. Another group found that no H-*ras* mutations were induced by DMH, but 66% of the colon carcinomas expressed K-*ras* point mutations (Jacoby et al, 1991). The same type of mutation was observed in 20% of the premalignant colonic mucosal samples 15 or more weeks after carcinogen administration. Studies of rats treated with the carcinogen methylnitrosourea (NMU) revealed that 33% of carcinomas and 3% of adenomas had detectable K-*ras* mutations but no H-*ras* alterations (Jacoby et al, 1992). Because the low incidence of *ras* mutations in these tumors contrasts with other animal models in which NMU induces a high incidence of point mutations, it is likely that activation of other oncogenes may predominate in this particular model. To examine this possibility, Alexander et al (1992) extracted DNA from NMU induced colon tumors and transfected this into NIH 3T3 cells. Most samples induced transformed foci and subsequently induced tumors in nude mice. They found no evidence for H-*ras*, K-*ras*, N-*ras*, *neu, raf, fms, met,* or *hst* genes, suggesting that another, perhaps unidentified, oncogene is activated in colon tumors induced with NMU.

Some other ventures at genetic alteration of mice have been made that are relevant to colonic carcinogenesis. A strain of mutagenized mouse has been described which was derived from ethylnitrosourea treated male C57BL/6J animals that were bred to AKR/J females (Moser et al, 1990). In attempting to breed offspring that exhibited circling behavior, it was observed that adult onset anemia appeared in some progeny as an autosomal dominant trait. It was subsequently found that the anemia was secondary to blood loss from multiple intestinal adenomas. These occur as broad based polyps one to three mm across which are often too numerous to count, particularly in the small intestine. Another line of mice that has been described recently is a transgenic pedigree that has an absent p53 tumor suppressor gene (Donehower et al, 1992). This gene is absent or mutated in the majority of humans with colon cancer. In the mice, 74% of homozygotes develop tumors by six months of age; although many tumors of various organs have been observed no intestinal tumors were described.

Immunodeficient Animals for Colon Cancer Studies

The use of immunodeficient animals allows the implantation of colon tumors from patients, implantation from other animals, or growth of cell lines to tumors *in vivo*. There are four types of immunodeficient animals that can be used for colon cancer studies. These include the nude rat and nude mouse, both of which are athymic and therefore produce no T lymphocytes. These animals are used most extensively for xenotransplantation of tumors. The third strain is the SCID (severe combined immune deficient) mouse which produces no T or B lymphocytes. The final strain is the Nu-bg-xid (nude-beige-x-linked immunodeficient) mouse, sometimes referred to as the NIH triple deficient strain which lacks T lymphocytes, T-independent B cells, and NK cells. All of these strains of immunodeficient rodent have been used successfully for colon cancer studies. One practical problem in studying diet effects on colon carcinogenesis in these animals is that immunodeficient animals are fed autoclaved diets and semipurified diets generally do not hold up well to sterilization; another approach used with success in nude mice is to feed the test diets and treat animals with combinations of antibiotics, but this clearly alters the gut flora and it may not be adequate for more severely immunocompromised strains. Irradiation of diets may prove best for sterilization in studies with these animals.

Although the choice of immunodeficient animal may not be critical, since all strains allow the majority of tumors to grow, the site for implantation of tumor material may be a significant variable in determining the results of a study. Implantation of human colon tumor cell suspensions, tumor fragments, or cell lines has been done by: subcutaneous injection; subcutaneous injection into a polyurethane sponge matrix; injection under the renal capsule; intraperitoneal injection; injection into the bowel wall, usually the cecum; and injection into the spleen, liver, or specific blood vessels. The last option of injecting into specific organs is suitable for studying growth and treatment of metastatic lesions. Although subcutaneous injection is the easiest technique in the list above, it is probably the least comparable to the situation that we wish to model. Fidler (1991) has shown that orthotopic implantation of human colon carcinomas into the wall of the cecum in nude mice resulted in consistent formation of metastatic lesions in liver and spleen while injection at other sites did not yield this result. This work showed that the organ environment determined the metastatic potential of these tumors and that ectopic locations did not provide the appropriate milieu. An interesting approach to this question is the use of vascularized polyurethane sponge matrices implanted subcutaneously one to two weeks prior to inoculation of tumor cells (Thiede et al, 1988). Several human colon cancer cell lines were tried as were a variety of tumors derived from other sites. Eighty-eight per cent of the colon tumors grew in these matrices. The number of cells necessary to induce tumor growth was significantly lower than with injection into the subcutis. While none of the tumors that developed from subcutaneous injection metastasized, up to 41% of the animals with sponge matrices developed metastatic lesions. Most metastases were to a second sponge or to the skin. One advantage of this system is the ability to easily monitor the growth of the tumors over time. An example of the potential problems in interpreting results of human colon cancer growth subcutaneously in nude mice can be found in the publication by McGarrity et al (1991). They compared three groups of mice fed: low fat, low fiber; high fat, low fiber; and high fat, high fiber. In the mice fed high fat and low fiber, two human colon cancer cell lines yielded significantly increased tumor DNA and ornithine decarboxylase, and nonsignificant increases in tumor volume and weight. However, the animals in this group weighed significantly more than either of these other two groups. It has been shown consistently that caloric intake is a critical mediator of colonic tumor growth (Klurfeld et al, 1987; Reddy et al, 1987). If factors in the colon lumen are thought to be involved in the initiation and/or promotion of colonic carcinomas, does it make sense to study colon tumors implanted at sites other than the colon? Another variable that must be considered in studies of transplanted tumors, whether derived from fresh surgical resections or cell lines, is if the tumors induced maintain the architecture and other characteristics of the primary tumors. Ideally, one would want relatively well-differentiated cells that retained the structural traits of adenocarcinomas; in practice, this goal is often not achieved.

Potential Tissue Mediators of Colonic Carcinogenesis

There are an assortment of putative biological intermediates that are thought to be related to the development of colon cancer. In this discussion of animal models, it seems appropriate to consider those factors associated with the colonic mucosa. Many studies have shown in both humans and animals that cytokinetics of colonic mucosal growth is positively correlated with risk of tumor growth. One of the evolving areas of research is in the marker to be used for measurement of cell turnover. The gold standard in this technique has been the incorporation of ^{3}H-thymidine into DNA to quantitate the proportion of cells in the S phase. One approach has been to isolate tissue or DNA and quantitate the radioactivity recovered. The more informative method has been to prepare histologic sections and perform autoradiography to determine individual labeled cell positions within the crypts. The final variant of using radiolabeled thymidine incorporation into colonic epithelium is to dissociate the cells into a single cell suspension and quantitate S phase cells using flow cytometry. Another widely used technique is the crypt cell production rate. This method uses injection of colchicine or other metabolic inhibitor that causes dividing cells to arrest in metaphase. Dissociation into individual crypts allows quantitation of dividing cells per crypt and allows stoichiometric calculations of the number of cells produced per unit time. One weakness of this technique is that the denominator in these equations is the crypt and ignores differences in crypt depth or total number of crypt cells which can vary markedly with different treatments. In the last several years other techniques of labeling dividing cells have been developed that are supplanting thymidine uptake. These include the markers bromodeoxyuridine (BUdr) and proliferating cell nuclear antigen (PCNA). These markers allow the advantage of not requiring radioactive precautions and the attendant disposal problems. BUdr is a thymidine analogue and must be injected while the animal is still alive or by *ex vivo* incubation of viable tissue; quantitation is usually done microscopically. PCNA is an auxiliary protein of DNA polymerase and has the distinct advantage of requiring no antemortem administration of any marker that must be taken up by cells. This antigen is highly conserved evolutionarily and is found in most species from yeast to plants to mammals. Results with PCNA correlate highly with those of thymidine uptake although PCNA stains a larger population of cells than those in the S phase.

Another potential mediator that has received great interest in the last few year is the aberrant crypt assay described by Bird (1987). These appear in rodent colons shortly after administration of carcinogens and respond to some compounds that are considered chemopreventive agents (Pereira and Khoury, 1991).

Nuclear aberrations that occur as a result of carcinogen administration have also been suggested as a short term marker of susceptibility of the colonic mucosa to various nutritional and pharmacologic modalities.

Alterations in the quality and/or quantity of intestinal mucin is one potential mediator of colonic carcinogenesis that merits further research. Since mucin serves as the intestinal lubricant and as the barrier between the lumenal contents and the epithelium, subtle changes in this layer could have important long term consequences. It has been shown that dietary fiber feeding alters the production rate of mucin found in the gut (Vahouny et al, 1985).

An important group of potential mediators that has received little attention from the diet and carcinogenesis area is peptide growth factors. These compounds have been shown to modulate growth in many types of tumors and a number have been implicated in controlling growth of colon carcinomas including peptide YY, gastrin, enteroglucagon, and others (Klurfeld, 1992). Schaudies et al (1990) have reported that wheat bran feeding to rats specifically reduces colonic epidermal growth factor (EGF) content. We have shown that reduced energy intake decreases both insulin and insulin-like growth factor-I (IGF-I) plasma levels (Ruggeri et al, 1989a); we have also reported that tumors from energy restricted rats abnormally regulate receptors for these growth factors while receptors in normal tissues are minimally affected (Ruggeri et al, 1989b).

Conclusions

The rodent models of human colon cancer are far from perfect but, given an understanding of the limitations of any animal model, it must be acknowledged that these paradigms are of use in understanding how human tumors might respond to a variety of stimuli. While they cannot replace clinical trials, many studies can be performed on animals that would be precluded from being conducted on people. At this point in time, orthotopic transplantation of human colon tumor fragments into immunodeficient animals appears to be the model that most closely approximates the human disease and affords the opportunity to determine effects of diet, cellular and molecular changes, and therapy.

Acknowledgments

This work was supported, in part, by grant CA 43856 from the National Institutes of Health.

References

Alexander, R. J., Grate, S. J., Raicht, R. F., and Buxbaum, J. N., 1992, Detection of transforming oncogenes in rat colon tumors induced by direct perfusion with N-methyl-N-nitrosourea, *Cancer Letters*. 61:119.
Barthold, S. W., 1981, Relationship of colonic mucosal background to neoplastic

proliferative activity in dimethylhydrazine-treated mice, *Cancer Res.* 41:2616.

Bird, R. P., 1987, Observation and quantification of aberrant crypts in the murine colon treated with a colon carcinogen: preliminary findings, *Cancer Letters.* 37:147.

Clapp, N. K., Lushbaugh, C. C., Humason, G. L., Gangaware, B. L. and Henke, M. A., 1985, Natural history and pathology of colon cancer in Saguinous oedipus oedipus, *Dig. Dis. Sci.* 30:107s.

Donehower, L. A., Harvey, M., Slagle, B. L., McArthur, M. J., Montgomery, C. A. Jr., Butel, J. S., and Bradley, A., 1992, Mice deficient for p53 are developmentally normal but susceptible to spontaneous tumors, *Nature.* 356:215.

Druckrey, H., Preussmann, R., Matzkies, F., and Ivankovic, S., 1967, Selektive Erzeugung von Darmkrebs bei Ratten durch 1,2-Dimethylhydrazin, *Naturwissenschaften.* 54:285.

Fidler, I. J., 1991, Orthotopic implantation of human colon carcinomas into nude mice provides a valuable model for the biology and therapy of metastasis, *Cancer Metastasis Rev.* 10:229.

Fischbach, W., Rubsam, B., Mossner, J., Wunsch, H. P., Seyschab, H., and Hohn, H, 1991, DNA aneuploidy and proliferation in spontaneous human and dimethylhydrazine-induced murine colorectal carcinogenesis, *Z. Gastroenterol.* 29:533.

Guillem, J. G., Hsieh, L. L., O'Toole, K. M., Forde, K. A., LoGerfo, P., and Weinstein, I. B., 1988, Changes in expression of oncogenes and endogenous retroviral-like sequences during colon carcinogenesis, *Cancer Res.* 48:3964.

Jacoby, R. F., Llor, X., Teng, B. B., Davidson, N. O., and Brasitus, T. A., 1991, Mutations in the K-ras oncogene induced by 1,2-dimethylhydrazine in preneoplastic and neoplastic rat colonic mucosa, *J Clin Invest.* 87:624.

Jacoby, R. F., Alexander, R. J., Raicht, R. F., and Brasitus, T. A., 1992, K-ras oncogene mutations in rat colon tumors induced by N-methyl-N-nitrosourea, *Carcinogenesis.* 13:45.

Kitamura, Y. and Fujita, J., 1986, Inbred and mutant mice and rats available in Japan with unique contributions to cancer research, *Jpn J. Cancer Res.* 77:1169.

Klurfeld, D. M., 1992, Dietary fiber-mediated mechanisms in carcinogenesis, *Cancer Res.* 52:2055s.

Klurfeld, D. M., Weber, M. M., and Kritchevsky, D., 1987, Inhibition of chemically induced mammary and colon tumor promotion by caloric restriction in rats fed increased dietary fat, *Cancer Res,* 47:2759.

Lorenz, E. and Stuart, H. L., 1941, Intestinal carcinoma and other lesions in mice following oral administration of 1,2,5,6-dibenzanthracene and 20-methylcholanthrene, *J. Natl. Cancer Inst.* 1:17.

McGarrity, T. J., Peiffer, L. P., Kramer, S. T., and Smith, J. P., 1991, Effects of fat and fiber on human colon cancer xenografted to athymic nude mice, *Digest Dis Sci.* 36:1606.

Moser, A. R., Pitot, H. C., and Dove, W. F., 1990, A dominant mutation that predisposes to multiple intestinal neoplasia in the mouse, *Science.* 247:322.

Miyamoto, M. and Takizawa, S., 1975, Colon carcinoma of highly inbred rats, *J. Natl. Cancer Inst.* 55:1471.

Pereira, M. A. and Khoury, M. D., 1991, Prevention by chemopreventive agents of azoxymethane-induced foci of aberrant crypts in rat colon, *Cancer Letters.* 61:27.

Pozharisski, K. M., 1973, Tumours of the intestines, In: "Pathology of Tumours in Laboratory Animals, Vol. I, Part 1," V. S. Turusov, ed., Intern. Agency Res. Cancer, Lyon (1973).

Reddy, B. S., Wang, C.-X., and Maruyama, H., 1987, Effect of restricted calories intake on azoxymethane-induced colon tumor incidence in male F344 rats, *Cancer Res.* 47:1226.

Ruggeri, B. A., Klurfeld, D. M., Kritchevsky, D., and Furlanetto, R. W., 1989, Caloric restriction and 7,12-dimethylbenz(a)anthracene-induced mammary tumor growth in rats: alterations in circulating insulin, insulin-like growth factors I and II and epidermal growth factor, *Cancer Res.* 49:4130.

Ruggeri, B. A., Klurfeld, D. M., Kritchevsky, D., and Furlanetto, R. W., 1989, Growth factor binding to 7,12-dimethylbenz(a)anthracene-induced mammary tumors from rats subject to chronic caloric restriction, *Cancer Res.* 49:4135.

Schaudies, R. P., Satchithanandam, S., and Calvert, R. J., 1991, Alteration in levels of immunoreactive epidermal growth factor in the gastrointestinal mucosa of Fischer rats fed a diet containing 10% wheat bran, *J Nutr.* 121:800.

Squire, R. A., Goodman, D. G., Valerio, M. G., Frederickson, T., Strandberg, J. D., Levitt, M. H., Lingeman, C. H., Harshbarger, J. C., and Dawe, C. J., Tumors, *in*: "Pathology of Laboratory Animals, Vol. II," Benirschke, K., Garner, F. M., Jones, T. C., eds., Springer-Verlag, New York (1978).

Thiede, K., Momburg, F., Zangemeister, U., Schlag, P., and Schirrmacher, V., 1988, Growth and metastasis of human tumors in nude mice following tumor-cell inoculation into a vascularized polyurethane sponge matrix, *Int J Cancer.* 42:939.

Tulchin, N., Ornstein, L., Guillem, J., O'Toole, K., Lambert, M. E., and Weinstein, I. B., 1988, Distribution of the c-myc oncoprotein in normal and neoplastic tissues of the rat colon, *Oncogene.* 3:697.

Vahouny, G. V., Le, T., Ifrim, I., Satchithanandam, S., and Cassidy, M. M., 1985, Stimulation of intestinal cytokinetics and mucin turnover in rats fed wheat bran or cellulose, *Am. J. Clin. Nutr.* 41:895.

van den Berghe, J., ver Heyen, A., Lauwers, S., and Geboes, K., 1985, Spontaneous adenocarcinoma of the ascending colon in Wistar rats: the intracytoplasmic presence of a Campylobacter-like bacterium. *J. Comp. Pathol.* 95:45.

Yasui, W., Sumiyoshi, H., Yamamoto, T., Oda, N., Kameda, T., Tanaka, T., and Tahara, E., 1987, Expression of Ha-ras oncogene product in rat gastrointestinal carcinomas induced by chemical carcinogens, *Acta Pathol Jpn.* 37:1731.

Summary Report of Dietary Fiber Analysis Workshop

Judith A. Marlett

Department of Nutritional Sciences
University of Wisconsin-Madison
1415 Linden Drive
Madison, WI 53706

Introduction

Workshop participants focused on three topics: Methods for analysis of dietary fiber in foods and concentrated fiber sources; criteria for selection of a method for fiber analysis; and physiologically relevant aspects of fiber analysis.

Methods for analysis of dietary fiber

The basic steps to fiber analysis were reviewed. All procedures begin with a sample that is dried and ground to a suitable particle size without heat damage. Lipid is extracted if present at concentrations of greater than 5 to 10% (dry wt.). All methods extract starch by incubation of the sample with enzymes. A variety of amylases are used and each method usually employs two enzymes. A protease is utilized in some procedures to extract protein; this step is usually not completely effective. Most methods either measure soluble and insoluble fractions of dietary fiber or have been modified to do so.

Several caveats were provided by the "seasoned" fiber analysts attending the workshop to those participants who were interested in learning about the basics of fiber analysis. These included the recognition that technical experience was necessary to conduct most of the analyses reproducibly. Second, all methods have evolved, undergoing a variety of modifications designed to improve the procedure. All publications about a method should be thoroughly reviewed before a particular method is attempted. Third, the distinction between soluble and insoluble fiber is made by the method of analysis. Generally, those methods with more extractive steps disrupt the plant matrix more, resulting in the recovery of a greater proportion of the total fiber in the soluble fraction.

Criteria for selection of a method for fiber analysis

Workshop participants agreed that several methods of analysis had merit, provided that the strengths and limitations of the procedure were recognized. These include the chemical methods developed by Southgate (1969, 1981), Theander (Theander and Aman, 1979; Theander and Westerlund, 1986; Theander et al., 1990) and Englyst (Southgate et al., 1978; Englyst, 1981; Englyst and Cummings, 1990), and the gravimetric procedures developed by Asp (Asp et al., 1983) and Mongeau (Mongeau and Brassard, 1986; 1990), and the neutral detergent fiber (NDF) method originally developed by Van Soest (Van Soest and Wine, 1967; Robertson and Van Soest, 1981) for animal feed analysis and the procedure developed by a committee primarily for food labeling known as the AOAC (Association of Official Analytical Chemists Method) (Prosky et al., 1984; 1985; 1992). Workshop participants were referred to a recent publication that reviews and compares these and other methods of dietary fiber analysis (Asp et al. 1992).

Purpose and resources determine what method will be used for fiber analysis. Regulatory reasons for measuring food composition were promulgated originally to protect the consumer; more recently, they are developed to inform the consumer (Asp et al. 1992). The aim of fiber analysis for research should be to learn as much as possible about the fiber source in order to understand the basis for the effect of fiber. Current methods of analysis provide information about the primary polysaccharide structure but not about the secondary or tertiary structures. Generally more resources are required to conduct chemical analyses than to perform gravimetric methods. However, as gravimetric analyses are modified to provide more information and as chemical methods are simplified to make them less costly and time consuming, the differences in resources needed to perform the various methods are disappearing.

Physiologically relevant aspects of fiber analysis

Most analytically determined characteristics of dietary fiber do not appear to be simply translated into determinants of physiological behavior. Relationships between analytical or in vitro and in vivo behaviors need to be defined before a physiologically relevant analysis or definition of dietary fiber can be developed. Workshop participants began to develop a list of issues closely aligned to dietary fiber analysis that are relevant to this gap in our knowledge. These included the bioavailabilities of starch and protein in fiber foods, the fraction of fiber that functions as soluble fiber in the upper gastrointestinal tract, and the characterization of the fermentable substrate supply, including mucin, that reaches the colon. Time constraints prevented further development of this list of issues and their discussion.

References

Asp, N-G., Johansson, C-G., Hallmer, H., and Siljestrom, M., 1983, Rapid enzymatic assay of insoluble and soluble dietary fiber. J. Agric. Food Chem. 31:476-482.

Asp, N-G., Schweizer, T. F., Southgate, D. A. T., and Theander, O., 1992, Dietary fibre analysis, in: "ILSI Europe Workshop: Dietary Fibre—A Component of Food—Nutritional Function in Health and Disease," T. F. Schweizer and C. Edwards, eds., Springer Verlag, New York.

Englyst, H. N., 1981, Determination of carbohydrate and its composition in plant materials, in: "The Analysis of Dietary Fiber," W. P. T. James and O. Theander, eds., Marcel Dekker, New York.

Englyst, H. N. and Cummings, J. H., 1990, Non-starch polysaccharides (dietary fiber) and resistant starch, in: "New Developments in Dietary Fiber," I. Furda and C. J. Brine, eds., Plenum Press, New York.

Mongeau, R. and Brassard, R., 1986, A rapid method for the determination of soluble and insoluble dietary fiber: comparison with AOAC total dietary fiber procedure and Englyst's method. J. Food Sci. 51:1333-1336.

Mongeau, R., and Brassard, R., 1990, Determination of insoluble, soluble, and total dietary fiber: collaborative study of a rapid gravimetric method. Cereal Foods World 35:319-324.

Prosky, L., Asp, N-G., Furda, I., DeVries, J. W., Schweizer, T., and Harland, B., 1984, Determination of total dietary fiber in foods, food products, and total diets: interlaboratory study. J. Assoc. Off. Anal. Chemists 67:1044-1052.

Prosky, L., Asp, N-G., Furda, I., DeVries, J. W., Schweizer, T. F., and Harland, B., 1985, Determination of total dietary fiber in foods and food products: collaborative study. J. Assoc. Off. Anal. Chemists 68:677-679.

Prosky, L., Asp, N-G., Schweizer, T. F., DeVries, J. W., and T. Furda, 1992, Determination of insoluble and soluble dietary fiber in foods and food products: collaborative study. J. Assoc. Off. Anal. Chemists 75:360-366.

Robertson, J. B. and Van Soest, P. J., 1981, The detergent system of analysis and its application to human foods, in: "The Analysis of Dietary Fiber in Food," W. P. T. James and O. Theander, eds., Marcel Dekker, New York.

Southgate, D. A. T., 1969, Determination of carbohydrates in foods. II. Unavailable carbohydrates. J. Sci. Food Agric. 20:331-335.

Southgate, D. A. T., 1981, Use of the Southgate method for unavailable carbohydrates in the measurement of dietary fiber, in: "The Analysis of Dietary Fiber in Food," W. P. T. James and O. Theander, eds., Marcel Dekker, New York.

Southgate, D. A. T., Hudson, G. J., and Englyst, H., 1978, The analysis of dietary fiber: choices for the analyst. J. Sci. Food Agric. 19:979-988.

Theander, O., and Aman, P., 1979, Studies on dietary fibres. 1. Analysis and chemical characterization of water-soluble and water-insoluble dietary fibres. Swedish J. Agric. Res. 9:97-106.

Theander, O., and Westerlund, E., 1986, Studies on dietary fiber. 3. Improved procedures for analysis of dietary fiber. J. Agric. Food Chem. 34:330-336.

Theander, O., Aman, P., Westerlund, E., and Graham, H., 1990, The Uppsala method for rapid analysis of total dietary fiber, in: "New Developments in Dietary Fiber," I. Furda and C. J. Brine, eds., Plenum Press, New York.

Van Soest, R. J., and Wine, R. H., 1967, Use of detergents in the analysis of fibrous feeds. IV. Determination of plant cell-wall constituents. J. Assoc. Off. Anal., Chemists 50:50-55.

Fiber and the GI Microflora

Abigail A. Salyers
Department of Microbiology
University of Illinois
Urbana, Illinois 61801

Current Problems

There are two types of questions that can be asked about the interaction between the human diet and the bacterial microflora of the human colon: How does the composition of the human diet affect the colonic microflora, and how do interactions between the diet and the microflora affect the host? Most scientists who work in this area would agree that very little progress has been made toward answering either of these questions during the past two decades. The goal of the workshop was to understand why there has been so little progress and how the barriers to progress can be removed.

Interactions Between the Diet and the Colonic Microflora.

Types of interactions. In theory, the diet could affect the colonic microflora in three ways: by changing the total number of bacteria, by changing the species composition of the microflora, or by changing bacterial products and activities. Of these three possibilities, only the first has been established with any certainty. That is, numerous studies have shown that diets high in fermentable fiber cause an increase in the total number of bacteria excreted. The second and third possibilities remain controversial and were discussed at some length in the workshop.

Diet and species composition. Many attempts have been made to test the hypothesis that changes in the diet can alter the species composition of the colonic microflora, but there is still no convincing proof either for or against this hypothesis. Some investigators have found no significant differences in microflora despite quite drastic differences in diet (for some examples, see Salyers, 1986), whereas others have reported significant changes associated with a single additive (A. Rao, this volume). Studies which have claimed to show significant differences in microflora often disagree about which groups of bacteria are affected (Salyers, 1986).

Disagreements about whether changes in diet change the species composition of the colonic microflora can be traced directly to limitations and uncertainties inherent in the methods that are currently used to define the species composition of the microflora: plating dilutions of fecal suspensions on agar media and identifying the species or genus of isolated colonies by classical microbiological techniques which rely on phenotypic rather than genotypic traits. Such methods work well for extensively-studied facultative bacteria such as *E. coli*, but when applied to the genera of obligate anaerobes that comprise over 95% of the colonic microflora, they are unreliable. First, plating efficiencies of the obligate anaerobes have not been rigorously determined and could vary considerably from genus to genus or from one lot of medium to another. Second, recovery of organisms varies with the length of time fecal specimens are stored prior to analysis and extent to which strict anaerobiosis is maintained throughout the dilution and plating procedure. Third, there are no well-validated selective or differential media for rapid and accurate identification of most genera of colonic anaerobes, and even the more laborious identification schemes based on fermentation tests are not completely reliable.

The most reliable methods for identifying colonic anaerobes are nucleic acid-based approaches; partial sequencing of 16S rRNA and species-specific or genus-specific DNA probes. Surprisingly, most nutritionists who study the colonic microflora have not followed research on molecular identification methods and are unaware that both 16S rRNA partial sequencing and DNA probe techniques have now been made simple enough for routine use on large numbers of isolates. The nucleic acid-based procedures have two important advantages over classical techniques. First, they are the gold standard for species identification and are much more reliable than phenotypic tests. Second, they can be applied directly to bacterial fractions from fecal specimens, thus bypassing the need to grow the bacteria. DNA probes for some species of colonic anaerobes have been available for years. In fact, use of a DNA probe-based method for enumerating fecal bacteria without growing them was described nearly 6 years ago (Kuritza et al., 1986). Today, this type of approach could be made much easier by taking advantage of technical advances made since 1986.

Not everyone who attended the workshop agreed with the assertion (by the workshop leader) that classical enumeration methods are artifact-prone and need to be replaced by new methods based on modern molecular techniques. Not surprisingly, those who had done numerous studies using the old techniques expressed confidence in these techniques. It was clear, however, that groups using these techniques have not applied to their media and identification procedures the rigorous standards of validation that have been applied routinely to isolation and identification procedures used in clinical laboratories. Such validation is essential to increase compatibility of results from different laboratories and to prevent those with a vested interest in a particular type of outcome from taking advantage of methodological grey areas. Despite disagreement about the accuracy of classical techniques, there was general unanimity on the need for a simpler method of characterizing the colonic microflora.

Diet and bacterial activities. A number of activities of the colonic microflora have now been studied in detail. These include: breakdown of dietary and host polysaccharides (Salyers, 1988), breakdown of proteins (Macfarlane et al., 1988), modification of xenobiotic compounds (Rowland and Mallett, 1988; Rafii et al., 1991), modification of bile acids and sterols (Story and Furumoto, 1988), and production of fecal mutagens (Kingston et al., 1990). Synthesis of many of these enzymes has been shown to be regulated. Thus, the predominant species of colonic bacteria are capable of considerable flexibility in adapting to changes in substrate availability or levels of toxic compounds. This may explain the remarkable stability of the colonic microflora, and raises the question of whether changes in diet afffect colonic bacteria mainly by changing their activities rather than by changing relative numbers of different species. To date, however, there has been no attempt to determine if the activities of the MAJOR GENERA of human colonic bacteria change with changes in diet.

Despite the lack of direct evidence for an effect of diet on bacterial activities, there was general agreement that the metabolic activities of the colonic microflora are likely to be more informative than its species composition. The measurement of bacterial enzyme activities in fecal extracts has been used to characterize the response of the colonic microflora to changes in diet (see, for example, Rowland and Mallett, 1988). The problem with investigations of this type is that the choice of enzymes to be assayed was based on those used in toxological studies rather than on information about known activities of the major colonic bacterial genera. This approach assumes that certain classes of xenobiotics, such as nitroaromatic compounds, are physiologically significant in the human colon. However, there is no evidence that these particular compounds are present in appreciable levels in the normal human colon or are associated in any direct way with the etiology of intestinal disorders such as colon cancer, which are thought to be diet-related. Given the toxicological orientation of such studies, there were some surprising omissions in the list of activities measured. One such omission was production of fecapentaenes, a class of mutagen that has actually been found in human feces and shown to be produced by bacteria (Kingston et al., 1990). Also omitted were enzymes associated with modification of bile salts, despite the fact that bile salts are thought to be tumor promoters.

Another criticism of this approach, as it is currently used, is that too little is known about the origin of the activities being measured. It is not known what groups of bacteria produce each activity, whether more than one enzyme contributes to each activity, whether the genes encoding the enzymes are regulated, or (most important) whether the activities have any real physiological significance. Such information is essential if results of the assays are to be interpretable. In is instructive to note that when an attempt was made to identify the bacteria responsible for fecal nitroreductase activity, it was found that this activity was the result of multiple enzymes produced by different species of bacteria, most of which were minor components of the colonic microflora (Raffi et al., 1991).

Based on what is known about the activities of the numerically predominant groups of bacteria, it is now feasible to design a set of assays that would at least indicate metabolic activities of the predominant genera of colonic bacteria. This set of assays would include not only measurements of enzyme activities (e.g., polysaccharidases, proteases, bile salt dehydrolases) but also of bacterial metabolites (e.g., short chain fatty acids, methane, ammonia sulfides). Whatever the assays chosen, each should be justified either as an indicator of levels of the major genera or as an activity with a demonstrable impact on the host.

There was some disagreement among workshop participants about the utility of the toxicologically-oriented enzyme assay approach. Some people (including the workshop leader) felt that this approach as it is currently constituted is worthless as a method for assessing the effect of dietary additives (other than xenobiotics) on the intestinal microflora. Others felt that some useful information was obtained, but agreed that a new look needs to be taken at the choice of enzyme activities. There seemed to be general agreement that this type of approach, i. e., the use of enzyme activities to characterize the state of the colonic microflora, is promising and merits further attention.

Effects of the Microflora on the Host

The main reason for wanting to know how dietary fiber and other dietary components affect the colonic microflora is that some types of bacterial activities may affect the host. A knowledge of what bacterial activities have the greatest effects on the gastrointestinal mucosa would make it much simpler to design tests for assessing the relevant characteristics of the colonic microflora. Unfortunately, virtually nothing is known about how bacterial products affect the gastrointestinal mucosa, and until this situation is remedied decisions about what bacterial activities are important will continue to be based entirely on guesswork. It has been shown that colonization of germfree animals with a normal microflora causes significant changes in mucosal architecture, turnover of mucosal cells and intestinal motility (Abrams, 1983), but nothing is known about the basis for these changes or what aspects of mucosal cell function are specifically affected. One hypothesis connecting bacterial activities and colonic function has been much discussed of late, i.e., the hypothesis that butyrate and possibly other short-chain fatty acids stimulate mucosal turnover. This is an interesting hypothesis, but one for which the evidence, based largely on studies of cell cultures or on unphysiological perfusion experiments, is inadequate. Clearly, investigations of the impact of bacterial products on the mucosa need to be undertaken. Such investigations are particularly timely because recent advances in molecular and cell biology of the gastrointestinal tract and beginning to provide a sound scientific basis for defining effect on the mucosa.

Some bacterial products are known to be toxic, at least to cells in culture. These include ammonia (from urease action or fermentation of hexosamines in mucin) and methanol (from fermentation of pectin). However, the question remains whether such compounds ever reach toxic levels in the intestines of people eating a normal diet and whether they have the same effect on cells in intact tissue as they do on cultured cells. There are some bacterial products which might have an effect on the mucosa but which have not been investigated. These include sulfides (from sulfate reducing bacteria), hormone-like compounds produced by bacteria, polyamines and subsymptotmatic levels of bacterial toxins. Of particular interest are fecal mutagens such as the fecapentaenes (Kingston et al., 1990). Fecapentaenes are produced by *Bacteroides* species from a plasmologen precursor and are excreted by many people in the population (Van Tassell et al., 1990). The fact that fecapentaenes cause mutations in DNA makes them particularly relevant to investigations of the possible role of bacteria in the etiology of colon cancer because recent research on colon cancer has shown that colon tumors are the result of a succession of point mutations and genetic rearrangements which disrupt normal control of colonocyte cell cycle (Fearon, 1992). Given this, it was surprising that there was no coverage of fecal mutagens in any session of the conference. Even more surprising was the fact that a poll of workshop participants revealed that only a few had even heard of fecal mutagens. This was one of many indications that the dietary fiber community has become too ingrown.

A factor that needs to be kept in mind when investigating the effect of bacterial activities on the host is the importance of using intact animals eating "real" foods. Cell cultures should be avoided where possible because cells in culture have undergone major genetic rearrangments and no longer express many of the messages expressed in the intact tissue. Also, perfusion with solutions of pure compounds may give a distorted picture of the effects of bacterial products. Some recent studies from M. Eastwood's laboratory, in which labeled plant cell walls were fed to laboratory rodents and the distribution of label monitored in the animal, were reported in the workshop and serve as an example of a more physiologically relevant approach to determining the fate of bacterial products in an animal.

Future Research Needs

Methods for Monitoring the Species Composition and Activities of the Colonic Microflora

Given the numerous shortcomings of current methods for characterizing the colonic microflora, it is clear that new methods are needed. The ideal method would be simple enough to allow reproducible processing of hundreds of samples and would be amenable to automation. It should not require fresh fecal specimens or growth of bacteria. It should be designed so that validation is straightforward and the same results are obtained when the same sample is processed in different laboratories. Although methods that measure metabolic activities of colonic bacteria are preferable to methods that measure species composition, it is doubtful that a rational activity-based method can be developed until more is known about what bacterial products have the greatest impact on the host. There is an acute need for such research. In the meantime, it would be desirable to pursue methods for determining the species or genus composition of the microflora because such tests could at least be used to determine if dietary additives were exerting a major effect on the population structure of the microflora. Such a method should be based on nucleic acid sequence, or on some other constant phylogenetically meaningful trait.

There are two promising, but largely untried, technologies that might be used as the basis of a simple method for crude monitoring of the genus composition of the microflora. One is a long chain fatty acid profiling, an approach which takes advantage of the fact that different genera of bacteria often have unique membrane lipids. This approach has been successfully used to identify pure cultures, and might be made to work on a bacterial fraction taken directly from feces. The problem with this approach is the complexity of the lipid profile that would be obtained from the bacterial mixture in the colon. However, if only lipids with phylogenetic significance were monitored, this problem might be overcome. A second technology that might be useful for characterizing the population structure of the colonic microflora is polymerase chain reaction (PCR). A mixture of DNA segments, each representing a different group in the colonic population, might be obtained by PCR amplification of highly conserved genes or operons. Such a pattern would provide a "fingerprint" of the population.

In Vivo Models for Colonic Fermentation

Workshop participants agreed on the need to develop and validate good in vitro systems for predicting the response of colonic bacteria to dietary components. Many such model systems have been proposed, ranging from diluted fecal specimens or simple batch cultures inoculated with human feces to complicated, multistage chemostats (for a recent review, see Rumney and Rowland, 1992). The relative merits of these models have been much debated, but the debate has been largely irrelevant because it is based on guesses about the nature of the colonic environment which may have little foundation in fact. In assessing different in vitro systems, the following questions should be asked: To what extent does the in vitro system reproduce the genus or species composition of the colonic microflora and the bacterial products detected in colon contents? How stable is the species composition or metabolic activity profile of the bacterial population in the system? The in vitro system need not be (and probably will not be) a perfect replica of the colonic microflora, but it is important for interpretation of results to know how far the population deviates from that found in the human colon. Obviously, development of simple well-validated methods for characterizing the microflora would help to solve the problem of how to assess in vitro systems.

If rational experimental criteria are applied, there could be some surprises. For example, it could prove to be the case that simple batch cultures, with appropriately chosen media, would resemble the colonic bacterial population as closely as a chemostat. In fact, a type of batch culture called a biphasic culture provides a reasonably good approximation of a chemostat in the case of pure cultures. Particular attention should be given to formulation of media, with a view toward excluding such unphysiological substrates as glucose and limiting growth rates to those likely to be experienced by bacteria in the colon (i.e., less than 5 hours per generation). Whatever the system chosen, it should be rigorously standardized and validated so that results from different laboratories can be compared with each other.

Animal Models for Studying Microflora-Fiber-Host Interactions

In vitro systems may be able to predict whether a particular type of fiber or food additive will be fermented by the human colonic microflora, but such systems cannot provide information about the effects of bacterial activities on the host. For this, an animal model is needed. Mice or rats are the animals of choice in the sense that these animals are small, easy to maintain and well-characterized physiologically. Also, most of the transgenic animals that might ultimately be of interest to nutritionists will be mice or rats. It has become fashionable in recent years to dwell on the characteristics of mice and rats that make them poor models for human dietary studies (e.g., coprophagy, presence of a cecum). However, this type of quibbling serves no useful purpose since it is entirely negative and leads ultimately to the conclusion that all animal models are inadequate.

In every fast-moving area of modern biology, from immunology to cancer research, animal model development has proceeded along more constructive lines. Instead of asking what is wrong with rodents as a model for humans, workers in these areas have been asking how rodent models can be improved to make them better approximations of humans. For example, immunologists have implanted human immune tissue in immune-deficient mice. A similar approach might be applied to developing an animal model for studying microflora-diet-host interactions. Perhaps the biggest problem with mice, aside from coprophagy, is that their colonic microflora is so different from that of humans. A solution to this problem would be to colonize a germfree mouse or rat with human feces. Mallett et al. (1987) reported colonizing germfree rats with human feces. The enzyme activities they measured in feces from the colonized rats resembled those in human feces, but no attempt was made to assess the composition of the resulting bacterial population. Recently, Rowland's group has begun a partial characterization of the bacterial genera in these animals and preliminary results, presented in the workshop, indicated that the microflora may be a reasonable approximation of that in the human colon. As with the in vitro systems, the question of validation and laboratory-to-laboratory comparability of whatever animal model is chosen needs to be addressed early and thoroughly. Also, the microflora of colonized animals need not be a perfect replica of the human microflora for the animals to be a useful model system.

Training and Mindset of People Working in the Area

It was clear from discussions in the workshop and in the general sessions where workshop summaries were given that many senior scientists who have been past leaders in dietary fiber research remain hostile to modern technologies, especially molecular biology. This hostility, which arises largely from a lack of training in the new areas, is unfortunate because some of these new technologies, properly adapted, might make a substantial contribution to solving some of the problems that have not been solved by classical techniques. In fact, it could be argued that the single greatest future challenge in the area of dietary fiber-colonic microflora interactions will be to overcome attitudes among nutritionists that have prevented development of innovative aproaches and critical evaluation of existing procedures.

Acknowledgements
This work was supported by grant AI17876 from the National Institute of Health.

References

Abrams, G. D., 1983, Impact of the intestinal microflora on intestinal structure and function, *in* "Human Intestinal Microflora in Health and Disease," D. Hentges, ed., Academic Press, New York.

Fearon, E. R., 1992, Genetic alterations underlying colorectal tumorigenesis, *in* "Tumor Suppressor Genes: The Cell Cycle and Cancer," Imperial Cancer Research Fund, London.

Kingston, D. G., Van Tassell, R. L., and Wilkins, T. D., 1990, The fecapentaenes, potent mutagens from human feces. *Chem. Res. Toxicol.* 3:391.

Kuritza, A. P., Shaughnessy, P., and A. A. Salyers, 1986. Enumeration of polysaccharide degrading *Bacteroides* species in human feces using species-specific DNA probes, *Appl. Environ. Microbiol.* 51:385.

Macfarlane, G. T., Allison, C., Gibson, S. A., and Cummings, J. H. 1988, Contribution of the microflora to proteolysis in the human large intestine, *J. Appl. Bacteriol.* 64:37.

Rafii, F., Franklin, W., Heflich, R. H., and Cerniglia, C. E. 1991, Reduction of nitroaromatic compounds by anaaerobic bacteria isolated from the human gastrointestinal tract, *Appl. Environ. Microbiol.* 57:962.

Rowland, I. R., and Mallett, A.. K., 1988, The influence of dietary fiber on microbial enzyme activity in the gut, *in* "Dietary Fiber: Chemistry, Physiology, and Health Effects," D. Kritchevsky, C. Bonfield, and J. W. Anderson, eds., Plenum Press, New York.

Rumney, C. J., and Rowland, I. R., 1992, In vivo and in vitro models of the human colonic flora, *Crit. Rev. Food Sci. Nutr.* 31:299.

Salyers, A. A., 1986, Diet and the Colonic Environment: Measuring the Response of Human Colonic Bacteria to Changes in the Host's Diet, *in:* "Dietary Fiber: Basic and Clinical Aspects," G. V. Vahouny and D. Kritchevsky, eds. Plenum Press, New York.

Salyers, A. A., 1988, Activities of polysaccharide-degrading bacteria in the human colon, *in* "Dietary Fiber: Chemistry, Physiology, and Health Effects," D. Kritchevsky, C. Bonfield, and J. W. Anderson, eds. Plenum Press, New York.

Story, J. A., and Furumoto, E. J. 1988, Dietary fiber and bile acid metabolism, *in:* "Dietary Fiber: Chemistry, Physiology, and Health Effects," D. Kritchevsky, C. Bonfield, and J. W. Anderson, eds. Plenum Press, New York.

Van Tassell, R. L. Kingston, D. G., and Wilkins, T. D. 1990, Metabolism of dietary genotoxins by the human colonic microflora: the fecapentaenes and heterocylic amines, *Mutation Res.* 238:209.

Dietary Fiber and Gastrointestinal Function

Martin A. Eastwood

Wolfson Gastrointestinal Laboratory
Western General Hospital
Edinburgh, EH4, 2XU
United Kingdom

The workshop discussed the influence of fibre on:

1. The lumenal contents of the gastrointestinal tract.
2. Intestinal motility.
3. Events outside the wall within the body.

Unfortunately time did not allow discussion other than the lumenal events.

Interactions of Dietary Fiber Polysaccharides

The physical properties of digesta will depend predominantly on the interactions of polymeric constituents (fiber, protein, and starch). These will, of course, be altered by cooking, by depolymerisation during enzymic digestion and fermentation, by changes in pH and water content along the gastrointestinal tract, and by non-polymeric materials present in the food or produced by polymer dissimilation.

Cooking may open unmasked groups, e.g., debranching pectin by beta elimination of side chains and also

1. splitting aggregates
2. changing primary structure
3. altering cellular structure

The main types of interaction can be classified as follows:

1. Space occupancy

Dissolved polysaccharides present in the digesta as disordered coils will, at comparatively low concentrations (typically less than 0.5%, w/v), interpenetrate to form an entangled, viscous network. Insoluble fibers, or swollen food particles, will make a significant contribution to viscosity only at much higher concentrations (when their combined volume exceeds about 50% of the total).

2. Non-specific adhesion

Solid particles will have a general tendency to form weak associations by non-specific (Van der Waals and dipolar) attractions. Much stronger association may arise from electrostatic attraction (e.g., between a negatively-charged polysaccharide, such as pectin, and proteins at a pH below their isoelectric point). Associations of this type may either exist in the food as it is eaten, or be induced by changes in luminal pH. It is possible that the action of pancreatic enzymes is affected by the presence of fiber. This, however, is difficult to prove since it is necessary to separate the enzymes from the fiber to estimate them.

3. Specific adhesion

Food structure (natural and manufactured) is often generated by polymer chains packing together into long, ordered assemblies stabilized by co-operative arrays of (individually weak) non-covalent bonds. These assemblies normally involve chains of one type (homotypic), although a few examples of specific heterotypic adhesions are known. They may either hold chains together in insoluble fibers or crosslink hydrated networks.

Fiber and other constituents of the gastrointestinal tract or best regarded as contributing to a sequence of physical chemical interactions which are complicated by the loss of small molecular weight molecules following dissimilation by enzymatic digestion or fermentation.

4. Covalent bonding

In addition to non-covalent packing, the polymeric constituents of plant tissue (particularly legumes) may be linked covalently. For example, extensin acts as a crosslink between proteins and polysaccharides.

5. Ion binding

Charged polymers attract an 'atmosphere' if ions of opposite charge. Counterions may also be incorporated as an integral part of ordered polymer assemblies. In particular, pectin chains in plant tissue are held together by arrays of bound calcium ions. These may be desorbed at gastric pH and re-absorbed in the ore alkaline environment of the duodenum. Copper is especially susceptible to binding.

6. Binding of small molecules

Certain antinutrients (e.g., tannins) are absorbed and preferentially extracted by salivary glycoproteins and proteolytic enzymes, in man and other animals. This is a detoxifying system; phenolics in berries and red wine are dealt with similarly.

Other examples of specific interactions between small molecules and polymeric components of food include the binding of bile salts to charged polysaccharides and the formation of inclusion complexes between amylose and lipids.

Immobilization of Water and Dissolved Nutrients

The water content of digesta may be classified as:

1. Bulk water, which will contain within it small molecules and dissolved polymers.
2. Water trapped within swollen particles (which will again include dissolved material).
3. A tightly bound sheath of water molecules onthe surface of polymer chains or polymeric assemblies. The amount bound in this way is small (typically 3–4 molecules per sugar in polysaccharides), and will therefore be neglible until the solids content approaches that in faeces.

Absorption from the lumen will be affected by

1. the concentration of osmotically-active species (e.g., dissolved nutrients, bile salts, and the products of digestion and fermentation)
2. the partition of water (and hence of nutrients dissolved within it) between the continuous, bulk phase and the dispersed phase of hydrated food particles (since nutrients trapped within parti cles cannot be absorbed)
3. the mobility of the bulk phase, and hence the ease of transport of nutrients to the musocal surface. This is normally discussed in terms of viscosity but, when the polymer content is high, solid-like (elastic) properties may dominate. These may be distinguished from viscous flow by oscillatory (rather than rotational) measurements of digesta rheology.

Experimental studies may be complicated by dilution of gut contents to offset deliberate attempts to generate extremely high viscosities. This biological feed-back mechanism may have important implications for the physiological action of dietary fiber, and merits substantial further investigation.

Colonic Fermentation

There is immense species variation, dependent on different anatomy. This is further complicated in the rat by coprophagy. The caecum is a displaced rumen. There seems to be variation in the use of the word caecum. In animal anatomy it almost always refers to the blind sac which corresponds to the vermiform appendix in humans. The distinction is important because a true caecum has no true flow and must empty pulsatively via the route of entry. This factor can perturb transit measurements in animals like pigs. Retention time, and hence fermentation rate, are important. The microbial yield per unit of carbohydrate in inversely related to the retention time in the caecum. Butyrate is important in maintaining colonic tissue turnover and growth but in this respect may be regarded as physiological nutrient.

The fermentation products may be different in different animals (e.g., starch can be converted to lactic acid in the rumen and to butyrate in the human colon). The ratio of short chain fatty acids generated is very important. A proportion of energy is taken up by bacteria and this is dependent on time of exposure and the needs of the caecal and colonic flora. This difference between rumen and colon probably exists because rapidly degadable starches are removed prior to the colon probably exists because rapidly degradable starches are removed prior to the colon. In the rumen only rapidly fermentable starches give lactate. However, this might occur in humans if there was malabsorption of carbohydrate.

Carbon dioxide is reduced to methane. This dictates the ratio of acetate to propionate. If less methane is produced, then electrons are removed as hydrogen or propionate. In methane-producers, more acetate is found in the blood.

Therefore, in decreasing order of facility, the ratio of acetate to propionate is the most readily affected, H S production from sulphur is important, and the production of methane occurs more slowly. There is important microbial interdependence in these reactions, which is called yntropic.

Overall Picture

It is important to see the meal as a hydrated polymeric mass, restricting the mobility of water and small molecules (including the products of hydrolysis and fermentation). The effect of such a polymeric meal is

1. to slow gastric emptying
2. to be involved in enteric mixing and entrapment of materials of low molecular weight and to retard absorption in the jejunum and ileum
3. immobilization of water in the small intestine.
4. influencing the effectiveness of pancreatic and other enzymes
5. to facilitate conditions in the colon wherein bacteria can ferment polymers
6. to influence stool weight by virtue of the residual polymeric mass, bacteria, and the immobilization of water and solutes (hydrophilic and hydrophobic).

Such modulations will have consequences for intestinal and colonic muscle-activity, the metabolic turnover rate of absorbed nutrients, and endocrine hormone activity. Transit time and rate of movement along the gastrointestinal tract is important. This is relevant in the colon where pectin is readily fermented in the caecum, ispaghula slowly fermented along the colon, and wheat bran is dissimilated much more slowly. The hierarchy is reversed for water immobilization.

Conclusions

The gastrointestinal tract may be likened to two dialysis bags in tandem, with each having different membrane properties. Physical contents have the same overall properties.

A. In the upper intestine, the whole meal consists of protein, fat and carbohydrate polymers; these are dissimilated by endogenous enzymes and the end products are absorbed.

B. The remaining polymer molecules, whether they be protein or carbohydrate, pass into the ileum where they may affect bile acid reabsorption and hence influence the enterohepatic circulation and sterol metabolism.

C. The residue that passes into the caecum is dissimilated by bacteria. Soluble fermentation-products are absorbed; the gases produced may be either absorbed or expelled. Water is immobilized by residual fiber and bacteria and by the osmotic activity of fermentation products and other remaining small molecules. The hydrated residue is expressed as feces.

Here the "dialysis bag" may be protective as well as absorptive.

Design of Human Studies to Determine the Effect of Fiber on Serum Lipids in Relation to Blood Lipids, Fecal Bulking, Glycemic Control or Bodyweight

David J. A. Jenkins, Ph.D., M.D., D.Sc.
Department of Nutritional Sciences
Faculty of Medicine
University of Toronto
Toronto, Ontario
M5S 1A8

This meeting was attended by some of the most active minds at the conference. Consequently, there was no clear consensus but many important issues were raised.

Purpose of the Studies

Was the purpose of the study: 1) to satisfy government regulatory requirements; 2) to satisfy academic curiosity; or 3) to screen potentially useful food ingredients by the food industry? In many instances, a fairly simple protocol would be required which would allow standardized comparisons to be made. However, the vehicle in which the ingredient was incorporated may play as significant a role in the success of the exercise as the fiber source tested. Furthermore, if the final product were for consumption by the general public, a comparatively small lipid reduction may have broad public health implications. At the same time, the product should be nutritionally sound bearing in mind that vulnerable groups, e.g., the young and the elderly, may also consume this product which must have a nutrient profile at least as good as the food it may displace.

Fibers for use in therapeutic situations would have the caveats mentioned above but greater potency may be sought. With this, possible untoward side effects may increase. Again, the vehicle for fiber administration was important. Gel forming fiber in capsules was not enough to be a good idea in view of the possible esophageal impaction, swelling and possible rupture. On the other hand, it was important to test the actual product since the fiber effect may be greatly modified by the other ingredients and the processing which the product underwent.

For mechanistic studies to define the mode of action of fiber selection was also difficult since it was recognized that fiber may alter blood lipids by several mechanisms. Different fibers may have different effects. It may be necessary to test a range of fibers with different viscosities, digestabilities, bile acid trapping ability and fermentability.

Different types of information will be obtained from different types of trials. Valuable data have been derived from ad libitum and metabolic studies in both normal and hyperlipidemic individuals. Initial leads on the health benefits of fiber came from population studies and these will lead to more useful information in the future. Data are needed in prospective studies where the effects of dietary intervention are studied on large groups of individuals and in smaller secondary intervention studies of patients with pre-exisiting coronary heart disease (CHD) where regression is the goal.

Fiber Sources

Fiber may be studied in a number of forms: as purified fiber; concentrated fiber source; single food; and mixed diet. The fiber sources acknowledged as having lipid lowering properties include the viscous materials such as pectin, guar, tragacanth, locust bean gum, psyllium and β-glucans. However, although these may have a role as in purified form pharmacological pharmacological agents, it was considered important to investigate food sources such as beans and oats and fiber enriched foods which would have application to the general population.

Adverse Effects. There was little discussion of such problems as vitamin, mineral and trace elements deficiencies with lipid lowering diets since, in general, the lipid lowering fiber sources, sometimes referred to as the soluble fibers, appear to be well tolerated in this respect. Concern was raised over other aspects such as the long-term effects of increased bile acid losses in the feces and the worry that in some situations fecal bile acid concentrations might rise. Similarly, there was concern that, although certain types of fermentation may be "healthy" for the colonic mucosa (e.g., through the production of butyrate), other types of fermentation may not have these properties. These matters remain to be resolved.

Conclusion. It was agreed that fiber had lipid lowering potential worthy of investigation. It was suggested that 4–6 weeks was an adequate study duration for most of the lipid lowering effects to be seen. Investigation of other actions of fiber may require longer studies. However, it was also agreed that this complex topic required to be debated further at the next conference.

Short-Chain Fatty Acids—
Research and Clinical Updates

John L. Rombeau, M.D. and Jonathan A. Roth, B.A.

Harrison Department of Surgical Research
Department of Surgery
Hospital of the University of Pennsylvania
Philadelphia, PA 19104

Many recent advances have occurred in the investigative and clinical aspects of short chain fatty acid (SCFA) metabolism since this topic was reviewed previously for the Vahouny Conference (Rombeau, 1988). This review provides an update on this topic, with specific emphasis upon the metabolic and clinical aspects of acetate, propionate, and butyrate. These SCFA will be discussed as to their production, extraction and analysis, absorption, metabolism, physiologic effects, intestinal effects, and future considerations. Proceedings from a conference discussing these issues has recently been published (Tenth Ross Conference, 1991). For purpose of this discussion, SCFA will be defined as the C-1-6 organic fatty acids.

Production

In the human, approximately 200 mmol of SCFA are produced daily contingent upon the amount and quality of ingested and secreted polysaccharide. Most SCFA are produced by anaerobic glycolysis mediated by bacterial enzymatic fermentation of colonic polysaccharide (Embden-Meyerhof Pathway). Extensive research has been performed during the past five years on identifying the many determinants of SCFA production. Broadly speaking, these determinants may be placed into three categories: l) substrate precursors, 2) microorganisms, and 3) other host factors.

Substrate Precursors

The most important determinant in the production of SCFA is the presence of substrate precursors for microbial fermentation. Substrates available for fermentation in the human colon exist in three main forms —unabsorbable carbohydrate, nitrogen, and endogenous polysubstrate sources. The amount of substrates fermented on a daily basis is largely contingent upon the amount of unabsorbed carbohydrate entering the cecum and ascending colon. The amount of colonic carbohydrate varies tremendously among different ethnic populations, dietary intakes, and endogenous microflora. A summary of the substrates available for fermentation in the human colon is shown in Table 1. A major recent finding has been the identification of substantial amounts of undigested starch reaching the cecum. Heretofore, nearly all ingested starch was presumed to have been digested in the upper gastrointestinal tract. The fraction of starch that escapes digestion is called "resistant starch" (Englyst, 1987). Starch may be resistant to digestion for several reasons. Firstly, starch is often physically resistant to digestion. Factors contributing to this physical resistance include the milling of grains and seeds, in addition to natural composition of foods such as corn and beans. Secondly, starch may exist as un-gelatinized granules. These granules, in turn, undergo varying degrees of crystallinity. The degree of crystallinity, in turn, determines digestibility. For example, crystalline

Table 1. Substrate available for fermentation in the human colon

Substrate (g/day)	Amount
Carbohydrate	
Resistant starch	8–40
Nonstarch polysaccharides (dietary fiber)	8–18
Unabsorbed sugars and sugar alcohols	2–10
Oligosaccharides (n = 3 tp 10)	2–10
Chitin and amino sugars	2–6
Synthetic carbohydrate-lactulose, lactitol, polydextrose, etc.	*a
Food additives: substituted celluloses, etc.	*
Therapeutic agents: ispaghula, sterculia	*
Nitrogenous	
Dietary protein	3–9
Pancreatic enzymes and other GI secretions	4–6
Urea, nitrate	0.5
Others	
Mucus	2–3
Bacterial recycling	?
Sloughed epithelial cells	?
Organic acids	?

a Small on average but variable in individuals (from Cummings, 1991).

Type A starch granules are present in cereals and are readily digested; however, Type B, present in bananas and potatoes, is relatively resistant to digestion. Finally, the process of retrogradation influences the resistance of starch to digestion. When starch gels are heated, and subsequently cooled or dried, re-crystallization occurs, which in turn leads to resistance to pancreatic amylase. It is estimated that approximately 12–14 g of resistant starch enter the human cecum each day in individuals consuming a standard Western diet (Englyst, 1987). However, individuals in developing countries consuming large amounts of starch, may have up to 40 g of resistant starch entering the colon daily. Thus, approximately half of the unabsorbable carbohydrate entering the human colon in individuals living in developing countries exists in the form of resistant starch.

Non-starch polysaccharides (NSP) (dietary fiber) is the largest contributor to the production of SCFA in many individuals. Interestingly, the type of NSP may influence the pattern of SCFA production. For example, the soluble fiber pectin is fermented to approximately 80% acetate, and only minimal amounts of butyrate, whereas guar gum produces less acetate and larger amounts of butyrate (Cummings, 1991). Oligosaccharides (n=3–10) is the remaining major carbohydrate available for fermentation in the human colon. Types of oligosaccharides reaching the cecum include raffinose and stachyose, and fructans. Oligosaccharides have different physiologic and biochemical properties from NSP and resistant starch, which in turn provide unique therapeutic possibilities (Cummings, 1991). Nitrogenous sources may also serve as precursors for the production of SCFA. In particular, the branch-chain fatty acids contribute to this process. Finally, additional fermentable substrates include colonic and intestinal mucus, the recycling of bacteria and sloughed intestinal epithelial cells. The amount that these substrates contribute to the total fermentation process is unknown, however, it is probably small in the absence of intestinal inflammation.

Colonic Microflora

The colonic microflora is an important determinant of SCFA production. The preponderance of anaerobic, saccharolytic bacteria in the human colon provide an important milieu for the fermentation process. Bacteria such as C-perfringens increase lactate production and decrease acetate production, thereby enabling bacteria to maximize energy. The frequent prescription of broad spectrum antibiotics to hospitalized patients may in turn significantly reduce the fermentation process. Whether the provision of exogenous, encapsulated bacteria to enhance fermentation in these individuals will be of value remains to be confirmed.

Additional Host Factors

Remaining host factors influencing the fermentation process include intestinal transit time and the administration of medications such as narcotics, and broad spectrum antibiotics. Finally, previous colonic resections may decrease this process by altering the microflora and reducing intestinal transit.

Analysis

The extraction and analyses of SCFA are indeed difficult and complex. The extraction process includes possible use of various solvents, steam, and cold vacuum methodologies. In a comparison of vacuum distillation and steam distillation extraction methods, the prior method was found to be superior with a recovery range of 90–110% for all SCFA in standard solutions. Analytical measurements include the use of either the gas liquid chromatograph or high performance liquid chromatograph. Most investigators use the former, due to improved sensitivity and specificity of analyses. Measurements of SCFA are often reported with reference to three denominators 24 hour production, weight of enteric contents, and volume of enteric contents. Each of these reference points have potential utility depending upon the research question asked and the indication for measurement. Because of the variability of production and considerable ranges in the daily weight of enteric contents, the volume of measured contents is often the preferred denominator (Holtug, 1988).

Absorption

Although predominantly absorbed in the cecum and ascending colon, SCFA may be absorbed throughout the gastrointestinal tract. Extensive research is ongoing to identify the mechanisms of the absorptive process. Current thinking concludes that the SCFA absorptive process is most likely passive and concentration-dependent (Von Engelhardt, 1991). Furthermore, absorption tends to occur transcellularly across the apical cell membrane and not via a paracellular pathway. Absorption of SCFA is, in turn, dependent upon factors such as the sodium-hydrogen exchange and the site of colon in which SCFA are produced. The availability of sodium in the proximal colon enhances the absorption of SCFA. Moreover, absorption occurs to a far greater extent in the ascending colon than the descending colon or rectum. Interestingly, in animal models, absorption tends to occur independent of pH, at least within ranges of 5–9 (Von Engelhardt, 1991).

Metabolism

The metabolism of SCFA differs for acetate, propionate, and butyrate. Acetate, despite being produced in the largest concentration, is only minimally metabolized by the colonocyte, and in turn enters the portal system to serve as an energy source for the periphery, synthesis of long-chain fatty acids, and production of ketone bodies by the liver. Interestingly, the increased concentration of plasma acetate in turn decreases utilization of glucose by skeletal muscle. Acetate may in turn be an important precursor for lipogenesis in the absence of adequate carbohydrate intake (Fahey, 1991). Recent studies in humans have demonstrated a significant increase in plasma acetate levels following starvation, thereby demonstrating the importance of endogenous production (Cummings, 1991). Propionate is metabolized in part by the colonocyte, however, it is primarily metabolized by the liver. An important regulatory effect of propionate is the reduction of cholesterol synthesis with ensuing hypocholesterolemia (Chen, 1984). The mechanism for the cholesterol-lowering effect of propionate is unclear. It may result, in part, from the redistribution of cholesterol from plasma to the liver. Butyrate, despite being produced in the least amount in the human colon, is the most important fuel for the colonocyte. As a major environmental factor that interacts with the genetic events of tumorgenesis and modifies neoplastic progression through the various stages, butyrate facilitates and may directly stimulate the proliferation of normal epithelium (Young, 1991). Other SCFA are less effective in inducing such cellular changes as: arresting cell growth, inducing those genes coding for cell differentiation, modifying cell morphology and ultrastructure (by organizing actin and vimentin filaments), and suppressing cancer-specific properties of transformed cells, including cytoskeleton deorganization (Kruh, 1991).

Physiologic Effects

The varied physiologic effects of SCFA have been highlighted in many recent publications (Katoh, 1991; Roediger, 1991; Sakata, 1991; Von Englherdt, 1991; Yajima, 1991). Effects with potential clinical utility include enhancement of sodium absorption, stimulation of blood flow, and regulation of carbohydrate and lipid metabolism. As mentioned previously, the absorption and transport of SCFA is in part related to the absorption of sodium. It is hypothesized that the increased availability of SCFA in turn promotes increased absorption of sodium and water from the colon, thereby perhaps lessening amounts of fecal solute. Studies in animals (Kvietys, 1981; Demigne, 1985) and humans

(Hoverstad, 1982; Hoverstad, 1986) have demonstrated enhancement of colonic blood flow due to increased concentrations of SCFA. Animal studies indicate that acetate produces a greater increase in blood flow than propionate or butyrate. In-vitro studies in humans have demonstrated that SCFA improves peripheral artery dilatation by reducing resistance in the colon (Mortensen, 1990).

As mentioned, recent developments have indicated that SCFA may play a role in reducing levels of serum cholesterol. The mechanisms by which this effect occurs is unknown. It is probably unrelated to inhibition of cholesterol synthesis, and a suggested mechanism is the shifting of cholesterol from the plasma to the liver. Although butyrate is not normally available to the liver, isolated hepatocytes have shown high rates of butyrate oxidation. Butyrate does have a sparing effect on glucose and glutamine metabolism. Labeling of butyrate also reveals that glucose and glutamine do not diminish the entry of fatty acid carbon into the tricarboxylic acid cycle. The proportional contribution of butyrate to total oxygen consumption is 70% for cell oxidation, indicating that fatty acid is the premier fuel for colonic epithelial cells (Roediger, 1991).

Intestinal Effects

Significant interest has accrued concerning the effects of SCFA, particularly butyrate, on intestinal proliferation and differentiation. These investigations have included studies of malignant cell lines and normal human epithelial cells. Butyrate inhibits DNA synthesis and reduces growth of in-vitro cultured tumor cells in the Gl phase of the cell cycle (Toscani, 1988). Despite the presence of butyrate, cell viability remains, due to only marginal inhibition of RNA and protein synthesis. Butyrate also induces differentiation of many tumor cell types. This in turn leads to an expression of a phenotype typically associated with a mature, functional cell line (Whitehead, 1986). Investigators have examined the effects of intraluminal butyrate infusions upon intestinal epithelial growth and function (Kripke, 1989). Intracolonic infusions of butyrate are trophic to colonocytes and surprisingly have similar, though less beneficial, effects on the small intestine. The mechanism(s) by which intestinal epithelial growth is stimulated is unknown. Possible pathways of trophism include provision of energy, enhancement of intestinal blood flow, enhanced production of enterotrophic gastrointestinal hormones, and increased production of pancreatic and biliary secretions (Figure 1). Several reports have identified potential benefits in humans due to intracolonic infusions of SCFA. A controlled trial from the United States in patients with diversion colitis demonstrated enhanced morphology and healing due to SCFA enemas (Harig, 1989). A prospective, randomized trial in European patients with diversion colitis failed to confirm the American results (Guillemot, 1989). Preliminary, uncontrolled investigations in patients with distal ulcerative colitis, in whom rectal irrigations of SCFA were infused, suggested possible therapeutic benefits (Breuer, 1991). A recent study investigating the effect of butyrate enemas on 10 patients with distal ulcerative colitis, unresponsive to standard therapy, showed that inflammation (measured endoscopically and histologically) was ameliorated. Furthermore, stool frequency decreased, and blood discharge ceased in 9 of 10 patients receiving intra-colonic butyrate (Scheppach, 1992).

Future Investigations

There are many interesting research and clinical challenges for the would-be investigator in SCFA metabolism. More information is needed on the effects of specific SCFA, and their different concentrations, on isolated epithelial cells. These studies are needed in both the normal and diseased epithelium. Studies concerning the possible mechanisms of butyrate stimulation of cell growth in malignant colonic epithelial cells should be performed. Investigations should be directed toward evaluation of SCFA on cellular and organ function, in addition to morphology. The interaction of SCFA with expression of cytokines and growth factors from epithelial cells is needed. Intracolonic administration of SCFA is technically difficult in many instances. Studies are needed

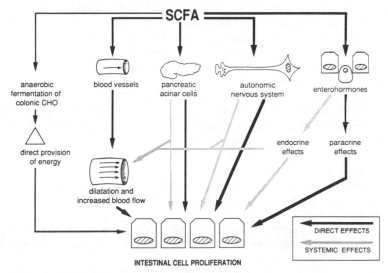

Figure.1. Possible mechanisms of enterotrphic effect in SCFA.

comparing the efficacy of intravenous administration to intralumenal delivery. Finally, potential clinical applications include the provision of SCFA as enterotrophic agents for short bowel syndrome, inflammatory bowel disease, and antibiotic-associated diarrhea. Controlled clinical trials are needed to investigate these therapeutic possibilities.

ACKNOWLEDGMENT

The authors gratefully acknowledge the secretarial assistance of Ms. Renee Seto.

References

Breuer, R. L., Buto, S. K., Christ, M. L., et al, 1991, Preliminary report: rectal irrigation with short-chain fatty acids for distal ulcerative colitis, Dig. Dis. Sci., 36:185.

Chen W-JL., Anderson, J. W., and Jennings, D., 1984, Propionate may mediate the hypocholesterolemic effects of certain soluble plant fibers in cholesterol fed rats, Proc. Soc. Exp. Biol. Med., 175:215.

Cummings, J. H., 1991, Production and metabolismof short-chain fatty acids in humans, in: "Short-Chain Fatty Acids: Metabolism and Clinical Importance," E. Silverman, ed., Ross Laboratories, Columbus.

Demigne, C., and Remesy, C., 1985, Stimulation of absorption of volatile fatty acids and minerals in the cecum of rats adapted to a very high fiber diet, J. Nutr., 115:53-60.

Englyst, H. N., Trowell, H., Southgate, D. A. T., and Cummings, J. H., 1987, Dietary fiber and resistant starch, Am. J. Clin. Nutr. 46:873-874.

Fahey, Jr., G. C. and Garleb, K. A., 1991, Production and metabolism of short-chain fatty acids by ruminants, in: "Short-Chain Fatty Acids: Metabolism and Clinical Importance," E. Silverman, ed., Ross Laboratories, Columbus.

Guillemot, F. Neut, C., Colombel, J. F., et al, 1989, Treatment of diversion colitis with short-chain fatty acids irrigation, Gastroenterology, 96:A188.

Harig, J. M., and Soe:gel, K. H., 1989, Treatment of diversion colitis with short-chain fatty acid (SCFA) irrigation, N. Eng. J. Med., 320:23-28.

Holtug, K., Rasmussen, H. S., and Mortensen, P. B., 1988, Short-chain fatty acids in inflammatory bowel disease. The effect of bacterial fermentation of blood, Scand. J. Clin. Lab. lnvest., 48:667-671.

Hoverstad, T., 1986, Studies of short-chain fatty acid absorption in man, Scand. J. Gastroenterol., 21:257260.

Hoverstad, T., Bohmer, T., and Fausa, O., 1982, Absorption of short-chain fatty acids from human colon measured by the '4C02 breath test, Scand. J. Gastroenterol., 17:373-378.

Katoh, K., 1991, The effect of short-chain fatty acids on the pancreas: endocrine and exocrine, in: "ShortChain Fatty Acids: Metabolism and Clinical Importance," E. Silverman, ed., Ross Laboratories, Columbus.

Kripke, S. A., Fox, A. D., Berman, J. M., et al, 1989, Stimulation of intestinal mucosal growth with intracolonic infusion of short-chain fatty acids, J. Parenter. Enter. Nutr., 13:109.

Kruh, J., 1991, Defer, N., Tichonicky, L, 1991, Molecular and cellular effects of sodium butyrate, in: "ShortChain Fatty Acids: Metabolism and Clinical Importance," E. Silverman, ed., Ross Laboratories, Columbus.

Kvietys, P. R., and Granger, N. D., 1981, Effect of volatile fatty acids on blood flow and oxygen uptake by the dog colon, Gastroenterology, 80:962-969.

Mortensen, F. V., Neilsen, H., Hesor, I., 1990, Short-chain fatty acids dilate human colonic resistance arteries, J. Parenter. Enter. Nutr. Supp., 14(1):9S.

Roediger, W. E., 1992, Cellular metabolism of short-chain fatty acids on colonic epithelial cells, in: "ShortChain Fatty Acids: Metabolism and Clinical Importance," E. Silverman, ed., Ross Laboratories, Columbus.

Rombeau, J. L., Kripke, S. A., and Settle, R. G., 1990, Short-chain fatty acids: production, absorption, metabolism, and intestinal effects, in: "Dietary Fiber," D. Kritchevsky, C. Bonfield, and Anderson, J., eds., Plenum Publishing Corporation, New York.

Sakata, T., 1991, Effects of short-chain fatty acids on epithelial cell proliferation and mucus release in the intestine, in: "Short-Chain Fatty Acids: Metabolism and Clinical Importance," E. Silverman, ed., Ross Laboratories, Columbus.

Scheppach, W., Sommer, H., Kirchner, T., Paglanelli, G. M., Bartman, P., Christl, S., Richter, F., Dasel, G., and Kasper, H., 1992, Effect of butyrate enemas on the colonic mucosa in distal ulcerative colitis, Gastroenterology, 103:51-56.

Toscani, A., Soprano, D. R., Soprano, K. J., 1988, Molecular analysis of sodium-butyrate growth arrest, Oncogene. Res., 3:223.

Engelhardt, W. von, Busche, R., Gros, G., and Rechkemmer, G., 1991, Absorption ofshort-chain fatty acids: mechanisms and regional differences in the large intestine, in: "Short-Chain Fatty Acids: Metabolism and Clinical Importance," E. Silverman, ed., Ross Laboratories, Columbus.

Whitehead, R. H., Young, G. P., and Bhathal, P. S., 1986, Effects of short-chain fatty acids on a new human colon carcinoma cell line (LIM1215), Gut, 27:1457.

Yajima, T., 1991, Sensory mechanisms of motor and secretory responses to short-chain fatty acids in the colon, in: "Short-Chain Fatty Acids: Metabolism and Clinical Importance," E. Silverman, ed., Ross Laboratories, Columbus.

Young, G. P. and Gibson, P. R., 1991, Contrasting effects of butyrate on proliferation and differentiation of normal and neoplastic cells, in: "Short-Chain Fatty Acids: Metabolism and Clinical Importance," E. Silverman, ed., Ross Laboratories, Columbus.

Bile Acids

Jon A. Story
Department of Foods and Nutrition
Purdue University
West Lafayette, IN 47907

Introduction

The interaction of dietary fiber and bile acids has been an important physiological relationship suggested as a part of the explanation of the dietary fiber hypothesis. Specifically the relationship among dietary fiber, daily bile acid excretion, fecal bile acid concentration and cardiovascular disease and colon cancer have been most often discussed.

Increased excretion of bile acids in response to sources of dietary fiber which were observed to lower blood cholesterol levels was suggested to be a part of the mechanism responsible for these changes (Story and Kritchevsky, 1976). More recent examination of this relationship has led to the conclusion that this relationship, i.e., increased bile acid excretion as a mechanism for lowered blood cholesterol levels, is not true for all sources of dietary fiber and is not consistent for all sources of dietary fiber which have been found to reduce serum cholesterol levels (Anderson et al., 1990). Some sources of dietary fiber which lower blood cholesterol consistently increase bile acid excretion (e.g., oat bran and psyllium) while others do not (e.g., beans).

An increase in the concentration of bile acids in the colon has been related to increased susceptibility to colon cancer in a variety of circumstances (Hill, 1982). Further investigation of this relationship suggests that the effects of dietary fiber on bile acid concentration do not consistently correspond to the predicted effects on colon cancer susceptibility in experimental animals. These results are further confounded by variation in animal models used for study of experimental carcinogenesis and by differences in other dietary components. Results from human experiments relating dietary fiber to bile acid metabolism and markers for colon cancer susceptibility have appeared in the literature (DeCosse et al., 1989; Alberts et al., 1990). They suggest interesting effects of some sources of dietary fiber, primarily wheat bran, but disagreement still exists concerning the validity of the markers for colon cancer risk used in these experiments.

The importance of the relative amounts of bile acids excreted and their pool sizes has emerged as a corollary to these hypotheses. Changes in the relative size of the bile acid pools has been suggested as a mechanism by which blood cholesterol levels might be modified by dietary fiber (Story and Thomas, 1982) while the ratio of lithocholic acid to deoxycholic acid excreted in feces has been related to colon cancer risk (Owen et al., 1983).

From this brief summary of the status of the relationship between dietary fiber and bile acids it is apparent that a great deal of work remains to be done. Our workshop group made the following suggestions concerning future efforts aimed at furthering our understanding of this relationship and its importance in human nutrition.

Recommendations

•It is important to recognize that alteration of bile acid excretion is not associated with all hypocholesterolemic effects of dietary fiber. As was noted above, it is important for some but apparently unimportant for others. We need to continue to clarify these relationships and educate both the public and the scientific community concerning this variability.

•Many questions still exist concerning the validity of the relationship between fecal bile acid concentration and colon cancer risk. Are bile acid concentrations increased in patients with polyps and colon cancer after surgery to correct these conditions? How can we explain the differences in response to bile acids in experimental models for colon cancer? Are these animal models for colon cancer valid? What markers for colon cancer risk in humans are valid for examination in relation to bile acids? Until we understand these relationships, it is difficult to make any conclusions concerning dietary fiber and its interactions with other diet components.

•An integrated approach toward improving our understanding of bile acid metabolism and investigating the effects of dietary fiber on bile acid metabolism and the mechanisms responsible for these changes is needed.

•Attention to use of up-to-date and appropriate methodology is essential. Species employed and experimental conditions influence the methods used to measure bile acid concentrations and enzyme activities. Newer, more precise measures of changes in bile acid metabolism (e.g. stable isotopes in humans) should be employed to increase the quality and quantity of information derived from an experiment.

•Experimental designs need to consider a number of related factors which might influence their outcome and incorporate the latest information available. For example gender differences in bile acid metabolism may influence results as well as changes in our understanding of the metabolism of other dietary components.

References

Alberts, D. S., Einspahr, J., Rees-McGee, S., Ramanujam, P., Buller, M. K., Clark, L., Ritenbaugh, C., Atwood, J., Pethigal, P., Earnest, D., Villar, H., Phelps, J., Lipkin, M., Wargovich, M., and Meyskens, F. L., 1990, Effects of dietary wheat bran fiber on rectal epithelial cell proliferation in patients with resection for colorectal cancers, *J. Natl. Cancer Inst.* 82:1280.

Anderson, J. W., Deakins, D. A., Floore, T. L., Smith, B. M., and Whitis, S. E., 1990, Dietary fiber and coronary heart disease, *Crit. Rev. Food Sci. Nutr.* 29:95.

DeCosse, J. J., Miller, H. H., and Lesser, M. L., 1989, Effect of wheat fiber and vitamins C and E on rectal polyps in patents with familial adenomatous polyposis, *J. Natl. Cancer Inst.* 81:1290.

Hill, M. J., 1982, Bile acids and human colorectal cancer, *in:* "Dietary Fiber in Health and Disease," G.V. Vahouny and D. Kritchevsky, eds., Plenum Press, New York.

Owen, R. W., Dodo, M., Thompson, M. H., and Hill, M. J., 1983, The faecal ratio of lithocholic acid to deoxycholic acid may be an important aetiological factor in colorectal cancer. *Eur. J. Cancer Clin. Oncol.* 19:1307.

Story, J. A. and Kritchevsky, D., 1976, Dietary fiber and lipid metabolism, *in:* "Fiber in Human Nutrition," G. A. Spiller and R. J. Amen, eds., Plenum Press, New York.

Story, J. A. and Thomas, J. N., 1982, Modification of bile acid spectrum by dietary fiber, *in:* "Dietary Fiber in Health and Disease," G. V. Vahouny and D. Kritchevsky, eds., Plenum Press, New York.

Resistant Starch

Alison M. Stephen

Division of Nutrition and Dietetics
College of Pharmacy
University of Saskatchewan
Saskatoon, SK S7N 0W0
Canada

Resistant starch is the sum of starch and products of starch degradation not absorbed in the small intestine of healthy individuals.[1] It is emerging as an important component of the diet in relation to a number of physiological processes and risk for certain diseases.[2-5] The intent of the workshop on resistant starch was that it should focus on several aspects:

1. Measurement of resistant starch.
2. Factors influencing the amount:
   a) *intrinsic*—physical properties of food and preparation and processing of food prior to consumption.
   b) *extrinsic*—physiological characteristics which influence the amount of starch resistant to digestive enzymes.
3. Importance of resistant starch for health.

Although there is considerable interest and a growing number of research publications on these aspects, the definition and measurement of resistant starch was the focus of the workshop, specifically whether or not resistant starch should be included in the definition and measurement of dietary fiber. An early solution to this controversy is desirable since continuing discussion on only this aspect may hinder progress in the investigation of the role of resistant starch in human health. Many consider preoccupation with the definition of dietary fiber to have hampered progress on investigations of other aspects of fiber consumption, and it would be unfortunate if the same were to occur for resistant starch.

Figure 1 shows the intake of carbohydrate components in the diet and that proportion of each which enters the colon.[6] This diagram exemplifies the controversy and was the focus of much of the discussion at the workshop. Those who wish to include resistant starch in the definition and measurement of dietary fiber do so because it enters the colon and is available for fermentation as are the non-starch polysaccharides of dietary fiber. Such a proposal ignores, as shown in Figure 1, other sugars which may also reach the colon and are available for fermentation, but which have not been put forward as components of dietary fiber, even though on the inclusion criteria for resistant starch they would clearly qualify. Those who do not believe that dietary fiber and resistant starch should be defined and analyzed together, suggest that these two dietary components are distinct chemically and therefore must be analyzed separately. Moreover, they challenge the physiological aspect of the definition of dietary fiber, i.e., its ability or not to enter the colon, as an out-of-date description of a food component which is now well characterized chemically, and which should be defined in chemical terms like all other constituents of food.

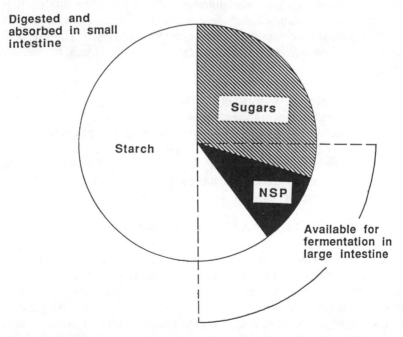

Figure 1. Carbohydrate intake in the human diet and the availability of its subfractions for colonic fermentation.[2]

Because of this controversy, the workshop did not reach discussions of the recent literature on new research on the effects of starch in the colon, including fecal bulking, fermentation products and the effects of these and other changes occurring as a result of starch fermentation.[7]

The particular issues which were raised in relation to definition and measurement were:

1. Historical definition of dietary fiber

   Two aspects were discussed here:
   a) the physiological definition and whether or not it should continue.
   b) the inclusion in the original definition that the polysaccharides of dietary fiber came from "plant cell wall material" which would not include starch.

   Clearly there are different aspects of the historical definition which are open to question.

2. Equating different analytical procedures for dietary fiber, when some contain some resistant starch and others contain none.

3. Whether or not there is a need to know the content of resistant starch and non-starch polysaccharides in foods separately.

4. Measurement of starch, resistant starch and dietary fiber in other species. Emphasis is presently concentrated on the overlap of effects of resistant starch and dietary fiber in the human gastrointestinal tract; in other species, particularly ruminants, starch and non-starch polysaccharides behave very differently and the content of each in foods or forage must be known separately.

5. Consideration of components other than resistant starch and non-starch polysaccharides which enter the colon, specifically sugars, oligosaccharides and protein. These will also be available for fermentation.

In Vitro Nutritional Classification of Starch

In 1987, Englyst and Cummings developed an in vitro nutritional classification of the various subcomponents of starch in the diet.[1] They now describe five distinct fractions of starch in the diet.[8] Two of these are completely digested in the small intestine, but at different rates, readily digestible starch (RDS), being rapidly digested, slowly digestible starch (SDS), as its name indicates, being more slowly digested. Three categories of resistant starch were described as shown in Figure 2. More recently, Englyst et al. have developed an analytical procedure for these

5 fractions and are using this scheme to characterize the starch-containing foods in the western diet.[7,9,10]

The workshop on resistant starch discussed this classification and the analytical procedure which was developed to measure the different fractions. The points of discussion were:

1. What types of starch should come under the name of "Resistant Starch." When originally described, the term referred only to retrograded amylose, that component first being identified as analyzing along with non-starch polysaccharides. Today, retrograded amylose is considered only one component of resistant starch, RS_3, other components being starch resistant to digestion through reasons of physical inaccessibility for digestive enzymes, or because of resistant (uncooked) granules.[9]

2. The relationship between the in vitro classification and in vivo results. Some questions were raised about whether the in vitro classification reflects what happens when starch is consumed.

3. The analytical procedure, and the choice of times to terminate digestion to describe each fraction of starch in a food.

Findings from Epidemiological Studies

One of the fields where an appropriate measure for resistant starch and dietary fiber is vital is in epidemiological work, for comparison of relationships between intake of certain nutrients and incidence of or mortality from certain diseases. At the workshop, those in this field discussed the importance of starch in epidemiological studies, indicating

Type of starch	Example of occurrence	Probable digestion in small intestine
RAPIDLY DIGESTIBLE STARCH	Freshly cooked starchy food	Rapid
SLOWLY DIGESTIBLE STARCH	Most raw cereals	Slow but complete
RESISTANT STARCH		
1. Physically inaccessible starch	Partly milled grains and seeds	Resistant
2. Resistant starch granules	Raw potato and banana	Resistant
3. Retrograded starch	Cooled, cooked potato, bread and cornflakes	Resistant

Figure 2. In vitro nutritional classification of starch.[8,9]

that in some recent studies, starch intake appeared to be an important factor in relationship to disease, yet in many investigations cereals do not appear to be protective. This is in contrast to fruits and vegetables, which invariably are shown to be protective against, for example, colon cancer. Since fruits and vegetables are not a major source of starch, the question of the importance of resistant starch for health was raised.

Conclusion

As indicated earlier, there was little discussion of factors affecting the content of resistant starch in foods or diets, or the importance of this component for health. The recent studies investigating effects of starch in the gastrointestinal tract were not considered, including recent investigations of small intestinal effects and recognition that the rate and extent of starch digestion in the small intestine may have important implications for health,[7,9] nor the recent work on fermentation of starch, and the repeated finding of an increased production of butyrate, compared to fermentation of non-starch polysaccharides.[11-13] These are important areas of research and cannot be ignored. Some resolution of the definition and measurement controversy is essential. In 1987–88, a series of letters in the *American Journal of Clinical Nutrition* set forth the arguments on either side at that time.[14-16] Since then, there have been a number of important publications which have demonstrated quite different properties for starch compared to non-starch polysaccharide. It is clear that continued work in this area will provide further information on the role of resistant starch in the gastrointestinal tract. It would appear that the time to consider all substrates for fermentation as a single entity is over. A stage has arrived for carbohydrate comparable to the period when consideration of different types of fat, or of individual fatty acids became apparent to enable progress on the role of fat in disease causation. The lumping of all components together, whether to give "total fat" or "dietary fiber," without further detail, provides little information. Like fat, the different components of our carbohydrate intake may have individual effects in the body and be of varying importance for our health. Surely the time has come to investigate these in depth.

References

1. European Flair—Concerted Action on Resistant Starch (EURESTA), Physiological implications of the consumption of resistant starch in man, Flair Concerted Action No. 11, *Newsletter III* (1991).
2. H. N. Englyst and J. H. Cummings, Resistant starch, a 'new' food component: a classification of starch for nutritional purposes, *in*: "Cereals in a European

Context," I. D. Morton, ed., First European Conference on Food Science and Technology, Ellis Horwood, Chichester, England (1987).

3. A. M. Stephen, Starch—the nutrient of the 90's, Kellogg Nutrition Symposium, Toronto, Ontario, March, 1992 (in press).

4. J. R. Thornton, A. Dryden, J. Kelleher and M. S. Losowsky, Does super efficient starch absorption promote diverticular disease?, *Br Med J.* 292:1708-1710 (1986).

5. J. R. Thornton, A. Dryden, J. Kelleher and M. S. Losowsky, Super-efficient starch absorption—a risk factor for colonic neoplasia?, *Digestive Diseases and Sciences.* 32:1088-1091 (1987).

6. H. N. Englyst, Personal communication, February, 1992.

7. A. M. Stephen, ed., Starch in human nutrition, *Can J Phys Pharm.* 69:53-136 (1991).

8. H. N. Englyst and S. M. Kingman, Dietary fiber and resistant starch. A nutritional classification of plant polysaccharides, *in*: "Dietary Fiber," D. Kritchevsky, C. Bonfield and J. W. Anderson, eds., Plenum Publishing Co., New York, (1990).

9. H. N. Englyst, S. M. Kingman and J. H. Cummings, Classification and measurement of nutritionally important starch fractions, *Eur J Clin Nutr.* (In press)

10. British Nutrition Foundation, Complex carbohydrates in foods, "The Report of the British Nutrition Foundation's Task Force," Chapman & Hall, London, England, (1989).

11. H. N. Englyst and G. T. Macfarlane, Breakdown of resistant and readily digestible starch by human gut bacteria, *J Sci Food Agric.* 37:699-706 (1986).

12. W. Scheppach, C. Fabian, M. Sachs and H. Kasper, The effect of starch malabsorption on fecal short-chain fatty acid excretion in man, *Scand J Gastroent.* 23:755-759 (1988).

13. G. A. Weaver, J. A. Krause, T. L. Miller and M. J. Wolin, Cornstarch fermentation by the colonic microbial community yields more butyrate than does cabbage fiber fermentation; cornstarch fermentation rates correlate negatively with methanogenesis, *Amer J Clin Nut.* 55:70-77 (1992).

14. H. N. Englyst, H. Trowell, D. A. T. Southgate and J. H. Cummings, Dietary fiber and resistant starch, *Amer J Clin Nut.* 46:873-74 (1987).

15. N. G. Asp, I. Furda, J. W. Devries, T. F. Schweizer and L. Prosky, Dietary fiber definition and analysis, *Amer J Clin Nut.* 48:688-690 (1988).

16. H. Trowell, Dietary fiber definitions, *Amer J Clin Nut.* 48:1079-1080 (1988).

Dietary Fiber and Body Weight Management

Charles T. Bonfield

Astra Associates, Inc.
1834 Woodgate Lane
McLean, Virginia 22101

Introduction

A workshop was convened during the Fourth Vahouny Fiber Symposium to discuss scientific support for the potential benefit of dietary fiber as an adjunctive aid in weight loss and weight maintenance programs. An increasing number of papers are being published in scientific journals reporting results of clinical studies evaluating the effects of various dietary fiber materials as aids in weight management. The workshop participants discussed aspects of conducting clinical studies of dietary fiber materials as aids in weight management and considered some of the possible mechanisms of action which have been proposed for dietary fiber's role in this process.

Clinical Studies

Major findings from 40 clinical studies which evaluated 50 high fiber foods or supplements were reviewed (Table 1). Several studies investigated more than one fiber material. Seven of these studies employed calorie restricted diets composed of natural fiber rich foods. Only a few of these studies used a control group. Another nine studies evaluated fiber enriched foods such as breads, crackers, or bars containing additional fiber isolates which were then consumed as a part of the normal diet. A few of these studies used an acceptable non-fiber control group but others had no control. Twenty four clinical studies assessed the effect of fiber supplements such as tablets, powders or crackers. All of these studies employed a non-fiber placebo control group. In most cases these experimental materials were consumed in addition to a prescribed diet. In all, 35 of the 40 studies used some form of control group.

Thirty three of the fifty materials (66%) evaluated in these studies produced a statistically significant or appreciable ($\geq$ 0.5 pounds per week) weight loss when compared to the control group or compared to baseline. Thus, approximately two thirds of these materials produced significant or appreciable weight loss. Seventeen of the materials studied were soluble fibers—eleven of these produced significant/apprec-

Table 1. Published Clinical Studies

SIGNIFICANT / APPRECIABLE WEIGHT LOSS	NOT SIGNIFICANT WEIGHT LOSS	TOTAL
SOLUBLE FIBER		
Yudkin, 1959 (Methylcellulose)	Duncan, 1960 (Methylcellulose)	
Evans, 1975 (Guar Gum)	Jenkins, 1979 (Apple)	
Evans, 1975 (Methylcellulose)	Hylander, 1983 (Psyllium)	
Jenkins, 1979 (Pectin)	Stevens, 1987 (Psyllium)	
Jenkins, 1979 (Guar)	Dodson, 1981 (Guar)	
Valle-Jones, 1980 (Sterculia & Guar)	Krotkiewski, 1985a (Psyllium)	
Tuomilehto, 1980 (Guar)		
Walsh, 1984 (Glucomannan)		
Krotkiewski, 1985a (Psyllium)		
Krotkiewski, 1984 (Guar)		
Lakhdar, 1989 (Guar)		
Subtotals 11	6	17
INSOLUBLE FIBER		
Macrae, 1942 (Wheat Bran)	Weinreich, 1977 (Wheat Bran)	
Mickelson, 1979 (Cellulose)	Henry, 1978 (Wheat Bran)	
Krotkiewski, 1984 (Wheat Bran)	Jenkins, 1979 (Wheat Bran)	
Dodson, 1979 (Wheat Bran)	Hylander, 1983 (Wheat Bran)	
	Stevens, 1987 (Wheat Bran)	
	Astrup, 1990 (Cellulose)	
Subtotals 4	6	10
MIXED FIBER		
Anderson, 1982 (Foods)	Russ, 1985 (Foods)	
Weinsier, 1982 (Foods)	Baron, 1986 (Foods)	
Solum, 1983 (Barley/Citrus Tablet)	Russ, 1986 (Foods)	
Weinsier, 1983 (Foods)	Schlamowitz, 1987 (Barley/Citrus Tablet)	
Anderson, 1984 (Foods)	Rossner, 1988 (Barley/Citrus Tablet)	
Ryttig, 1984 (Barley/Citrus Tablet)		
Anderson, 1985 (Foods)		
Ehmann, 1985 (Barley/Citrus Tablet)		
Krotkiewski, 1985a (Oat Bran)		
Krotkiewski, 1985b (Oat Bran)		
Krotkiewski, 1985c (Oat Bran & Dates)		
Stevens, 1985 (Oat Bran)		
Rossner, 1987a (Barley/Citrus Tablet)		
Rossner, 1987b (Barley/Citrus Tablet)		
Solum, 1987 (Barley/Citrus Tablet)		
Birketvedt, 1988 (Barley/Citrus Tablet)		
Ryttig, 1989 (Barley/Citrus Tablet)		
Rigaud, 1990 (Barley/Citrus Tablet)		
Subtotals 18	5	23
Totals 33	17	50

iable weight loss, whereas six did not. Another ten materials were insoluble fibers. Four of these were positive and six were not. Twenty three of the materials tested were mixed fibers (containing both soluble and insoluble fibers). Eighteen of these materials produced significant/appreciable weight loss, whereas five did not. Overall, the majority of dietary fiber materials tested in these studies produced the expected benefit regardless of experimental design, investigator or study location.

Workshop members discussed a number of important factors that need to be considered when preparing clinical study designs and when reviewing clinical study reports of dietary fiber materials as aids in weight management programs. Some of these factors are as follows:

1. Subject compliance in protocol requirements may be a problem. High fiber diets, fiber enriched foods and many supplements are often not pleasingly palatable and may not be consumed as required, especially in non-institutionalized conditions, so many subjects may not follow the prescribed dietary program. Also, overweight individuals are notorious for cheating on meal plans. Monitoring for dietary compliance is, therefore, a very important element of study design.

2. Time of administration of fiber supplements or consumption of fiber enriched foods may be a very important factor, depending on which possible mechanism may play a role in the expected benefit.
   —It may be critical that the fiber be taken just before or as an integral part of the meal to exert its maximum effect.
   —It may also be important to consider that fiber may exert a delayed effect (e.g., three to six hours after ingestion of the fiber) so fiber meals or supplements should be taken well in advance if this is thought to be a major effect.

3. Fiber type is not predictive of weight loss effectiveness. Of the 33 materials which produced significant or appreciable weight loss in the 40 studies reviewed, 18 were mixed fibers, 11 were soluble fibers and 4 were insoluble fibers. Well designed clinical studies are therefore required to determine efficacy of any fiber material and predictions about potential efficacy of untested fiber materials are not appropriate.

4. Data from the 40 studies reviewed and from the general literature do not provide sufficient information to predict either responders or nonresponders of fiber treatment so it is not possible, at this time, to predict which person may or may not respond to dietary fiber treatment in weight management programs.

5. Expectations among overweight individuals, the general population and even scientists may impose an unfair bias against fiber materials. An average weight loss of 0.5 to 1.0 pound per week (0.25–0.5 kilogram) is a healthy, safe and reasonable weight loss goal. Overweight individuals are impatient with such small weight loss amounts and many other individuals, including scientists, consider these amounts trivial. Fiber treatment may, therefore, not be able to satisfy general expectations of weight loss even though it may provide a reasonable and healthy benefit.

6. The long-term effectiveness of fiber treatment in weight management has not been determined.

7. Fiber's effect is subtle and may be more useful in weight maintenance than it is in weight loss.

The workshop concluded that it is very difficult to design, recruit appropriate subjects and conduct clinical studies of dietary fiber materials as aids in weight management programs.

Mechanisms of Action

Since the scientific literature does support the premise that some dietary fiber materials are effective aids in weight management, a number of possible mechanisms of action have been proposed for this effect. Unfortunately, very few mechanism of action studies have actually been conducted; however, results of clinical studies which have been conducted for other purposes give some insight to a few of these proposed mechanisms. Each of the following mechanisms was discussed at the workshop:

1. Chewing

It has been proposed that many fiber rich foods require longer chewing times because they are bulky and have a rigid architecture. Blundell and Burley (1990) have proposed that longer chewing times may then lead to earlier sensations of satiety and, therefore, bring an early termination to the eating process. McCance (1953) conducted a crossover study comparing wholemeal bread to white bread. Eating times averaged 45 minutes for wholemeal bread and 34 minutes for white bread. Haber (1977) evaluated eating time for equi-caloric meals of whole (diced) apples, pureed apples and apple juice. It took an average of 17.2 minutes to eat the whole apples, 5.9 minutes for the apple puree and 1.5 minutes to drink the apple juice. Duncan (1983) found that eating time of a low energy dense diet (rich in fresh fruits and vegetables) was 42%

greater than for a high energy dense diet (rich in meats and desserts). These findings are interesting and may provide some support for this premise; however, the workshop consensus was that even if this mechanism was a factor it would only be a supportive one.

2. Stomach Distention

A number of investigators have observed that fiber materials, particularly the viscous polysaccharides, tend to absorb considerable quantities of water and thereby swell to large volumes. It has been proposed that when these materials are consumed and swallowed they expand in the stomach, causing stomach distention and thereby produce sensations of satiety. There is very little evidence in the literature to support this hypothesis (see review by Strickler and Verbalis, 1990). Firstly, the clinical methodology for measuring stomach distention in humans is not well developed, and secondly, clinical studies of viscous polysaccharides which are known to absorb the greatest volumes of liquid (e.g., glucomannan, psyllium) have not shown a satiation effect. Attendees of the workshop concluded that this is not likely an important mechanism for the benefit of fiber in weight management.

3. Stomach Emptying

Clinical studies have confirmed that a number of viscous polysaccharides delay stomach emptying. A review of clinical studies evaluating stomach emptying properties of 25 fiber materials showed that 12 delayed stomach emptying, 4 accelerated stomach emptying and 9 had no effect. Single doses of 10g or more of pectin and 2g or more of guar gum consistently delay stomach emptying. The workshop felt that this was likely one of the important mechanisms of effectiveness; at least for the viscous polysaccharides.

4. Nutrient Absorption

A number of investigators have shown that certain fiber materials when consumed with a meal, produce a more gradual absorption of carbohydrates and lipids from the small intestine. This results in lower and more favorable blood glucose levels and, therefore, more controlled rates of insulin secretion (see review by Jenkins, et al, 1990). Excess blood nutrient and blood insulin levels both promote lipogenesis (fat deposition) so moderation of these factors may lessen the propensity for weight gain. The effect of certain fiber materials on carbohydrate and lipid absorption is well documented, however, the possibility that this may then aid in weight management still needs to be confirmed. Even so, the workshop felt that this may be a worthwhile benefit of a diet rich in high fiber materials.

5. Gastrointestinal Hormones

Fiber materials do not seem to have an effect on gastric hormones such as CCK, gastrin, motilin or glucagon, some of which have been associated with hunger and satiety feelings. There is some evidence, however, that certain fiber materials have either a direct or indirect effect on several hormones in the small intestine. Selected fiber materials carry lipids into the ileum and the cecum. Spiller (1984, 1988) found that perfusion of lipids into the ileum resulted in an increase in plasma concentration of enteroglucagon, neurotensim and peptide YY. Peptide YY and perhaps other neurotransmitters have been found to delay stomach emptying. This action could then promote satiation (see discussion under Ileal Brake).

6. Ileal Brake

Spiller (1984, 1988) found that infusion of partially digested lipid into the ileum resulted in a slowing of small bowel transit time. Read (1984), at about the same time, showed that infusion of lipid into the ileum caused a reflex delay of stomach emptying and a slowing of small bowel transit. This phenomenon has been called the ileal brake. The mechanisms for this effect have not been worked out, but it is thought that the presence of lipid in the ileum may stimulate secretion of enteroglucagon, neurotensin and peptide YY, which may then cause a reflex delay in stomach emptying and a slowing of small bowel transit. The role that dietary fibers play in stimulating secretion of intestinal neurotransmitters and in initiating the ileal brake needs to be confirmed and defined in greater detail; however, attendees at the workshop thought that these potential mechanisms may play an important role in dietary fiber's possible benefit in weight loss and weight maintenance programs.

7. Caloric Excretion

A number of investigators have proposed that some fibers carry nutrients into the large intestine where they will be fermented and used as energy by the colonic microflora or be excreted in the feces. Read, Jenkins and Spiller have confirmed that guar gum given with a meal increases the caloric load in the ileostomy reservoir of ileostomy patients. In either case this will result in loss of available caloric material to the host and thereby possibly contribute to long term weight management. Heaton reviewed studies of fecal energy loss after administration of dietary fiber materials and found an average energy loss of 100 to 200 kcal/day. This is a small but perhaps important mechanism of action in the benefit of fiber rich diets over the long run. The workshop felt that further investigation of this possible mechanism was warranted and its relative importance needs to be better defined.

Conclusion

The workshop concluded that there was substantial evidence that certain dietary fiber rich foods and fiber isolates may provide supportive benefits in weight management programs but that further research into possible mechanisms of action would vastly contribute to a better understanding of the process.

References

Burley, V. J. and Blundell, J. E., (1990), Action of dietary fiber on the satiety cascade, in: Dietary Fiber—Chemistry, Physiology And Health Effects, D. Kritchevsky, C. Bonfield and J. Anderson, ed., Plenum Press, New York, p. 227.

Duncan, K., Bacon, J. and Weinseir, R., (1983) The effects of high and low energy density diets on satiety, energy intake and eating time of obese and non-obese subjects, Am. J. Clin. Nutr., 37:763.

Haber, G. B., Heaton, K. W. and Murphy, D., (1977) Depletion and distruption of dietary fiber: effects on satiety, plasma and serum insulin, The Lancet, 2:679.

Jenkins, D. J. A., Jenkins, A. L., Wolever, T. M. S., Vuksan, V., Brighenti, F., Cunnane, S., Rao, A. V., Thompson, L. and Josse, R. G., (1990) Lente carbohydrate or slowly absorbed starch: physiological and therapeautic indications, in: Dietary Fiber—Chemistry, Physiology And Health Effects, D. Kritchevsky, C. Bonfield and J. Anderson, ed., Plenum Press, New York, p. 247.

McCance, R. A., Prior, K. M., and Widdowson, E. M., (1953) A radiological study of the rate of passage of brown and white bread through the digestive tract of man, Br. J. Nutr., 53:98.

Read, N. W., MacFarlane, A., Kinsman, R., Bates, T., Blackhall, N. W., Farrar, C. B. J., Hall, J. C., Moss, G., Morris, A. P., O'Neill, B. O., Welsh, I., Lee, Y. and Bloom, S. R., (1984) Effect of infusion of nutrient solutions into the ileum on gastrointestinal transit and plasma levels of neurotensin and enteroglucagon, Gastroenterology, 86:274.

Spiller, R. C., Trotman, I. F., Adrian, T. E., Bloom, S. R., Misiewicz, J. J. and Silk, D. B. A., (1988) Further characterization of the ileal brake reflex in man—effect of ileal infusion of partial digests of fat, protein and starch on jejunal motility and release of neurotensin, enteroglucagon and peptide yy, GUT, 29:1042.

Spiller, R. C., Trotman, I. F., Higgins, B. E., Ghodei, M. A., Grimble, G. K., Lee, Y. C., Bloom. S. R., Misiewicz, J. J. and Silk, D. B. A., (1984) The ileal brake-inhibition of jejunal motility after ileal fat perfusion in man, GUT, 25:365.

Strickler, E. M. and Verbalis, J. G., (1990) Control of appetite and satiety: insights from biologic and behavioral studies, Nutr. Rev., 48:49.

Food Industry Perspective: Functional Properties and Food Uses of Dietary Fiber

Mark L. Dreher

M&M/MARS
Division of MARS, INC.
800 High St.
Hackettstown

Background

Dietary fiber generates a great deal of interest among adult consumers, food processors, ingredient suppliers, and health professionals. Over 80% of American adults are concerned about the effects of diet, such as the consumption of dietary fiber on their future health (International Food Information Council, 1991). Since interest in dietary fiber tends to grow with increasing consumer age, fiber-rich foods will continue to gain visibility in the marketplace as the American population ages. The most recent U.S. Department of Agriculture "Nationwide Food Consumption Survey" reveals that Americans eat considerably lower amounts of dietary fiber than the recommended 20 to 35 grams per day (Wright et al., 1991). Further, as the benefits of increased dietary fiber in the diet, from the standpoints of health maintenance and reduction in risk of certain chronic diseases, become better understood more fiber-rich food labeling and marketing opportunities are expected.

Americans should consume more dietary fiber (from food products). One way to increase fiber is by eating naturally occurring fiber-rich foods such as whole grain cereals, legumes, fruits, and vegetables. Another way involves the use of food science to develop fiber-rich processed foods that are either much higher in dietary fiber, more available and convenient foods, or different in form than the natural sources. Although breakfast cereal manufacturers are the most visible in developing and advertising their fiber-rich products, other food manufacturers such as the baking industry have also been active. Over the past 20 years the sales of variety breads or dietary fiber supplemented breads have increased from a few percent to about 35% of total bread sales (Vetter, 1988). The number of fiber-enriched food products in the marketplace has significantly increased since 1984 when the Kellogg Company (R) began an advertising and labeling campaign that linked dietary fiber with cancer.

The availability of new dietary fiber sources (for use as food ingredients) has intensified the interest in understanding food functionality (all those parameters that make a food acceptable for processing and to the consumer). Food functionality includes organoleptic, microstructural, mechanical/physical, and chemical properties (Table 1). The factors affecting fiber functionality are composition (e.g., hexoses, pentoses, and uronic acid), cell wall matrix characteristics, functional groups, surface area, cellulose crystallinity, surface characteristics, ionic linkages, noncovalent bonds, and structure (e.g., glycosidic linkages and degree of branching). Usually the addition of high levels of dietary fiber to foods has an adverse effect on food texture and flavor but when the functionality of fiber is understood or improved the chances of it being successfully incorporated into foods is greatly enhanced.

Usually fiber containing foods need at least 2 to 3 grams of dietary fiber to be considered a good source. New fiber-enriched products include breakfast cereals, breads and rolls, crackers, snacks, cookies, bakery dry mixes, beverages, and frozen entrees. Food uses of dietary fiber range from bulking agents to fat substitutes (Table 2). Since consumers usually prefer products that taste good to products that are nutritious and taste bad, it is critical to understand fiber functionality.

Table 1. Parameters related to food functionality[1]

Parameters	Examples
Sensory	Gumminess
	Hardness
Physical	Density
	Viscosity
Microstructural	Porosity
	Crystallinity
Functional	Water binding
	Emulsification

[1] Adapted from Stanley (1986).

Dietary fiber is a heterogenous mixture of materials that are the structural and some of the non-structural components of all plants. These components are resistant to digestion by enzymes produced by humans. The components of dietary fiber include: cellulose, hemicellulose, lignins, pectins, and a variety of gums and mucilages. All except lignins are polysaccharides. The composition of dietary fiber components varies with the type and maturity of plant tissue. The heterogeneity of dietary fiber is the primary reason for the diversity of its functional properties in food systems.

Total dietary fiber (TDF) is the analytical term for dietary fiber. It includes both insoluble dietary fiber and soluble dietary fiber. Insoluble fiber consists mainly of cell wall components such as cellulose, lignins, and hemicellulose. Soluble fiber consists of noncellulosic polysaccharides such as pectin, gums, and mucilages. About 75% of the dietary fiber in goods is in the form of insoluble fiber. Products frequently referred to as soluble or insoluble fibers are actually sources of both types of fiber. The dietary fiber sources in this chapter are subdivided into three classes: soluble fibers (primarily of soluble fiber; e.g., gums), insoluble fibers (mostly of insoluble fiber; e.g., wheat bran), and composite fibers (blends of soluble and insoluble fibers; e.g., oat bran).

Dietary Fiber Sources and Properties

A wide variety of dietary fiber sources are available to the food industry. Since the early 1980's, the number and availability of dietary fiber sources has increased dramatically. Almost every conceivable fiber source has been considered as a potential ingredient for fiber-enriched foods. These fiber sources range from purified cellulose to cocoa flour, cereal brans to sunflower hulls, and guar gum to konjac flour. Not all of these sources of dietary fiber, however, have made it to the marketplace as mainstream commercial ingredients; there has been a gradual sifting out of these materials based on functionality, economics, or other reasons (Vetter, 1988).

Dietary fiber sources can vary widely in their composition and physicochemical properties. The TDF content is highly variable; for

Table 2. General food uses for dietary fiber

Dietary fiber supplements
Bulking agent
Fat replacer
Reduce oil uptake during frying
Hydrocolloid properties
Anticaking/Antisticking

example, oat bran and powdered cellulose have 16 and 99%, respectively. The gums are completely dispersible in water, whereas powdered cellulose is completely insoluble in water and oat bran fiber is only about 50% water soluble. The calorie content of dietary fiber sources relects the TDF level; powdered cellulose is noncaloric whereas wheat bran is about 2 kilocalories per gram. Fiber comes in a wide variety of colors such as white from cellulose, cream from soy fiber and corn bran, tan/brown from apple fiber and wheat bran and brown from cocoa flour. The flavor of fiber can range from bland to fruity, nutty, malty, chocolate, or mild. The bulk density of fiber can range from about 12 lbs/cu. ft. to over 45 lbs/cu. ft. Additionally, particle size and water binding capacity (WBC) vary widely within sources. Fiber functionality is greatly effected by its composition and physicochemical properties. Dietary fiber components are classified as either soluble (or dispersible), insoluble, or composite (mixtures of soluble and insoluble fibers). The most common class of soluble fibers are gums (hydrocolloids). Gums have the basic properties of thickening or adding viscosity and gelling foods. They are used extensively in foods at low levels (less than 2%) to suspend particles, emulsify fat, inhibit ice crystallization, inhibit syneresis, form films, and mimic the properties of fat; their usage at high levels (greater than 10%) tends to be limited with only a few exceptions. Insoluble fibers consist of fiber sources that are rich in cell wall content such a most cereal brans (e.g., wheat and corn bran), oilseed hulls (e.g., sunflower seed and soybean hulls), and purified cellulose. Their usage in food systems is often improved by pretreatments which improve functionality. Insoluble fibers are most often used to control calories, add bulk, or provide a health benefit. Some fiber sources are a mixture of both soluble and insoluble fibers such as oat bran, legumes, and fruit fibers. The functionality of these fibers is a function of the type and level of soluble and insoluble fiber.

Soluble Dietary Fiber (Gums)

A major class of soluble fiber ingredients is the hydrocolloids, frequently referred to as gums (Dziezak, 1991). These compounds are long-chain polymers which dissolve or disperse in water to give a thickening or viscosity. Hydrocolloids are also used for secondary effects which include stabilization of emulsions, suspensions of particulates, control of crystallization, inhibition of syneresis, encapsulation, and the formation of a film. Additionally, a few hydrocolloids form gels.

The United States Food and Drug Administration regulates hydrocolloids. They are classified as either food additives or "generally recognized as safe" (GRAS) substances. Regulations of specific hydrocolloids are outlined in Title 21 of the Code of Federal Regulations in Parts 172.580-172.874 and Parts 182.1480-184.1724, respectively.

Hydrocolloids are generally used at levels of less than 2 percent to achieve desired properties in food systems. Although using gums can sometimes be tricky, understanding several critical factors will help in their selection (Dziezak, 1991). For example, while some gums go readily into solution, others require extra care to prevent clumping. Often clumping can be controlled by mixing the gum with a diluent such as sugar, then gradually pouring the blend into a vigorously stirred solution. Another point to consider is the gum's compatibility with other ingredients and the order of ingredient mixing; for example, a CMC solution will have a higher viscosity if acid is added to it but a lower viscosity if it is added to an acid solution. In addition, there are other criteria to consider when choosing a gum that will help safeguard against making a wrong choice; these include: (a) effects of temperature, pH, and mechanical stress on solubility and dispersibility, rheological characteristic, and emulsification and product stability, (b) synergism with other gums; (c) effect of the color, odor, and taste on the finished product; (d) microbiological stability, (e) regulatory status for the targeted application, and (f) cost effectiveness.

Food gums are obtained from a variety of sources. Gums usually come from: (1) plant materials such as seaweed, seeds, roots and tree exudates, (2) microbial biosynthesis, and (3) chemical modification of natural polysaccharides.

Insoluble Dietary Fiber

Insoluble dietary fiber comes primarily from plant cell walls. There are two distinct types of cell walls—primary (immature) and secondary (mature). These cell walls consist of a heterogeneous mixtures of cellulose, noncellulose polysaccharides, and lignin that are crosslinked (to varying degrees) to form a complex matrix. The primary cell wall is formed after cell division and it is basically a matrix of cellulose fibrils, hemicellulose, and glycoproteins. Usually as the cell wall matures, lignin and inorganic materials become integrated into the cell wall. The secondary cell wall is formed by a thickening process after the cell has reached maturity. This is associated with a progressive increase in lignin and cellulose content which makes the cell wall hydrophobic and very rigid. These lignocellulose materials constitute a majority of the mature cell wall of the plant materials such as cereal brans, seed hulls, vegetables pulps, stems, and leaves.

Numerous insoluble dietary fibers are commercially available as supplements for use in foods such as bakery goods. Unfortunately, many of these sources result in gritty textures and degradation in functional properties when they are added to foods. One of the reasons for these functional problems is that these fiber sources tend to hydrate more completely on the particle surface than in the particle interior, reducing the extent to which the particle can soften and swell in food systems such as dough and cake mixes. Thus, insoluble fiber sources can cause undesirable changes in food flavor, texture, and mouthfeel. However, many of these functional problems can be overcome by modifying the source with chemical or physical treatments, selecting the appriopriate source for a specific application, using the isolated fiber components, or blending different sources. One example is the reduction of wheat bran particle size on water binding capacity (Table 3).

A number of treatments have been developed to improve the functionality of insoluble dietary fiber. These include:

(1) Partial delignification of lignocellulose by alkaline hydrogen peroxide treatment produces highly water absorbant, swellable, cellulosic products that can be used at high levels in food products such as bakery goods (Gould, 1987; Gould and Dexter, 1988). This treatment solublilizes a portion of the lignin present in the lignocellulosic matrix, leaving a cell wall material with higher water absorbency and improved softening and swelling characteristics.

(2) Modification of bran by extrusion to produce a more acceptable product. Bran is subjected to a high temperature, high shear extrusion in a counterrotating twin screw extruder, which modifies the structure of the bran to make it more readily millable (Fulger and Bradbury, 1984). Additionally, the invention allows the naturally present starch to coat the lignocellulosic bran material during the extrusion process. After milling, the modified bran has an acceptable mouthfeel with an absence of grittiness, a higher water binding capacity, and textural properties which are compatable with a wide variety of food products.

(3) Encapsulation of bran with soluble fiber to produce a product with better textural properties. Morley and Sharma (1986) coated cereal bran with soluble fiber to produce an improved low calorie food ingredient. The process works best with refined bran which has been chemically and/or enzymatically purified to provide a concentrated source of

Table 3. Effect of wheat bran particle size on water binding capacity (WBC)

Particle size (microns)	WBC (ml/g)
804	4.0
308	2.4

[1] Adapted from Cadden (1987).

insoluble fiber. This refined fiber is then coated with 1.5 to 8.0% soluble fiber (dry weight basis) to provide a smooth, non-fibrous texture and mouthfeel.

(4) Enzymatic modification of dietary fiber may improve sensory properties due to a change in chemical composition and physical properties (Caprez et al., 1987). Enzymatic treatments lead to an increase in soluble fiber content. The modified fiber sources show reduced water binding capacity, which is advantageous for technology purposes. Also, the enzyme treated fibers have a softer texture, which facilitates their use in food products.

Composite Dietary Fiber

Many dietary fiber sources cannot be classified as either strictly soluble or insoluble fiber. Although there is no universally accepted threshold for the ratio of insoluble to soluble fiber that results in a composite fiber, a level of about 10% soluble fiber appears to be a reasonable value with regard to functionality, This can be somewhat of a problem for certain fiber sources such as soy fiber because the solubility or insolubility can vary greatly depending on the analytical method which is use.

Consumer Awareness

Healthy-image fiber-rich food products are now mainstream. It started in the mid-1980s with the success of a Kellogg's All-Bran campaign that linked cancer prevention to dietary fiber intake. Not only did All-Bran sales improve dramatically, the campaign pulled along an entire high-fiber category into the food stores. A new era in diet consciousness and food marketing and manufacturing had begun. Reinforced by studies from the scientific community and recommendations about dietary fiber from the government and consumer organizations, fiber became a way for many food companies to enter the healthier-image food market.

One of the many factors affecting food choices is an individual's belief about the health benefits or harm associated with specific food choices (National Research Council, 1989). This factor is becoming more important in America. A 1990 Gallup survey concluded that over 80% of adults are concerned about the effect of diet on future health (International Food Information Council 1991). This concern tends to be higher among women, adults (31–49 years of age), and the college-educated. Males, younger adults (18–30 years) and those with less than a high school education tend to be less concerned.

Developments in the breakfast cereal market provide unique broad market averages for fiber consumption from cereal, the evidence suggests that producer advertising was a significant source of information on the potential benefits of fiber, in contrast to the government and general information sources during 1978–1984. Under reasonable assumptions we estimate that the 7% increase in fiber content of cereals implies that advertising caused approximately 2 million more households to consume high fiber cereals.

References

Cadden, A. M., 1987, Comparative effects of particle size reduction on physical structure and water binding properties of several plant fibers, J. Food Sci., 2(6):1595-1599.

Caprez, A, Arrigoni, E., Neukom, H., and Amado, R., 1987, Improvement of the sensory properties of two different dietary fibre sources through enzymatic modification, Lebensm.-Wiss. u-Technol., 20:245-250

Dziezak, J.D., 1991, A focus in gums, Food Tech., 45(3):116-132.

Fulgar, C. V. and Bradbury, A.G., 1985, Modification of bran by extrusion, General Foods Corp., U.S. Patent 4,500,558.

Gould, J.M., 1987, Alkaline peroxide treatment of non-woody lignocellulosics, U.S. Patent No. 4,649,113.

Gould, J.M., and Dexter, L.B., 1988, Modified plant fiber additive for food formulations, U.S. Patent 4,774,098.

International Food Information Council, 1991, How Americans are making food choices, Washington, D.C.

Morley, R.C. and Sharma, S.C., 1986, Dietary fiber products and method of manufacture, U.S. Patent 4,565,702.

National Research Council, 1989, Dietary intake and nutritional status: trends and assessment, in: "Diet and Health Implications for Reducing Chronic Disease Risk", National Academy Press, Washington, D.C.

Stanley, D. W., 1986, Chemical and structural determinants of texture of fabricated foods. Food Technology, 40:65-68.

Vetter, J. L., 1988, Commercial available fiber ingredients and bulking agents, AIB Technical Bulletin, X(5):1-5.

Wright, H. S., Guthrie, H. A., Qi Wang, M., and Bernardo, V., 1991, The 1987–88 nationwide food consumption survey: an update on the nutrient intake of respondents, Nutr. Today, May/June, pp. 21-27.

Future Research in Dietary Fibre?

Martin Eastwood

Gastrointestinal Unit
Department of Medicine
University of Edinburgh
Western General Hospital
Edinburgh EH4 2XU Scotland

Introduction

A number of questions still remain to be answered for our understanding of the action of dietary fibre in nutrition.

The first question to be posed is: Is dietary fibre an obligatory component of the diet? Is the evidence that has been provided by epidemiologists sufficient for us to suggest that our intake of dietary fibre should be increased to 30g per day? Should fibre be seen as an essential nutrient or a desirable modulator of events along the gastrointestinal tract?

There is undoubtedly a need to achieve a balance between what might be called paralytic idealism and an informed working system that has nutritional reality.

The action of dietary fibre may be regarded as acting on four major areas:

1. the modulation of nutrient absorption
2. altering sterol metabolism
3. affecting caecal metabolism
4. Affecting stool weight.

The biological properties of dietary fibre are those of a hydrated polymer passing along the gastrointestinal tract, altering the movement of water in the small bowel. There is dissimulation of some of the fibre in the colon and then a shift of water, to be absorbed in the colon, or bound to residual fibre or incorporated into bacteria.

Definition of Dietary Fibre

An important problem that has arisen in the dietary fibre field is that of nomenclature. We still do not know whether to call the material of our interest dietary fibre, non starch polysaccharides or complex carbohydrates. As Alice, in Alice in Wonderland, responded to the March Hare when he said "Then you should say what you mean" and Alice hastily replied "I do, at least I mean what I say—that's the same thing you know." "Not the same thing a bit" said the Hatter, "you might just as well say I see what I eat is the same thing as I eat what I see."

Measurement of Dietary Fibre

Another important problem is the measurement of dietary fibre. The measurements are chemically reasonable but have no predictive value for function. The emphasis on soluble and insoluble fibre has no real value. The fibres are not soluble in the plant cell wall and the designation of soluble and insoluble relates to extraction properties rather than possibly any properties that have any merit on the gastrointestinal tract.

Nevertheless, at the end of the day the method that is most likely to produce realistic results which have biological and physiological meaning is the Englyst method. This method, whilst not satisfying the more immediate needs of the statutory agencies, comes closest to meeting the more discerning requirements of the nutritionist.

Dietary Fibre in the Foregut

There are two important effects of fibre along the small intestinal tract. The first are physico-chemical properties which lead to stratification of flow from the stomach. Dietary fibre and other dietary macromolecules cause changes in convection characteristics in lumenal contents. This affects and release and subsequent absorption of nutrients in the upper small bowel and sterols in the ileum. One of the better studies areas is that which relates to the beneficial effects of a high fibre diet on nutrient absorption.

Sterol Metabolism

Less well understood is the influence of dietary fibre on sterol metabolism. The action of fibre on sterol metabolism may well be through the enterohepatic circulation of bile acids. Yet, the field is obscured by the possibility that it is associated polyunsaturated fats that reduce the serum cholesterol. As yet there has been no serious work looking at the effect of dietary fibres on the various steps involved in the synthesis or catabolism of cholesterol. Work on the adsorption of bile aids to fibre does not take cognizance of the fermentability of dietary fibre. The fibres which are most effective in influencing sterol metabolism are fermented in the colon. Those fibre which alter serum cholesterol such as gum arabic and raw carrot, are not necessarily associated with changes in faecal bile acid excretion but coincide with increases in breath hydrogen suggesting that fermentation in the colon is an important aspect of hypocholesterolaemic action. So that the importance of adsorption of bile aids to fibre is likely to be a small bowel and ileal loss effect rather than colonic and faecal loss.

Caecal Fermentation

In the colon colonic metabolism is inversely related to the efficiency of upper gut ingestion. Caecal metabolism involves the fermentation of a confluence of materials coming from the diet, from biliary secretion and intestinal secretion. The interplay between these substances is very complex. In the one instance bile secretions are converted from hydrophilic to hydrophobic substances. There is a production of nutrients from fibre, the precise chemistry and fate of which are not known or understood, but include short chain fatty acids. It is possible that nutrients arriving in the liver from the colon may be routed through different hepatic metabolic pathways to those nutrients which are absorbed in the jejunum. A major difference between jejunally-derived and caecally-derived nutrients is chemical. Jejunal nutrients will, in general, consist of the individual prime dietary constituents, amino acids, sugars and fats. In contrast colonically-derived nutrients will constitute a range of fermentation products which will include short chain fatty acids.

Stool Weight

There is a wide range of normal faecal output which seems to be independent of fibre intake. Therefore there is an individual response to fibre. This is both a feature of the normal and in individuals suffering from functional bowel disease. It is also not known why there is an increase in intracolonic pressure following ingestion of ispaghula materials.

Coronary Disease and Cancer

One of the perplexing problems is why there is an inverse relationship between coronary artery disease and colonic cancer. What is the role of dietary fibre in this?

The Future of Fibre Work

It is important to define the role of fibre in food and to see fibre as a component of food and not as an isolate. Fibre studies should be on food as it is eaten rather than on individual isolated fibre sources added to food. The mode of extraction, processing and cooking may well produce physical properties which are different from those of the raw fibre. It is also necessary for us to define the role of fibre in food.

Fibre Measurements

The present dilemma about the measurement of dietary fibre is a consequence of the indecision as to what is meant by fibre. This has led to great confusion. The best definition would be the use of a general umbrella term Complex Carbohydrate. This would include resistant starch, soluble starch, plant cell wall material, mucillages, gums and isolates identified by their plant origin.

Perhaps, however, an alternative would be to develop a measurement of function of fibre which records a defined activity per gram carbon, and to measure complex carbohydrates as nutritionally active physical phases in the intestine rather than hydrated voids passing along the intestine. Physiological equations which reflect the physico-chemical properties of fibre in the intestine are necessary and must be a major objective in the near future.

Function in the upper small intestine

Such function could be measured as rate of release of trapped nutrients from cohesive particles and would be increased proportionally to the concentration of the nutrient within the particles and decreases with increasing particle size.

Stool metabolism

It is possible to make a little progress in predicting the action of a fibre on sterol metabolism by physical chemical retardation methods. These look at the ability of fibres to retard the movement of bile acids from a suspension of the fibre within a dialysis bag to the outside. This only gives a partial indication of the ability of a fibre to influence cholesterol synthesis. This retardation effect may be important in the small bowel especially the ileum. It is possible that an additional mechanism whereby fibres affect faecal bile acids is a result of the fermentation of fibre. This may be mediated through:

1. release of volatile fatty acids
2. decreased caecal pH

3.   increased adsorption to fibre bacteria
4.   altered enterohepatic circulation of bile acids consequent upon
     2 and 3.

Caecal Fermentation

It is important to concentrate on the physiology of caecal fermentation rather than have a preoccupation with the effect of short chain fatty acids on mucosal stability. The evidence for an effect of butyric acid nonmucosal stability is somewhat sparse. The normal physiology of the colon mucosal turnover is not sufficiently understood for rudimentary knowledge to be extended into quite wide sweeping dietary recommendations.

It is also important to know what happens to caecal fermentation products once they have been absorbed.

The rate of fermentation and transit along the intestine may also be important so that pectin which is dissimulated quite rapidly in the caecum will have quite different colonic and nutritional effects to ispaghula which is fermented quite slowly along the colon.

Stool Weight

Why does stool weight vary so much in an individual? What is the physiology of the variation? It is important that a measure of colonic function is developed, something akin to the creating clearance for the kidneys.

Stool weight is dependent upon fermentation and the contribution to the stool of bacteria, the water holding capacity of the residual fibre and transit time. Stool weight reflects the residual dietary intake, the residual colonic water, biliary excretion of products more than 300 molecular weight, caecal metabolism and bacterial mass. The influence of fibre of stool weight may be expressed as a formula:

stool weight = $W_F (1 + H_F F) + W_B (1 + H_B) + W_M (1 + H_M)$
W = dry weight
F = residual fibre
H = water holding capacity
B = bacteria
M = osmotically active metabolites of fibre metabolism.

In summary, we are still in a state of indecision. A new technology is required to describe the events along the intestine.

The most important requirement for the future of fibre research is develop measurements which reflect function per gram carbon as carbohydrate. This can then be drawn into formulae which will reflect the fibre in its raw state, extracted state, processed form and as it is eaten as food.

To misquote from Thom Gunn:

On the Move
Men manufacture both machine and food
And use what they imperfectly control
To dare a future from the taken routes.

At worst, chyme is in motion: and at best
Reaching no absolute, in which to rest,
Absorption is always nearer by not keeping still.
It is part solution, part phases after all.

References

Kritchevsky, D., Bonfield, C., and Anderson J. W., eds. Dietary Fibre. Plenum Press, New York, 1988.

Eastwood, M. A. What does the measurement of dietary fibre mean? Lancet, 1487, 1986.

Eastwood, M. A. and Morris, E. R. Physical properties of dietary fiber that influences physiological function: a model for polymers along the gastrointestinal tract. Amer. Jnl. of Clinical Nutrition 55:436-442, 1992.

Index

absorption, 306
acidic steroid, 102
adaptational hyperplasia, 82
alimentary lipemia, 87
allium compounds, 208
7 alpha-dehydroxylase, 120
amino acid
    degradation, 63
    digestibility, 150
animal fat, 117
anticarcinogenic agents, 298
apo B100, 88
Apo B48, 88
apolipoprotein B, 141
appendicectomy, 17
arabinogalactan, 65
arabinose, 26
arachidonic acid, 116

bacterial fermentation, 349
beans, 126
bile acid excretion, 111
bile acids, 62, 121, 354
    interaction of dietary
        fiber, 450
Black diet, 14
    appendicitis, 15
    colon cancer, 15
    constipation, 14
    defecation frequency, 14
    fiber intake, 14
    stool size, 14
    transit time, 14

bladder cancer
    vegetables and, 193
body weight management, 459
bran, 90
breast cancer, 297
    estrogen, 166
    fiber, 165
broccoli, 194

cabbage, 194
cabbage fiber, 151
calcitonin, 392
calcium, 231
caloric excretion, 464
cancer
    nutritional deficiency, 175
    role of plant foods, 191
    vegetables or fruits, inverse
        association of, 192
cancer prevention, 159
cancer risk
    dietary factors in, 159
canned beans, 129, 131
carbohydrate metabolism, 137,
    360
β-carotene, 200
carotenoids, 198, 199
carrots, 194
cecotrophs, 331
cell wall organization, 30
cellulose, 28, 78, 81, 90, 98, 105,
    106, 118, 120, 126, 148
cereal fiber, 162

chitosan, 95, 96, 113
chitosan hydrolysates, 100,
    properties of, 96
cholecystokinin, 391
cholesterol, 88, 108, 128
cholesterol metabolism, 353
colon cancer, 17
    animal models of, 378
    cereal grain intake, 186
    clinical trials, 164
    cruciferous vegetables
       and, 193
    dietary fiber, epidemiologic
       evidence, 183
    fruit, 186
    vegetable intake, 186
colon carcinogenesis, 117
colonic crypt size, 122
colonic cytokinetics, 115
colonic fermentation, 61, 142,
    351, 360
colonic hyperplasia, 81, 83
colonic phospholipids, 116
colonocytes, 77
colorectal cancer
    fiber and, 161
comparative digestion, 326
constipation, 5, 16
coprophagy, 324
coprostanol, 355
coprostanone, 355
coronary heart disease, 17
coumarins, 205
coumestrans, 294
crypt depth, 73
cutin, 31

diabetes, 137, 138, 140
diadzein, 296
diet
    bacterial activities, 425
    colonic microflora, 423
dietary fiber, 26, 202, 231

fermentation of, 62
food uses, 469
future research, 477
insoluble, 473
mineral content, 278
net energy value, 49
physiological effects
    implications of structure
    for, 32
primary structure, 26
secondary structures, 27
soluble, 472
tertiary structures, 28
viscosity, 107
dietary fiber analysis, 361, 419
dietary mineral thresholds, 272
diethylstilbestrol, 298
digestive tract disorders
    dietary fiber, 237
dimethylhydrazine, 408
distal colon
    risk of cancer in, 121
dithiolthiones, 203
diverticular disease, 17
DNA synthesis, 75
dried beans, 129

ECP Intervention Study, 229
energy
    fiber as, 46
energy intake
    dietary fiber, 243
enzyme activities
    bacterial, 261
enzymic digestion, 40
equol, 295
European Cancer Prevention
    (ECP) organization, 226
experimental colon cancer
    genetic alterations, (32/4)

familial adenomatous
    polyposis, 164

fat cell number, 382
fats, 116
fecal bulk, 312
fecal flora, 262
fecal microflora, 260
fecal mutagens, 164
fecal neutral steroid, 102
fecal pH, 17, 118, 164
fecapenataenes, 427
fermentation, 132
    products of, 65
fiber fermentation
    in vitro, 367
fiber hypothesis, 15
fiber intact foods, 247
fiber requirements, 334
fiber types, 160
fiber viscosity, 365
fiber-supplemented foods, 245
flavonoids, 205
flaxseed, 294
folic acid, 201
foods, 37
    fiber in, 37
    fruit, 186
fruit, 194

galacto-mannans, 29
galactose, 27
galacturonic acids, 27
gall stones, 17
gamma ray spectroscopy, 282
gastric emptying, 59, 60, 132
gastrointestinal anatomies, 322
gastrointestinal disorders, 237
gastrointestinal function,
    dietary fiber, 433
gastrointestinal hormones, 464
gastrointestinal transit times, 161
genistein, 296
GI microflora, 423
glucose, 27
glucosinolates and indoles, 204

glucuronic acids, 27
gluomannan, 90
glycemic response, 306
glycemic index, 362, 370
goblet cells, 77
grain fiber
    colon cancer and, 162
gross energy, 47
guar gum, 29, 52, 60, 63, 65, 76–
    80, 89, 90, 106–110
gum arabic, 58
gut fermentation
    nonruminants, 325

haemorrhoids, 5
HDL cholesterol, 128, 130, 141
heats of combustion, 47
hepatic cholesterol, 110
high-density lipoprotein, 110
high-fiber lunch, 252
high-fiber/low fat diet, 231
high-fiber foods
    health benefits, 305
historical aspects, 3
HMGCoA reductase, 141
hormone-dependent cancers
    vegetable and fruit, 193
hydroxypropyl
    methylcellulose, 107
hypocholesterolemic effects
    of fiber
        proposed
            mechanism, 132
hypothalmus, 385

ileal brake, 253, 464
immunodeficient
    animals, 412
inhibition of cancer
    potential mechanisms, 179
inositol, 311
inositol hexaphosphate, 206
insulin, 131, 138, 393

intestinal adaptation
   physiological, 72
   pathological, 72
intestinal development, 72
intestinal microflora, 260
    metablic activity, 257
intestinal motility, 132
intestinal structure, 73
intestinal transit time, 132
intestinal villi, 73
isoflavones, 205, 294, 297
   breast cancer, 299
   mechanism of action, 300
isolated polysaccharides, 58
ispaghula, 63, 65
isthiocyanates, 204

jejunal hyperplasia, 83
jejunal villi, 76
jejunal villus development, 79

lactulose, 231
large bowel cancer
   diet and, 220
   environmental factors, 219
LDL cholesterol, 127–131, 141
LDL/HDL ratio, 131
lente carbohydrate, 138
lettuce, 194
lignans, 167, 294, 295
limonene, 208
linoleic acid, 117
lipid metabolism, 140, 353
lipoprotein lipase, 394
locust bean, 29
low density lipoprotein, 109
luminal pH, 116
lung cancer, 193
   carrots and, 193
   green leafy vegetables
     and, 193
lymphatic absorption
   cholesterol and fatty acids, 100

lymphatic flow rates, 132

maladaptation, 8
mammary carcinogenesis, 309
mannans, 28
mannose, 27
mannuronic acids, 27
micelle formation, 132
mineral absorption, 267
mineral bioavailability, 269
National Wheatmeal Loaf, 13
natural killer (NK) cell
   activity, 311
neutral polysaccharides, 29
non-starch polysaccharides
   heats of combustion, 47
nutrient absorption
   slowing of, 59
nutrients, absorption of insoluble
   fibers, 61

oat bran, 106, 126–130
oat fiber, 65
obesity, 378
   animal models, 378
   diet induced, 380
   adrenal steroids, 386
   genetic models of, 388
oleic acid, 102, 117
oncogenes, 411
ornithine decarboxylase
   activity, 74, 80

pancreas cancer
   vegetables and, 193
pancreatic enzyme activity, 132
pancreatic secretion, 132
pectin, 28, 73, 89, 90, 106, 118
phenols, 205
phytic acid, 13, 305
phytochemicals, 197
   anticarcinogenic, 198
phytoestrogens, 167, 294

plant polysaccharides, 58
plant sterols, 207
plasma cholesterol,
    control of, 341
plasma cholesterol, 111
    reduction, 109
plasma lipoproteins, 108
plasma phospholipids, 140
Polyp Prevention Trial, 219
    rationale and design, 219
polysaccharides
    dietary fiber
    interactions, 433
polysaccharides, 38, 46
    viscosity, 41
    molecular size, 41
postprandial lipemia, 88, 90
potatoes, 194
pregastic fermentation, 324
propionate, 142, 342
    cholesterol reduction, 341
propionic acid, 349
protease inhibitors, 207
protein digestibility, 147,149,
    153
protein digestion, 146
protein utilization, 147
proximal colon
    risk of cancer in, 121
psyllium, 133
psyllium husk, 90
psyllium seed hydrocolloid, 106

Recommended Dietary
    Allowances, 268
rectal cancer
    vegetables, 193
resistant starch, 453
resistant starches, 46
resorcylic lactones, 294
retinoic acid, 199
retinoids, 199
retinol, 199

reverse cholesterol transfer, 88
rhamnose, 27, 28

sacculated colons, 324
saponins, 206
satiety, 244
selenium, 202
serum cholesterol, 98, 126, 130,
    161
serum lipids, 312
serum lipoproteins, 127
serum total cholesterol, 129
sex hormones, 166
short chain fatty acids, 49, 62,
    118, 141, 441
    absorption, 444
    analyses, 444
    intestinal effects, 446
    metabolism, 444
    physiological actions, 65
    physiologic effects, 445
    precursors, 442
    production, 441
small intestine hyperplasia, 81
soy protein, 296, 297
starch digestibility, 361
stearic acid, 117
stomach cancer
    fruit and, 193
structure-function
    relationships, 39
suberin, 31

thermogenesis, 385
thiocyanates, 204
total cholesterol, 140
transit times, 5
transition-midpoint
    temperature, 39
triglyceride-rich lipoproteins, 87
triglycerides, 88, 116, 128, 140
triolein, 102

unavailable carbohydrate
   apparent digestibility, 52
   net energy values, 51
unsaturated fatty acids, 116
upper aerodigestive tract cancer
   fruit, lower risk, 193
uronic acid, 26
   polymers of, 28

vegetable fat, 117
   vegetables or fruits
      inverse association, 192
very low density lipoprotein, 109
viscous fibers, 60

vitamin A, 199
vitamin C, 200
vitamin E, 201
Vivonex liquid diet, 76–78
villus height, 73

water-holding capacity, 346
Western diseases, 5–7
wheat bran, 63, 65, 106, 120,
   126, 127, 151, 163, 312

xylans, 28
xylose, 26

Think Globally, Act Regionally

GIS and Data Visualization for Social Science and Public Policy Research

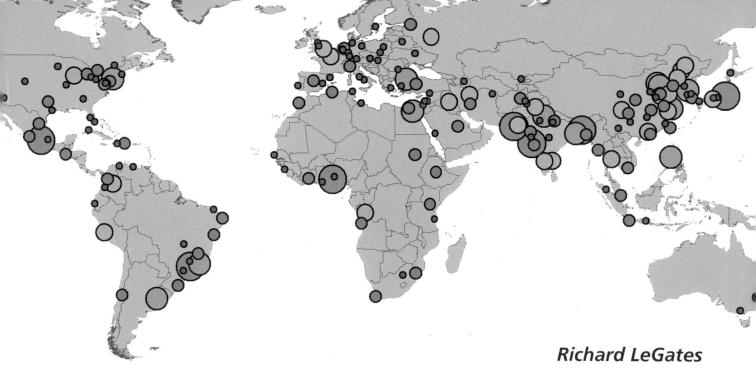

Richard LeGates

ESRI PRESS

REDLANDS, CALIFORNIA

ESRI Press, 380 New York Street, Redlands, California 92373-8100

Printed in the United States of America

Library of Congress Cataloging-in-Publication Data
LeGates, Richard T.
Think globally, act regionally : GIS and data visualization for social science and public policy research / Richard LeGates.—1st ed.
        p.   cm.
    Includes bibliographical references and index.
      ISBN 1-58948-124-0 (pbk. : alk. paper)
        1. Regional planning—Data processing. 2. Regional planning—United States. 3. Urban geography—Data processing.
      4. Urban ecology—Data processing. 5. Urban policy—Data processing. 6. Geographic information systems. 7. Visualization.
      8. Computer graphics. I. Title.
    HT391.L45 2005
    307.1′2′0285--dc22   2005010160

Ask for ESRI Press titles at your local bookstore or order by calling 1-800-447-9778. You can also shop online at www.esri.com/ esripress. Outside the United States, contact your local ESRI distributor.

ESRI Press titles are distributed to the trade by the following:

In North America, South America, Asia, and Australia:
Independent Publishers Group (IPG)
Telephone (United States): 1-800-888-4741
Telephone (international): 312-337-0747
E-mail: frontdesk@ipgbook.com

In the United Kingdom, Europe, and the Middle East:
Transatlantic Publishers Group Ltd.
Telephone: 44 20 8849 8013
Fax: 44 20 8849 5556
E-mail: transatlantic.publishers@regusnet.com

Cover design by Savitri Brant
Book design and production by Savitri Brant
Copyediting by Tiffany Wilkerson
Print production by Cliff Crabbe